# Modern Statistical Methods in Chronic Disease Epidemiology

# Modern Statistical Methods in Chronic Disease Epidemiology

EDITED BY

**Suresh H. Moolgavkar**

**Ross L. Prentice**

Proceedings of a Conference sponsored by
**SIAM Institute for Mathematics and Society**
and supported by the
**Department of Energy**

**A Wiley-Interscience Publication**

**JOHN WILEY & SONS**

**New York Chichester Brisbane Toronto Singapore**

SIMS

The SIAM Institute for Mathematics and Society was established in 1973 by the Society for Industrial and Applied Mathematics. Its purpose is to develop, promote, support, and maintain research in the application of mathematics in the study and solution of social problems. To this end, SIMS conducts conferences relevant to its objectives, a transplant program wherein mathematicians are "transplanted" for two years into university interdisciplinary centers to work as members of a team on societal problems, and university research and education studies on statistics and environmental factors in health.



***Library of Congress Cataloging in Publication Data:***

Modern statistical methods in chronic disease epidemiology.

"A Wiley-Interscience publication."
Conference held in 1985 in Alta, Utah.
1. Chronic diseases—Research—Statistical methods—Congresses. 2. Epidemiology—Statistical methods—Congresses. I. Moolgavkar, Suresh H. II. Prentice, Ross L. III. SIAM Institute for Mathematics and Society. [DNLM: 1. Epidemiologic Methods—congresses. 2. Statistics—congresses. WA 950 M689 1985]
RA644.5.M63 1986 614.4 86-1597
ISBN 0-471-83904-3

Printed in the United States of America

10 9 8 7 6 5 4 3 2 1

*To the memory of Mark Kac,*
*enthusiastic founder and ardent supporter of SIMS,*
*this volume is affectionately dedicated*

Contents

# Foreword

In 1974 SIMS initiated a series of five-day Research Application Conferences (RAC's) at Alta, Utah, for the purpose of probing in depth societal fields in light of their receptivity to mathematical and statistical analysis. The first nine conferences addressed ecosystems, epidemiology, energy, environmental health, time series and ecological processes, energy and health, energy conversion and fluid mechanics, environmental epidemiology: risk assessment, and atomic bomb survivor data: utilization and analysis.

These *Proceedings* are a result of the tenth conference "Modern Statistical Methods in Chronic Disease Epidemiology" which was held in 1985. Forty speakers and observers contributed their expertise in such disciplines as biometry, environmental medicine, epidemiology, genetics, mathematics, and statistics. Topics addressed were: issues in matching and covariate adjustment, choice of primary time variate and evolutionary covariates, design and analysis of prevention trials, problems involving auxiliary and incomplete covariate data, confidence region and model criticism, absolute and relative risk methods, methods in genetic epidemiology, models for carcinogenesis and cancer progression, and multivariate failure time methods.

Suresh H. Moolgavkar and Ross L. Prentice, both of the Fred Hutchinson Cancer Research Center (Seattle) and the University of Washington (Seattle) co-chaired the Conference. Donald R. Snow of Brigham Young University served as Assistant Conference Director.

The Conference was supported by the Department of Energy, Human Health and Assessments Division, Office of Health and Environmental Research, Office of Energy Research.

D.L. Thomsen, Jr.
President

August 1985

# Preface

The last quarter century, since the publication of Mantel and Haenszel's pioneering paper in 1959, has seen a veritable explosion of statistical methodology in chronic disease epidemiology. The central methodologic issues revolve around environmental and genetic risk assessment, and risk extrapolation. The tenth Research Application Conference held under the auspices of SIMS brought together experts from around the world to discuss the theory and applications of statistical methods in chronic disease epidemiology. This volume represents the proceedings of that conference.

Relative risk regression models provide flexible and powerful tools for the analysis of epidemiologic data. These models have been the objects of intense study in the past several years, and it seems reasonable to predict that relative risk regression methods will become a, or perhaps, the, central analytical tool in chronic disease epidemiology. Thus, a major emphasis of the conference was on relative risk regression, and various papers in this volume deal with time-dependent covariates, new study designs, multivariate failure time data, methods of model criticism, parameter transformations for optimal inference, and issues in matching, covariate adjustment, and incomplete and missing covariate information.

The relative risk regression models in current use are generalizations of a semi-parametric model for survival data analysis proposed by Cox in 1972. In the original model of Cox, the relative risk function was $\exp(\beta^t z)$, where $\beta$ is a vector of parameters and z is a vector of covariates. Estimation of $\beta$ proceeds via maximization of a partial likelihood. The original model has been generalized in two main directions. First, relative risk functions other than the exponential are being increasingly used. Second, the covariates are allowed to evolve over time. The large sample properties of such generalized models are now fairly well understood and elegant proofs using martingale theory are avaiable.

Nevertheless, the use of time-dependent covariates raises some technical problems. An approach to some of these is described in the paper by Andersen. The use of relative risk functions other than the exponential leads to problems in small to moderate sized samples. The use of parameter transformations to alleviate some of these problems is considered in the paper by Moolgavkar and Venzon.

Epidemiologic studies are largely observational in nature, and particular care needs to be exercised in their design. Often, the cost of processing information on a large number of study subjects is an important consideration. The issues arising in various designs for cohort studies are discussed in the paper by Prentice et al. A consequence of the observational nature of epidemiologic studies is that covariate information is sometimes missing and often measured with error. The impact and accommodation of covariates that are measured with error are discussed in the paper by Whittemore and Grosser. The impact, on various aspects of the data analysis, of the complete omission of certain 'balanced' covariates is discussed by Gail. Careful selection of controls is of crucial importance in epidemiologic studies. Often controls with the appropriate characteristics are difficult to find. Partial matching is discussed in the paper by Greenland.

There has recently been interest in the analysis of failure time data in which the response in subgroups of individuals may be correlated. This situation may arise, for example, in twin studies. The papers by Oakes and by Self and Prentice discuss the issues that arise in multivariate failure time data.

An important area of research is the development of methods of model criticism for the relative risk regression models used for the analysis of epidemiologic studies. While much work still remains to be done, some approaches are discussed in the papers by Lustbader and Davis et al.

Often, time measurements other than elapsed time on study, may be of importance in the analysis of cohort data. A "real time" approach to the analysis of cohort data, which does not require the rezeroing of time as subjects enter the cohort, is advocated in the paper by Arjas. Finally, papers by Breslow and Thomas discuss the fitting of certain non-standard relative and absolute risk models to epidemiologic data.

It is becoming increasingly clear that most chronic diseases are a complex interplay of heredity and environment. Genetic epidemiologists have devised powerful and flexible statistical tools for the analysis of pedigree and linkage data. Unfortunately, there is a paucity of dialogue between scientists whose primary interest is the environment and those whose primary interest is heredity. Such a dialogue could only benefit both groups. Papers on pedigree and path analysis by Elston and Rice, respectively, are valuable contributions to such interchange.

Often, the risk to human populations from exposures to low levels of various agents must be inferred from the results of experiments in which animals have been exposed to very high levels of the agent in question. Various statistical methods have been devised for such "low-dose extrapolation", and at least some of these methods are based on biologically derived models. A satisfactory solution to the extrapolation problem is not presently at hand. However, the paper by Krewski et al addresses the issue and describes some models currently in use.

Finally, in some cancers, early detection appears to improve prognosis. For example, screening for cervical cancer is now widespread. The statistical issues involved in large scale screening programs are the subject of the paper by Day and Walters.

The conference was characterized by excellent presentations and stimulating discussions. We feel that this collection of papers represents a timely and provocative discourse on some of the central statistical issues in chronic disease epidemiology.

Suresh H. Moolgavkar
Ross L. Prentice

Seattle, 1985

# Modern Statistical Methods in Chronic Disease Epidemiology

# SECTION 1
## Aspects of the Validity and of the Design of Epidemiologic Studies

A central issue in the interpretation of observational studies concerns the possible omission of important explanatory factors or covariates. Mitchell Gail considers the omission of a covariate that, by design, is not associated with the primary exposure variable in a cohort setting. His paper demonstrates that, except in certain special cases, such omission can be expected to bias parameter estimates that relate exposure level to disease occurrence. Even if such bias does not occur, standard tests of the absence of exposure effect may well be invalid.

Alice Whittemore and Stella Grosser consider problems that arise when the exposure variables of interest are measured inaccurately. This is a topic of obvious importance in observational studies, and one that has received limited attention in the context of odds ratio or relative risk methods that are commonly used in epidemiologic research. One wonders, for example, the extent to which an apparent lack of consistency of results relating intake levels of selected nutrients to the incidence of major chronic diseases may be attributed by important and highly correlated measurement errors among the estimated nutrient intakes. Whittemore and Grosser provide a quite general approach to the use of information on the covariate error distribution into regression analysis, along with several illustrations.

Literature on the role of matching in case-control studies is quite extensive. Issues of practicality and ease of conduct may compete with those of simplicity and efficiency of data analysis. The paper by Sander Greenland notes that much of the benefit of a fully matched, but possibly awkward, design can be retained by certain logistically advantageous 'partially matched' designs.

The time-matched case-control design has been advocated by a number of authors for relative risk regression in the context of a large cohort study. Possible 'case-control within cohort' designs are described in the paper by Prentice, Self and Mason, as is a case-cohort design. This latter design appears to have some efficiency advantages relative to corresponding case-control designs and is particularly useful in situations (e.g., large scale prevention trials) where it is useful to be able to identify the 'comparison group' prior to cohort follow-up.

# Adjusting for Covariates That Have the Same Distribution in Exposed and Unexposed Cohorts

*Mitchell H. Gail**

Abstract. We examine the effects of omitting a balanced covariate, namely a covariate, X, that has the same distribution among exposed and unexposed subjects, from regression analyses of cohort data. Except for models with linear or multiplicative regressions of the response variable on exposure and X, omission of a balanced covariate yields biased estimates of treatment effect. Moreover, even in cases where bias is not introduced, omitting X can lead to hypothesis tests for no exposure effect that have supranominal size, if the Fisher information is used to estimate required variances. A robust variance estimate is recommended, instead, which leads to tests of nominal size, but omitting X can still lead to substantial power loss. These ideas are discussed in relation to the following models (Table 1) for epidemiological cohort studies: normal linear, exponential multiplicative, exponential reciprocal, Bernoulli logistic, Bernoulli additive, Bernoulli multiplicative, Poisson multiplicative, Cox model, and the proportional hazards model for paired survival data.

## INTRODUCTION

The ready availability of computing facilities allows epidemiologists to perform a variety of linear and non-linear regression analyses in order to estimate the effects of exposure, to detect effect modification, and to adjust for potential confounding variables [3,5,17,20,23,31]. Which potential confounders or effect modifiers to include in a regression model is problematic, and this issue is a topic of continuing research and discussion [8, 10,22]. We shall consider the implications of discarding a covariate X that has the same distribution in the exposed and unexposed cohorts.

Recent publications show that estimates of treatment effect may or may not be changed by ignoring such a covariate, depending on the nature of the response measurement. For example, if the dis-

---

*Mitchell H. Gail, National Cancer Institute, Bethesda, Maryland 20892

tribution of X is the same in each of two exposure cohorts, a "valid" (i.e., asymptotically unbiased) estimate of relative risk may be obtained without adjustment on X, whereas adjustment on X is required to obtain a "valid" estimate of the odds ratio of disease [2,15,28]. The purpose of this paper is to describe more generally what happens to inference about exposure when a balanced covariate is omitted from the model.

The emphasis will be on cohort designs, which permit one to study a wide variety of possible response measures, rather than on case-control designs, which typically yield only the relative odds. The prospective risk models we use apply directly to cohort data, and much of the required theory has already been developed for randomized clinical trials in which the distribution of X is known to be independent of treatment, T [12,13].

In a cohort study we assume that the response variable, Y, for an individual with exposure T and covariate X, has a conditional density $f(Y|T,X)$. The likelihood is the product of such densities over all study participants. Clearly, no aspect of the inference on exposure will be altered by omitting X if $f(Y|T,X)=f(Y|T)$, namely if Y is conditionally independent of X, given T. We call this requirement NC1 (non-confounding specification 1). This is the strongest requirement for X to be a non-confounder. It is equivalent to model $\mathcal{E}$ in Samuels [26], who considers dichotomous responses. Other less stringent criteria of non-confounding may be utilized. For example, suppose $f(Y|T,X)$ is normal with conditional expectation $E(Y|T,X)=\mu+T\alpha+X\beta$ and conditional variance $\sigma^2$. Then, if $\beta\neq 0$, NC1 does not hold. Yet if X and T are independent, standard results in linear regression analysis show that estimates $\hat{\alpha}^*$ of $\alpha^*$ in the false model with X omitted, namely $E(Y|T,X)=\mu^*+T\alpha^*$, will converge to the true treatment effect, $\alpha$, for large samples. In epidemiological parlance, the estimate $\hat{\alpha}^*$ is "valid". We define non-confounder criterion NC2 to be the condition that estimates of the treatment effect with X omitted converge to the true treatment effect $\alpha$, and we apply this notion to a variety of response models. Yet another possible definition of non-confounder, NC3, is the condition that model-based score tests for no treatment effect retain nominal size when X is omitted. For most models this is not so, though the problem can be circumvented by replacing the Fisher information with a robust estimate of the variance of the score. Clearly NC1 implies both NC2 and NC3. However, we shall discuss models that satisfy NC2 but neither NC1 nor NC3, and models, like the logistic, that satisfy NC3 but neither NC1 nor NC2.

There are several epidemiological settings in which the covariate X and exposure indicator T might be statistically independent, or at least uncorrelated. The unexposed cohort (T=-1) might be chosen to have the same distribution of X as the exposed cohort (T=1). This could be accomplished by pair matching exposed and unexposed individuals on X or by randomly sampling unexposed individuals whose X values fall into various categories with probabilities defined by the conditional density $f(X|T=1)$. This latter procedure is called "frequency matching" [29]. Recently, Rosenbaum and Rubin [24,25] defined the "propensity score", $e(\tilde{X}) \equiv P(T=1|\tilde{X})$, where $\tilde{X}$ includes all possible covariates, and they showed that any component of $\tilde{X}$, such as X, is conditionally independent of T given $e(\tilde{X})$. Thus within strata defined by $e(\tilde{X})$, X and T are independent. Our results might also be of interest to the data analyst who has just compared the distributions of a number of covariates in the exposed and unexposed groups and has identified several covariates that are uncorrelated with T. Less commonly, an epidemiologist might have access to data from a randomized experiment. For example, Boice et al [1] studied the long term risk of leukemia in patients who had previously been randomly assigned to receive the alkylating agent, Semustine, for treatment of gastrointestinal cancer. The exposure to Semustine had been assigned at random, guaranteeing the independence of T and X. We shall use the phrases "X is independent of T" and "X is a balanced covariate" interchangeably. Although the results we present on bias and the NC2 criterion hold in each of these settings, our comments on hypothesis testing, power, "variance deflation" and the NC3 criterion pertain only to the last three situations, where it is reasonable to suppose that individuals are selected by simple random sampling from a defined population. As emphasized by Weinberg [29], frequency matching and pair matching induce variances that correspond to stratified random sampling, for which our results on the NC3 criterion are not directly applicable.

## RISK MODELS AND A SUMMARY OF RESULTS FOR BALANCED COVARIATES

We imagine two cohorts of individuals, one unexposed (T=-1) and one exposed (T=1). For simplicity we assume equal numbers in each cohort. We observe an individual in exposure group T with covariate X and subsequently measure his response Y. The response Y may be a quantitative measurement like blood pressure, or a categorical event, like whether or not he survived a fixed time interval. We suppose that the expectation of Y depends on T and X according to the regression model

$$E(Y|T,X) = h(\mu + T\alpha + X\beta) \qquad (2.1)$$

where h is a twice differentiable function. We assume that X is a scalar covariate, independent of T. Without loss of generality, we center X so that E(T)=E(X)=0. The response Y is assumed to depend on T and X only through the argument

$$\eta = \mu + T\alpha + X\beta \quad . \qquad (2.2)$$

Equation (2.1) defines what is meant by "treatment effect", $\alpha$. Note that this model does not include an interaction term for effect modification. Thus each subject has the same treatment effect, regardless of X. Model (2.1) is oversimplified in one important respect; it ignores the possible influence of other covariates $\tilde{X}$ that may or may not be independent of T. As Fisher and Patil [10] demonstrate, confounders should be evaluated jointly, but to do so requires specification of joint probability distributions and is beyond the scope of this paper. However, it is straightforward to extend results on a scalar X to a vector of covariates, all of which are independent of T [12,13].

We shall concentrate primarily on members of the exponential family

$$f(Y|T,X;\mu,\alpha,\beta)=f(Y|\eta)=\exp\{K(\emptyset)[Y\gamma(\eta)-g\{\gamma(\eta)\}+r(Y)]+\psi(Y,\emptyset)\} \quad (2.3)$$

where $\gamma(\eta)$ is the "natural parameter" linking X and T to Y, $g'\{\gamma(\eta)\}=E(Y|T,X)=h(\eta)$, and $K(\emptyset)$ is a positive scale factor that usually equals 1.0 in our models.

Some commonly used models are listed in Table 1. All but the Cox and paired survival models, which are defined in the next section, fall within the framework outlined at (2.3). In the next section, we shall discuss each of the models in Table 1 in relation to the following general results, most of which are taken from Gail, Wieand and Piantadosi [12] and from Gail, Tan and Piantadosi [13].

TABLE 1

Some Models Used in Epidemiological Cohort Studies†

| | $\gamma(\eta)$ | $h(\gamma)$ | Asymptotic Bias | Variance Deflation |
|---|---|---|---|---|
| Normal Linear | $\eta$ | $\eta$ | 0 | yes |
| Uncensored Exponential Multiplicative | $-e^{\eta}$ | $e^{-\eta}$ | 0 | yes |
| Uncensored Exponential Reciprocal | $-\eta$ | $\eta^{-1}$ | $\lvert\alpha\rvert<\lvert\alpha^*\rvert$ | yes |
| Bernoulli Logistic | $\eta$ | $e^{\eta}(1+e^{\eta})^{-1}$ | $\lvert\alpha^*\rvert<\lvert\alpha\rvert$ | no |
| Bernoulli Additive | $\log\{\eta/(1-\eta)\}$ | $\eta$ | 0 | no |
| Bernoulli Multiplicative | $\log\{e^{\eta}/(1-e^{\eta})\}$ | $e^{\eta}$ | 0 | no |
| Poisson Multiplicative | $\eta$ | $e^{\eta}$ | 0 | yes |
| Cox Model* | - | - | $\lvert\alpha^*\rvert<\lvert\alpha\rvert$ | no |
| Paired Survival* | - | - | $\lvert\alpha^*\rvert<\lvert\alpha\rvert$ | no |

†The scale factor $K(\emptyset)$ equals one in all these models except the normal, for which $\{K(\emptyset)\}^{-1}=\sigma^2$, the conditional variance. The term "bias" describes whether the estimate, $\hat{\alpha}^*$, with X omitted converges to the true treatment effect, $\alpha$.

*The theory requires some modification because conditional or partial likelihoods are used.

We estimate the treatment effect $\alpha$ under the correct model, $\eta=\mu+T\alpha+X\beta$, and under the false model, $\eta^*=\mu^*+T\alpha^*$ with X omitted. We shall be interested in the relationship in large samples between "estimates" $\hat{\alpha}$ and $\hat{\alpha}^*$, and the quantities $\alpha$ and $\alpha^*$, respectively. We say $\hat{\alpha}^*$ is a "valid" estimate if it is asymptotically unbiased, namely $\alpha^*=\alpha$. The estimators $\hat{\alpha}$ and $\hat{\alpha}^*$ are maximum likelihood estimates for models like (2.3) or maximum conditional or partial likelihood estimates for paired survival data or the Cox model. The condition that $\hat{\alpha}^*$ be "valid" is equivalent to the non-confounding specifications, NC2. The main results on bias, for independent X and T, are summarized as follows:

1. If $\alpha=0$, then $\alpha^*=0$, no matter what model is used.
2. Condition NC2 holds for uncensored data if and only if $h(\eta)=\eta$ or $h(\eta)=\exp(\eta)$. In other words, only additive and multiplicative regression models yield valid estimates $\hat{\alpha}^*$ when X is omitted.
3. For the family (2.3), the approximate asymptotic bias is given by
$$\alpha^*-\alpha = (Q/4)\{h''(\mu+\alpha)/h'(\mu+\alpha)-h''(\mu-\alpha)/h'(\mu-\alpha)\} \quad (2.4)$$
where $Q=\beta^2 \text{var}(X)$.
4. For randomly censored survival data with hazard proportional to $\exp(\eta)$, parametric models with known nuisance hazards yield conservative estimates, $|\alpha^*|<|\alpha|$, as does the Cox partial likelihood analysis.

We now consider hypothesis testing. Under the complete model, the one-sided score test for $\alpha=0$ is

$$U(n\hat{V})^{-1/2} > c \quad ,$$

where

$$U = \sum T\gamma'(\hat{\eta}_o)\{Y-h(\hat{\eta}_o)\} \quad , \qquad (2.5)$$

$$\hat{V} = \{nK(\emptyset)\}^{-1} \sum \gamma'(\hat{\eta}_o)h'(\hat{\eta}_o) \quad ,$$

summations are over the n subjects under study, and $\hat{\eta}_o=\hat{\mu}_o+X\hat{\beta}_o$ is the maximum likelihood estimate of $\eta$ under the hypothesis $\alpha=0$. The variance estimate $\hat{V}$ is $n^{-1}$ times the observed information calculated from the second derivative of the log-likelihood.

Under the false model with X omitted, (2.5) is replaced by

$$U^*(n\hat{V}^*)^{-1/2} > c \qquad (2.6)$$

where $\hat{\eta}_o^*=\hat{\mu}^*$. As discussed in [13], the model-based variance estimate $\hat{V}^* = \{nK(\emptyset)\}^{-1} \sum \gamma'(\hat{\eta}_o^*)h'(\hat{\eta}_o^*)$ is inconsistent, and asymptotically it differs from the true variance of $U^*n^{-1/2}$ by a "variance deflation factor", $k\neq 1$. Thus, omitting X may lead to an anticonservative significance test if the model-based variance estimate $\hat{V}^*$

is used. We call the model NC3 only if $k = 1$, namely there is no variance inflation or deflation. Under NC3, standard model-based significance tests for $\alpha = 0$ will have nominal size, even if X is omitted. Gail, Tan and Piantadosi [13] propose a robust, "empirical" variance estimate

$$V_e^* = (n-1)^{-1}\sum[\gamma'(\hat{\eta}^*)\{Y-h(\hat{\eta}_o^*)\}]^2 \tag{2.7}$$

which is consistent for $\mathrm{var}(U^* n^{-1/2})$ even though X is omitted. A similar variance estimate $V_e$ is available for the complete model, and $V_e$ and $V_e^*$ are to replace $\hat{V}$ and $\hat{V}^*$, respectively, in the score tests (2.5) and (2.6). These empirical variance estimates yield score tests of nominal size even when a variable X that is independent of T is inadvertently omitted from the model. Robust variance estimates are also available for censored survival data, provided the censoring distributions are the same in both treatment groups [13].

Even if one uses robust variance estimates to obtain a score test of nominal size, one loses power for testing $\alpha = 0$ if X is omitted. An approximate formula [13] for the asymptotic relative efficiency for the model with X omitted compared to the complete model is

$$\begin{aligned} \mathrm{ARE} = {} & \{\gamma'h'+0.5(\gamma'h'''+\gamma''h'')Q\}^2 \times \\ & \{\gamma'h'+0.5(\gamma'''h'+2\gamma''h''+\gamma'h''')Q\}^{-1} \times \\ & [\gamma'h'+0.5\{2(\gamma'')^2h'/\gamma'-\gamma'''h'+\gamma'h'''\}Q+K(\emptyset)(\gamma'h')^2Q]^{-1} , \end{aligned} \tag{2.8}$$

where $Q = \beta^2\mathrm{var}(X)$ and all functions are evaluated at $\mu$. Note that ARE reduces to 1.0 when $\beta = 0$ or $\mathrm{var}(X) = 0$. This formula only applies to uncensored data from members of the exponential family, (2.3).

Although we have not obtained characterization theorems to define the class of models that satisfy NC3, it is a matter of practical importance that all the Bernoulli models (Table 1) and the Cox analysis do satisfy NC3. However, if frequency matching is used, the variance estimate $\hat{V}^*$ will overestimate the variance of $n^{-1/2}U^*$, resulting in a conservative hypothesis test even for Bernoulli models.

## SPECIFIC MODELS

Normal Linear Model. The conventional methods of analysis of covariance [7] are based on the normal linear model, with conditional expectation $h(\eta) = \eta$, conditional variance $\sigma^2 = \{K(\emptyset)\}^{-1}$, and the identity link function $\gamma(\eta) = \eta$. This model might be applied, for example, to analyzing blood pressure, Y, one year after exposure, with adjustment for initial blood pressure, X. This model satisfies NC2 because $h(\eta)$ is linear; thus, omission of a balanced covariate, X, does not affect the validity of $\hat{\alpha}^*$.

The variance estimate $\hat{V}^*$ converges to $\sigma^2$, whereas, the true variance of Y with X omitted from the model is $\text{var}\{E(Y|X)\} + E\{\text{var}(Y|X)\} = \beta^2\text{var}(X)+\sigma^2$. Thus the variance deflation factor is $k = \{\beta^2\text{var}(X)+ \sigma^2\}/\sigma^2$. The reason that standard computer programs for analysis of covariance lead to valid tests of significance with X omitted is that $\sigma^2$ is usually taken to be unknown. Instead, the residual sum of squares is used to estimate $\sigma^2$ as in (2.7). This is equivalent to using the empirical variance estimate, $V_e^* = (n-1)^{-1}\sum(Y-\bar{Y})^2$, which converges to $\beta^2\text{var}(X)+\sigma^2$, as required.

The approximate ARE, computed from (2.8), is $\{1+\beta^2\text{var}(X)/\sigma^2\}^{-1} = \sigma^2/\{\sigma^2+\beta^2\text{var}(X)\}$, a classical result [7]. For $\sigma^2 = 1$, $\beta = 0.5$, $\text{var}(X) = 1$, we calculate ARE = 0.80. Unless stated otherwise, we shall treat the case $\beta = 0.5$, $\text{var}(X) = 1$ in subsequent examples for comparison. Indeed, we shall assume X is dichotomous with $P(X=-1)=P(X=1)=0.5$ for theoretical calculations of variance deflation and ARE. In all the remaining members of the exponential family (2.3) treated in this paper, the scale factor $K(\emptyset)=1$.

Uncensored Exponential Survival Data. First consider the exponential multiplicative model with conditional hazard $\exp(\eta)$ and conditional expectation $h(\eta) = \exp(-\eta)$. Because the expectation is multiplicative, $\hat{\alpha}^*$ is asymptotically unbiased. The link function for this model is $\gamma(\eta) = -\exp(\eta)$. With $\mu=0$, the variance deflation factor from omitting X is k=1.43 [13]. Thus, if standard computing packages, such as GLIM, are used, tests of $\alpha=0$ will be anticonservative if X is omitted. Simulations for $\mu=0$, $\beta=0.5$ and $P(X=1) = P(X=-1) = 0.5$ show a null rejection rate of 13.0%, instead of the nominal 5.0% level. If one uses the empirical variance $V_e^*$, to obtain a test of nominal size, the ARE is 0.70, which is slightly less than for the normal model.

The exponential reciprocal model, $h(\eta) = \eta^{-1}$, arises when one assumes that the hazard is linear in T and X. Suppose $\mu=1$, $\alpha=.5$, $\beta=0.5$, and $\text{var}(X)=1$. Then, from (2.4), the approximate bias is $\alpha^*-\alpha = (0.25/4) \times \{-2/1.5 + 2/0.5\} = .167$. This means that $\alpha^*$ is greater than $\alpha$ by approximately 33%. This example shows that omission of a balanced covariate can lead to overestimates of the treatment effect. The variance deflation factor for this model at $\mu=1$ is 1.50, and the simulated size for the score test (2.6) is 10.4%, rather than 5.0%. The corresponding ARE for the score test based on $V_e^*$ is 0.83.

Bernoulli Models. Suppose each member of a closed cohort is followed for a fixed time interval $[0,\tau]$, and at time $\tau$ it is determined whether a given event has occurred. For example, one might determine for each individual whether cancer had developed during the follow-up interval, and the response might be coded $Y=1$ if cancer did develop and $Y=0$ if not. We shall concentrate on this simple example, though the results are generally valid for Bernoulli responses.

The Bernoulli logistic model is widely used. Each subject has probability of response $P(Y=1|T,X)=E(Y|T,X)=\exp(\eta)/\{1+\exp(\eta)\}$. The link function for this model is the identity $\gamma(\eta)=\eta$. The data in Figure 1 conform to this model perfectly with $\mu=0, \alpha=\beta=0.5\log(9)=\log(3)=1.10$. Omitting X from the model corresponds to analyzing the pooled data. The odds ratio in the pooled data, 5.44, is less than the odds ratio in the separate strata defined by X. This is not surprising to those familiar with the following sufficient condition for NC2 in 2×2×2 tables [9,30]: either Y is conditionally independent of X given T or T is conditionally independent of X given Y. For the prospective risk model (2.3), Y is conditionally independent of X, given T, if and only if $\beta=0$, regardless of whether or not T and X are independent. We note as an aside that the conditional independence of Y from X, given T, and the independence of X and T together imply that T is conditionally independent of X given Y. Thus, for balanced data, $\beta=0$ is "doubly sufficient" to guarantee NC2 for the Bernoulli logistic model. In the present example, $\beta=\log(3)$, and the estimate of $\alpha^*$ from the pooled table is $0.5 \log(49/9)=0.85$. Thus $\hat{\alpha}^*$ is biased toward zero, with $\hat{\alpha}^*-\hat{\alpha}=0.85-1.10=-0.25$. The approximate bias formula (2.4) yields $\alpha^*-\alpha=-0.30$ in this case. Equation (2.4) also yields the useful result that $\hat{\alpha}^*$ is biased towards unity, $|\alpha^*|<|\alpha|$, when any kind of balanced covariate is omitted [12]. In particular, X may be a quantitative measurement.

| | | X=-1 | | X=1 | | Pooled | |
|---|---|---|---|---|---|---|---|
| | | T | | T | | T | |
| | | 1 | -1 | 1 | -1 | 1 | -1 |
| Y | 1 | 500 | 100 | 900 | 500 | 1400 | 600 |
| | 0 | 500 | 900 | 100 | 500 | 600 | 1400 |
| | | 1000 | 1000 | 1000 | 1000 | 2000 | 2000 |
| Odds Ratio | | 9 | | 9 | | 49/9=5.44 | |
| Risk Difference $P(Y=1\|T=1) - P(Y=1\|T=-1)$ | | 0.40 | | 0.40 | | 0.40 | |
| Relative Risk $P(Y=1\|T=1)/P(Y=1\|T=-1)$ | | 5.00 | | 1.80 | | 2.33 | |

Figure 2. Hypothetical data for Bernoulli logistic, additive and multiplicative models.

An attractive feature of the Bernoulli logistic model is that there is no variance deflation when a single balanced covariate, X, is omitted. Thus standard logistic computer programs yield valid tests of the null hypothesis, $\alpha=0$, and the score test (2.6) has proper size. If the correct model includes several balanced covariates, $X_1, X_2, \cdots, X_p$, only some of which are included in the analysis, slight variance deflation may arise, but the examples examined so far indicate that the variance deflation is minute and has no practical impact on size [13]. Losses of power from omitting X are slight, but detectable, and, in the previously treated case with $\beta=0.5$, $P(X=1)=P(X=-1)=0.5$, the exact ARE=0.94.

The Bernoulli additive model is defined by $h(\eta)=\eta$, and $\gamma(\eta) = \log\{\eta/(1-\eta)\}$. The data in Figure 1 also conform perfectly to this model with $\mu=0.5$, and $\alpha=\beta=0.2$. Because this is an additive model, omission of X yields a valid estimate of $\alpha$, namely 0.40/2=0.2 from the pooled data. Thus no bias is introduced, which is consistent with (2.4) because $h''=0$. Omission of X causes no variance deflation; thus standard tests for $\alpha=0$ have nominal size. If values of $X\beta$ are too large or small, estimates of $P(Y=1|T,X)$ fall outside the admissible interval [0,1]. Therefore, we consider the case $\beta=0.25$ instead of 0.5 as previously, and, for $\mu=0.5$, we find the exact ARE=0.75.

Next we consider the Bernoulli multiplicative model with $h(\eta)=\exp(\eta)$ and $\gamma(\eta)=\eta-\log\{1-\exp(\eta)\}$. The data in Figure 1 do not conform to this model because the relative risk is 5.00 when X=-1 and 1.80 when X=1. On this scale of response measurement, an interaction between T and X is required to fit the data. When the relative risk is constant across strata defined by X, the Bernoulli multiplicative model is appropriate. Siegel and Greenhouse [28] assume such a model and conclude that pooled estimates of the relative risk are unbiased either if the risk in unexposed persons does not vary with X (equivalent to our $\beta=0$) or if X is balanced.

This finding is in keeping with our general results that $\hat{\alpha}^*$ is valid for multiplicative models provided X is balanced or $\beta=0$. Omission of X does not produce variance deflation, so standard GLIM results may be used safely for testing $\alpha=0$. The asymptotic relative efficiency of the unadjusted analysis depends on the baseline proportion of those having events, say $\exp(\mu)$. For $\beta=0.5$, $P(X=1)=P(X=-1)=0.5$, the baseline rates $\exp(-4)=.018$, $\exp(-1)=0.368$, and $\exp(-0.6)=0.549$ correspond, respectively, to exact ARE's 0.99, 0.76 and 0.32. Thus, considerable power is lost by omitting X if about half the subjects have events. Fortunately, this model is more often used in the rare disease setting, where losses in efficiency are negligible.

The epidemiological literature on the "validity" of unadjusted estimates for dichotomous outcomes is voluminous [2,10,15,20,28,31] and covers treatment effects measured as the odds ratio, risk difference and relative risk. These analyses agree with the general results in [12] when applied, respectively, to the Bernoulli logistic, additive and multiplicative models. It may be demonstrated from formulas (2.20) and (2.21) in [13] that omission of a single balanced covariate does not induce variance deflation in Bernoulli models, no matter what scale of measurement of treatment effect, $h(\eta)$, is chosen. This means that routine likelihood methods based on the Fisher information may be safely used for testing $\alpha=0$. Approximate calculations of asymptotic relative efficiency may be obtained from (2.8). If the distribution of X is known, exact ARE calculations are feasible, and if multiple balanced covariates are included in the model, the ARE for partial adjustment may be calculated as in [13]. As mentioned in a previous section, if one ignores a stratification variable used for frequency matching, variance inflation will result, and hypothesis tests will have smaller size than nominal.

An extension of the multiplicative model allows one to treat dynamically stable cohorts [14,21] and other cases where exposure time varies, provided each individual's exposure time, $\log(\varepsilon)$, is known. Then, for low event rates, the probability of an event is given by $E(Y|T,X,\varepsilon) = \exp(\mu+T\alpha+X\beta+\varepsilon)$. If the exposure time, $\log(\varepsilon)$, is known for each subject, then the likelihood analysis in [12] is essentially unaltered because no new unknown parameters are introduced. Under the model with X omitted, the likelihood equations for estimating $\mu^*$ and $\alpha^*$ are, respectively,

$$\sum\gamma'(\hat{\eta}^*)\{Y-h(\hat{\eta}^*)\} = 0$$

$$\text{and} \qquad \sum T\gamma'(\hat{\eta}^*)\{Y-h(\hat{\eta}^*)\} = 0 \quad , \tag{2.9}$$

where now $\hat{\eta}^* = \hat{\mu}^*+T\hat{\alpha}^*+\varepsilon$. As in [12], these equations, and the independence of T from X and $\varepsilon$, imply the following relationships for large samples:

$$\exp(\mu+\alpha)E\{\gamma'(\mu^*+\alpha^*+\varepsilon)\exp(X\beta+\varepsilon)\} = \exp(\mu^*+\alpha^*)E\{\gamma'(\mu^*+\alpha^*+\varepsilon)\exp(\varepsilon)\} \tag{3.0}$$

and

$$\exp(\mu-\alpha)E\{\gamma'(\mu^*-\alpha^*+\varepsilon)\exp(X\beta+\varepsilon)\} = \exp(\mu^*-\alpha^*)E\{\gamma'(\mu^*-\alpha^*+\varepsilon)\exp(\varepsilon)\} \quad . \tag{3.1}$$

Dividing (3.0) by (3.1), we find that the coefficient of $\exp(2\alpha)$ on the left hand side equals that of $\exp(2\alpha^*)$ on the right hand side, provided $\varepsilon$ is independent of X as well as T. Thus, $\hat{\alpha}^*$ converges to $\alpha$ provided X, T and $\varepsilon$ are independent.

<u>The Multiplicative Poisson Model</u>. The multiplicative Poisson model with $E(Y|T,X,\varepsilon)=\exp(\mu+T\alpha+X\beta+\varepsilon)$ has been used for the analysis of cancer incidence data [4,11]. In this application, Y is the number of incident cancers in a fixed time period in a population with exposure T and covariate stratum X, and $\log(\varepsilon)$ is the known size of the population. The link function for this model is $\gamma(\eta)=\eta$. If all populations are the same size, the results of [12] apply directly to show that omitting

a balanced covariate X yields asymptotically unbiased estimates of $\alpha$. However, variance deflation and efficiency loss can be substantial. Assuming $\mu+\varepsilon=2$ for each population, so that the baseline expected count is exp(2)=7.38 in each population, and taking $\beta=0.5$, and $P(X=1)=P(X=-1)=0.5$ as before, we find variance deflation factor 2.78 and simulated size 23.1% rather than 5%. Thus standard significance tests for no exposure effect can be very misleading if a balanced covariate is omitted. The robust variance estimates (2.7) should be used instead. Manton, Woodbury and Stallard [18] and McCullagh and Nelder [19] discuss alternative methods to allow for extra-Poisson variation in the analysis of vital rates. Power loss from omitting X is considerable, and the score test with variance $V_e^*$ has exact ARE 0.36. Moreover, the variance deflation increases and the ARE decreases dramatically with increasing baseline rate. The argument presented at equation (3.0) shows that when the known population size, $\log(\varepsilon)$, varies, $\hat{\alpha}^*$ is still asymptotically unbiased for $\alpha$, provided T, X and $\varepsilon$ are independent.

Proportional Hazards Survival Models with Censored Data. Suppose the hazard for a subject with exposure T and covariate X is given by

$$\lambda_0(u)\exp(\mu+T\alpha+X\beta) \qquad (3.2)$$

where $\lambda_0(u)$ is a non-negative function of time, u. Parametric estimates of $\mu$, $\alpha$ and $\beta$ are easily obtained if $\lambda_0(u)$ is a known hazard function, like $\lambda_0(u)=1$ for the exponential distribution. Assuming a random censorship model and arbitrary known $\lambda_0(u)$, Gail, Wieand and Piantadosi [12] obtained expressions for $\alpha^*$ when a balanced covariate was omitted and found:

(1) In the absence of censorship, $\hat{\alpha}^*$ is asymptotically unbiased.

(2) With uniform entry and administrative censorship at the time of analysis, $\hat{\alpha}^*$ is biased toward zero, $|\alpha^*|<|\alpha|$.

(3) At the null hypothesis, $\hat{\alpha}^*$ is asymptotically unbiased for $\alpha=0$.

If, instead, (3.2) is analyzed via the partial likelihood of Cox [6], $\hat{\alpha}^*$ is biased toward zero even in the absence of censoring. This result was presented by J.D. Kalbfleisch and C. Struthers at the Columbus, Ohio Conference on Survival Analysis, 1981. See also [12]. At the null hypothesis, $\hat{\alpha}^*$ is asymptotically unbiased.

For testing the null hypothesis $\alpha=0$, Gail, Tan and Piantadosi [13] found that the variance deflation for the parametric analysis mentioned above for uncensored exponential data is substantially attenuated by censorship of 20% or more of the observations under the model (3.2). Even so, use of empirical variances, rather than the observed second derivative of the log likelihood, is recommended to insure tests of nominal size. The validity of empirical variances depends on the equality of the censoring distributions in the two exposure groups. In contrast, the score test for $\alpha=0$ based on the partial likelihood is robust, because omission of a balanced covariate does not cause variance deflation, and, as Lagakos and Schoenfeld [16] have shown, the size of the test is near the nominal 5% level when X is omitted. However, power loss can be substantial [16].

To summarize, parametric analyses with omission of a balanced covariate can result in less biased estimates of $\alpha$ than the partial likelihood approach for $\alpha \neq 0$. However, the partial likelihood method yields significance tests of nominal size when X is omitted, whereas, to obtain nominal size with a parametric score test requires use of an empirical variance estimate, $V_e^*$.

Paired Survival Data. Suppose an individual is selected at random from the set of exposed individuals; his exposure status is $T_1=1$. His propensity $e=P(T=1|X)$ is $e_1=e(X_1)$. Now suppose an unexposed individual with $T_2=-1$ is selected to have identical propensity, $e_2=e_1$. See [24,25] for details on propensity. By virtue of matching on propensity, T and X are conditionally independent. Therefore, given $e_1=e_2$, the covariates $X_1$ and $X_2$ are independent and identically distributed, each with marginal distribution $P(X|T=1)$. Suppose that an individual with exposure T, covariate X and propensity e has hazard

$$\lambda_o(u)\exp\{\mu+T\alpha+X\beta+Z(e)\} \tag{3.3}$$

where Z(e) is a real function and $\lambda_o(u)$ is a hazard function. The propensity e typically depends on X; thus $X\beta$ in (3.3) represents an association between response and X that is not controlled by matching. For simplicity assume no censorship. Let Y be an indicator variable with values Y=1 if the exposed individual dies first and Y=0 otherwise. Then Y is a Bernoulli variate with expectation

$$\exp(\alpha+X_1\beta)/\{\exp(\alpha+X_1\beta)+\exp(-\alpha+X_2\beta)\} \quad .$$

Note that Y, which characterizes the outcome for the pair, depends on covariates from both individuals. The log-likelihood is

$$\sum Y\{2\alpha+(X_1-X_2)\beta\} - \log\{\exp(\alpha+X_1\beta)+\exp(-\alpha+X_2\beta)\} - \alpha+X_2\beta \quad .$$

Equating the score equations under the true model and under the model with X omitted yields the asymptotic relationship

$$\{\exp(\alpha^*)-\exp(-\alpha^*)\}\{\exp(\alpha^*)+\exp(-\alpha^*)\}^{-1} =$$

$$E\{\exp(\alpha+X_1\beta)-\exp(-\alpha+X_2\beta)\}\{\exp(\alpha+X_1\beta)+\exp(-\alpha+X_2\beta)\}^{-1} \quad , \tag{3.4}$$

where the expectation is over the distribution of $X_1$ and $X_2$. Suppose $\alpha=1$, $\beta=1$ and $X_1$ and $X_2$ are independent, each taking on values 1 or -1 with probability 0.5. Then the right hand side of (3.4) is 0.622, and $\alpha^*=0.728$. Thus $\hat{\alpha}^*$ is biased toward zero for large samples.

The negative of the second derivative of the log-likelihood for the false model with X omitted has expectation n. The false score is $\sum(2Y-1)$, and the variance of this quantity is n times 4 var(Y). From $\mathrm{var}(Y) = E\{\mathrm{var}(Y|X_1,X_2)\} + \mathrm{var}\{E(Y|X_1,X_2)\}$, it may be shown that the false score also has variance n. Thus there is no variance deflation with this model. This analysis of paired survival data without censorship is a special application of the Cox model. However, asymptotic arguments to prove the absence of variance deflation for the Cox model have been based on the assumption of large risk sets [13,16].

## DISCUSSION

We have discussed the implications of omitting a balanced covariate X from the analysis of cohort studies. Many epidemiologists would not regard a balanced covariate as a confounder because, in some definitions, a confounder must satisfy "both of two conditions: (1) it is a risk factor for the study disease; and (2) it is associated with the study exposure but is not a consequence of exposure" [27]. We have seen that omission of a balanced covariate may result in biased estimates of the exposure effect. In principle, the bias may be either toward or away from zero, though in more important examples in Table 1 the bias is toward zero. In important applications with additive or multiplicative regression, there is no bias. Even so, omission of a balanced covariate can result in variance deflation, and hypothesis tests for no exposure effect may have supranominal size if standard variance calculations based on the Fisher information are used. Robust empirical variance estimates are recommended instead. Finally, even if hypothesis tests of nominal size are obtained, omission of a balanced covariate can result in substantial loss of power. Therefore, one cannot rely on various procedures for balancing, including matching on the propensity score, as substitutes for stratification or adjustment through regression on important determinants of disease outcome.

In practice, these issues are of less concern in two important cases. Standard analysis of covariance procedures for the linear model lead to unbiased estimates $\alpha$, and classical hypothesis tests based on the residual sum of squares already embody "robust variance estimates" when a balanced covariate is omitted. For rare diseases, the Bernoulli logistic and multiplicative models are virtually identical. Unbiased estimates of treatment effect and valid tests of the null hypothesis with high efficiency are obtained by standard likelihood methods, even when a balanced covariate is omitted from the model.

It would be interesting to examine the effect of omission of a balanced covariate, X, when the risk model includes other important covariates that may be associated both with T and X. When frequency matching is used and the matching factor is ignored, arguments similar to those in (29) demonstrate that the variance of the score test is overestimated, leading to hypothesis tests with infranominal size and loss of power. Quantitative evaluation of these phenomena would be useful. Another area requiring study is the application of these ideas to the case-control design.

Acknowledgements. I wish to thank Professor Nan Laird for discussions on propensity, Professors Ross Prentice and Alice Whittemore for helpful comments, and Mrs. Jennifer Donaldson for typing the manuscript.

## REFERENCES

[1] J.D. BOICE, M.H. GREEN, J.Y. KILLEN, S.S. ELLENBERG, R.J. KEEHN, E. McFADDEN, T.T. CHEN and J.F. FRAUMENI. Leukemia and pre-leukemia after adjuvant treatment of gastrointestinal cancer with Semustine (methyl-CCNU). New Engl. J. Med., 309, (1983), pp. 1079-1084.

[2] J.F. BOIVIN and S. WACHOLDER. Conditions for confounding of the risk ratio and of the odds ratio. Am. J. Epidemiol., 121, (1985), pp. 152-158.

[3] N. BRESLOW. Regression analysis of the log odds ratio: a method for retrospective studies. Biometrics, 32, (1976), pp. 409-416.

[4] N. BRESLOW and N.E. DAY. Indirect standardization and multiplicative models for rates, with reference to the age-adjustment of cancer incidence and relative frequency data. J. Chronic Diseases, 28, (1975), pp. 289-303.

[5] N. BRESLOW and W. POWERS. Are there two logistic regressions for retrospective studies? Biometrics, 34, (1978), pp. 100-105.

[6] D.R. COX. Regression models and life tables (with discussion). J. Royal Stat. Soc. Ser. B, 34, (1972), pp. 187-220.

[7] D.R. COX and P. McCULLAGH. Some aspects of analysis of covariance. Biometrics, 38, (1982), pp. 541-561.

[8] N.E. DAY, D.P. BYAR and S.B. GREEN. Overadjustment in case-control studies. Am. J. Epidemiol., 112, (1980), pp. 696-706.

[9] S.E. FIENBERG. The Analysis of Cross-Classified Data. The MIT Press, Cambridge, Mass., (1983).

[10] L. FISHER and K. PATIL. Matching and unrelatedness. Am. J. Epidemiol., 100, (1974), pp. 347-353.

[11] M.H. GAIL. The analysis of heterogeneity for indirect standardized mortality ratios. J. Royal Stat. Soc. Ser. A, 141, (1978), pp. 224-234.

[12] M.H. GAIL, S. WIEAND and S. PIANTADOSI. Biased estimates of treatment effect in randomized experiments with non-linear regressions and omitted covariates. Biometrika, 71, (1984), pp. 431-444.

[13] M.H. GAIL, W.Y. TAN and S. PIANTADOSI. The effect of omitting covariates on tests for no treatment effect in randomized clinical trials. Submitted, (1985).

[14] S. GREENLAND and D.C. THOMAS. On the need for the rare disease assumption in case-control studies. Am. J. Epidemiol., 116, (1982), pp. 547-553.

[15] L.L. KUPPER, J.M. KARON, D.G. KLEINBAUM, H. MORGENSTERN and D.K. LEWIS. Matching in epidemiologic studies: validity and efficiency considerations. Biometrics, 37, (1981), pp. 271-291.

[16] S.W. LAGAKOS and D.A. SCHOENFELD. Properties of proportional hazards score tests under misspecified regression models. Biometrics, 40, (1985), pp. 1037-1048.

[17] N. MANTEL and W. HAENSZEL. Statistical aspects of the analysis of data from retrospective studies of disease. JNCI, 22, (1959), pp. 719-748.

[18] K.G. MANTON, M.A. WOODBURY and E. STALLARD. A variance components approach to categorical data models with heterogeneous cell populations: analysis of spatial gradients in lung cancer mortality rates in North Carolina counties. Biometrics, 37, (1981), pp. 259-269.

[19] P. McCULLAGH and J.A. NELDER. Generalized Linear Models. Chapman and Hall, New York, (1983), pp. 130-133.

[20] O. MIETTINEN. Confounding and effect modification. Am. J. Epidemiol., 100, (1974), pp. 350-353.

[21] O. MIETTINEN. Estimability and estimation in case-referent studies. Am. J. Epidemiol., 103, (1976), pp. 226-235.

[22] O. MIETTINEN and E.F. COOK. Confounding: essence and detection. Am. J. Epidemiol., 114, (1981), pp. 593-603.

[23] R. PRENTICE. Use of the logistic model in retrospective studies. Biometrics, 32, (1976), pp. 599-606.

[24] P.R. ROSENBAUM and D.B. RUBIN. The central role of the propensity score in observational studies for causal effects. Biometrika, 70, (1983), pp. 41-55.

[25] P.R. ROSENBAUM and D.B. RUBIN. Reducing bias in observational studies using subclassification on the propensity score. J. Am. Stat. Society, 79, (1984), pp. 516-524.

[26] M.L. SAMUELS. Matching and design efficiency in epidemiologic studies. Biometrika, 68, (1981), pp. 577-588.

[27] J.J. SCHLESSELMAN. Case-Control Studies: Design Conduct, Analysis. Oxford University Press, Oxford, (1982), pp. 58.

[28] D.G. SIEGEL and S.W. GREENHOUSE. Validity in estimating relative risk in case-control studies. J. Chronic Dis., 26, (1973), pp. 219-225.

[29] C.R. WEINBERG. On pooling across strata when frequency matching has been followed in a cohort study. Biometrics, 41, (1985), pp. 117-127.

[30] A.S. WHITTEMORE. Collapsability of multidimensional contingency tables. J. Royal Stat. Soc. Ser. B, 40, (1978), pp. 328-340.

[31] T. YANAGAWA. Designing case-control studies. Environ. Health Perspect., 32, (1979), pp. 143-156.

# Regression Methods for Data with Incomplete Covariates

*Alice S. Whittemore* and Stella Grosser**

Abstract. Modern statistical methods in chronic disease epidemiology allow simultaneous regression of disease status on several covariates. These methods permit examination of the effects of one covariate while controlling for those of others that may be causally related to the disease. However they do not accommodate data in which one or more covariates are incomplete, e.g. missing or measured with error. This paper uses assumptions about the probability laws governing covariate incompleteness to obtain estimates of regression coefficients relating disease to the unobserved complete covariates. The estimates are obtained by maximizing the likelihood of the observed, incomplete data via the EM algorithm [1].

## INTRODUCTION

The multivariate procedures available for the analysis of epidemiological studies of chronic disease provide useful techniques for the control of confounding and evaluation of combined effects and interactions. However, application of these techniques is problematical when study subjects lack accurate or complete data on one or more potential risk factors to be tested in multiple regressions. The following examples illustrate several types of covariate incompleteness characteristic of epidemological data.

### Cervical Dysplasia and DES.

To examine any relationship between in-utero exposure to diethylstilbesterol (DES) and subsequent cervical dysplasia, a cross-sectional study ascertains indicators for the presence or absence of these two variables for a sample of women seen at a cervical cancer screening clinic. The women (or their mothers) may report prior DES exposure information incorrectly. Thus each woman has a probability of being misclassified into the wrong exposure category.

### Colorectal Cancer and Diet.

To examine any relationship between dietary intake of certain nutrients and cancers of the large intestine, a case control study ascertains estimates of frequency and amount of all foods eaten in the previous year, for a sample of cancer patients (cases) and nonpatients (controls). These data are reported with error.

---

*Department of Family, Community and Preventive Medicine, Stanford University School of Medicine, Stanford, CA 94305. Supported by NIH Grants CA-23214 and CA-34617 and by grants to the Society for Industrial and Applied Mathematics Institute for Mathematics and Society, from the Sloan Foundation, the Environmental Protection Agency, and the National Science Foundation.

Death Due to Breast Cancer and Extent of Disease.

To examine any relationship between weight-for-height and survival from breast cancer after adjustment for extent of disease at diagnosis, a prospective study ascertains age, height, weight and stage of disease from a sample of women with newly diagnosed breast cancer who are monitored for subsequent mortality. The medical records of a woman usually provide enough information to place her in exactly one of five stages. Occasionally a woman's stage is ambiguous due to her incomplete records, so that she is known only to be in one of two stages. Alternatively, she may be lacking the information to stage her at all, or she may be misclassified. Recent findings have shown poor survival among heavy breast cancer patients, relative to survival among those who are leaner [2]. These findings may not reflect an adverse effect of obesity per se, but rather a greater tendency for oncologists to understage obese women, for whom nodal involvement and tumor size may be more difficult to determine.

Adult Mortality and Childhood Asthma.

To examine any relationship between history of childhood asthma and subsequent mortality among a cohort of former college students, Whittemore *et. al.* [3] reviewed characteristics of youth as reported on physical examination at college entrance, as well as alumni characteristics obtained from questionnaires mailed in 1962 or 1966. Virtually complete mortality data were available from alumni records. Some individuals, however, lacked data on childhood asthma because this variable was not included in the physical exam for their college year. Others lacked data on alumni cigarette smoking history, because they died prior to questionnaire mailing.

In all of these examples, an individual's covariate vector may be incomplete. The incompleteness is due to partially observed, missing, or erroneously measured components. A common approach to such missing covariate data is to delete the individual from the analysis. This approach involves loss of information and possible bias. For example, deleting those alumni who died prior to 1960 restricts the study to those who survived, who may be less susceptible to the effects of smoking than those who died earlier. The alternate approach of omitting from analysis any incomplete covariate components can also lead to bias. Ignoring cigarette smoking can induce a spurious protective effect of childhood asthma, because asthmatics tend to smoke less.

The problem of measurement error applies especially to data from studies of adverse effects of exposures to air or water contaminants, and to data from case-control studies of chronic disease vs. diet, tobacco consumption, or energy expenditures in physical activity. This errors-in-variables problem has been studied extensively when covariates and disease response can be assumed to have a joint multivariate normal distribution (e.g., [4], Chapter 29; [5]). Prentice [6-8] has studied covariate error effects on the Cox regression model. There is need for further work to incorporate such errors into multivariate regressions when the response and/or covariates are nonnormal. The results of Gail *et al.*, in this volume and elsewhere [9], indicate biased estimates of treatment effect when omitting a balanced covariate. These results suggest more careful attention to incomplete covariates in both the design and analysis phase of epidemiological studies.

This paper develops and illustrates a general method for obtaining multivariate risk estimates using all of the available data. Computational aspects of the method are handled via the EM algorithm [1]. Section 2 defines assumptions about incomplete covariates and describes the general theory for dealing with them. It is shown that in many situations of practical utility, the EM algorithm provides a heuristically appealing and computationally simple method for obtaining maximum likelihood estimates of parameters relating disease to true covariates, based on the observed, incomplete data. At each iteration of the algorithm, an individual's incomplete covariates are replaced by their expected values, given his disease status, his observed covariates, and the current parameter estimates. Section 3 uses the first three examples outlined above to illustrate the general theory. Section 4 contains a discussion of issues in need of further work.

## GENERAL THEORY

Let the random variable Y represent response (e.g. time-to-disease or disease status), and let X be an m-dimensional vector of covariates that is observed incompletely. That is, components of X may be missing, truncated, censored, or measured with error, and one observes only a vector Z of incomplete covariates. Although some components of X may be fixed by design, we shall regard them all as random variables with (possibly degenerate) distributions.

We make the following assumptions: i) the observed covariate Z is incomplete because of some stochastic deletion mechanism D. That is, D is a random variable and $Z = \varphi(X,D)$ is a known function of X and D. Examples include a mechanism D that randomly deletes one or more components of X (e.g. [10]), or an error vector D with $Z = X + D$ (e.g. [5]); ii) conditional on X, Y and Z are stochastically independent random variables whose distributions depend on functionally independent parameters $\beta$ and $\tau$, respectively. In symbols,

$$f_{YZ|X}(y,z|x) = f_{Y|X}(y|x,\beta)f_{Z|X}(z|x,\tau); \tag{2.0}$$

iii) the parameter $\eta$ governing the marginal distribution of X is functionally independent of both $\beta$ and $\tau$.

Assumption (ii) would be violated in the first three examples of Section 1 if women with dysplasia report prenatal DES exposure more accurately than do those without it, if colorectal cancer cases recall their diet more accurately than controls, or if breast cancer patients with poorer prognosis are staged less accurately than those with more favorable prognosis. Assumption (ii) is violated by the asthma mortality data. Conditional on an alumnus' asthma and smoking status X, the probability that his observed covariate Z is complete depends on his time of death Y. The theory described below is therefore inappropriate for this data set, and we do not discuss it further.

We wish to make inferences about the parameter $\beta$ governing the relationship between response and the incompletely observed covariates. Assumptions (i)-(iii) imply that the joint ("complete data") distribution for X, Y and Z is

$$f_{XYZ}(x,y,z|\eta,\beta,\tau) = f_X(x,\eta)f_{Z|X}(z|x,\tau)f_{Y|X}(y|x, \beta) . \tag{2.1}$$

According to (2.1), X and Z are jointly ancillary for $\beta$ in the complete data distribution. That is, (X,Z) are jointly sufficient for $(\eta,\tau)$, and their joint distribution does not depend on $\beta$. Such ancillarity suggests that if the investigator could observe the value assumed by X, he should base inferences for $\beta$ on the distribution $f_{Y|X}$ of response conditional on that value [11].

The marginal distribution of the observed data (Y,Z) is

$$f_{YZ}(y,z|\eta,\beta,\tau) = \int f_X(x|\eta)f_{Z|X}(z|x,\tau)f_{Y|X}(y|x,\beta)dx , \tag{2.2}$$

obtained by integrating (2.1) with respect to the m components of X over the sample space of X. (Throughout the paper, summation replaces integration for discrete components of X.) The conditional distribution of response given the observed covariate Z is obtained by dividing (2.2) by the marginal distribution for Z:

$$f_{Y|Z}(y|z,\beta,\eta,\tau) = \int f_{X|Z}(x|z,\eta,\tau) f_{Y|X}(y|x,\beta)dx \ . \tag{2.3}$$

Note from (2.3) that Z is ancillary for $\beta$ in the observed data distribution (2.2) only if $f_{X|Z}$ is completely specified, i.e. with no unknown parameters. In the absence of such complete specification, inferences based on (2.3) may involve some loss of information for $\beta$. (See [12-15] for further discussion of information and ancillarity in the presence of nuisance parameters.)

We assume that $f_{X|Z}$ is specified by the investigator. Then given independent, identically distributed observations $(y_i,z_i)$, $i = 1,\ldots,n$, we can infer $\beta$ from the conditional loglikelihood

$$\begin{aligned} l(\beta) &= \sum \log f_{Y|Z}(y_i|z_i,\beta) &(2.4)\\ &= \sum \log \int f_{X|Z}(x|z_i) f_{Y|X}(y_i|x,\beta)dx \ . \end{aligned}$$

The second equality in (2.4) follows from (2.3) and the assumption that $f_{X|Z}$ involves no unknown parameters. Unless otherwise specified, all summations are taken over $i = 1,\ldots,n$.

We will need to evaluate the loglikelihood of the complete data $(x_i,y_i)$, conditional on the $z_i$, $i = 1,\ldots,n$. From (2.1) the probability density for a complete data point (x,y), given the observed covariate z, is

$$f_{XY|Z}(x,y|z) = f_{X|Z}(x|z) f_{Y|X}(y|x,\beta) \ .$$

Since $f_{X|Z}$ is assumed known, the loglikelihood kernel for the complete data is

$$l_0(\beta) = \sum \log f_{Y|X}(y_i|x_i,\beta) \ . \tag{2.5}$$

Of course (2.5) arises from the observed data loglikelihood (2.4) when each $f_{X|Z}(x|z_i)$ is degenerate, with all of its mass at $x_i = z_i$.

In this conditional setting, using the terminology of Dempster, Laird and Rubin [1], the complete data are the pairs (y,x). The observed data are the responses y, i.e. the x's are "missing."

Specifying $f_{X|Z}$ implies some knowledge of the marginal covariate distribution $f_X$, and of the deletion mechanism giving rise to $f_{Z|X}$. In some applications it may be more reasonable to specify only the distribution $f_{Z|X}$ of incomplete covariates, conditional on their actual values. Then efficient inferences for $\beta$ would be based on the joint distribution $f_{YZ}$ in (2.2), which involves the nuisance parameter $\eta$ governing $f_X$. In this unconditional setting, the observed data are the pairs (y,z), and the complete data are the triples (x,y,z). From (2.2) the observed data loglikelihood kernel would be

$$l^*(\beta,\eta) = \sum \log \int f_{XZ}(x,z_i|\eta) f_{Y|X}(y_i|x,\beta)dx \ , \tag{2.6}$$

and from (2.1) the complete data loglikelihood kernel would be

$$l_0^*(\beta,\eta) = \sum \log f_X(x_i|\eta) + \sum \log f_{Y|X}(y_i|x_i,\beta)dx . \quad (2.7)$$

Maximizing (2.7) with respect to $\beta$ and $\eta$ involves maximizing separately each of its two summands. The latter are often assumed to be functions with maxima available in closed form or via standard packaged programs. By contrast (2.4) and (2.6) are loglikelihood kernels for a collection of independent mixture densities, with "mixing parameters" $f_{X|Z}$ and $f_{XZ}$ dependent on the individual observed covariates $z_i$. The decreased tractability of the observed data kernels (2.4) and (2.6) relative to the complete data kernels (2.5) and (2.7) suggests using the EM algorithm to maximize the former.

The EM algorithm is an iterative procedure for maximizing the observed data loglikelihood kernel with respect to $\beta$. Each iteration consists of an expectation (E) step and a maximization (M) step. The E step uses a current estimate $\beta^c$ to compute the expected value of the complete data kernel with respect to the x's, given the data points (y,z), with $\beta = \beta^c$. Thus the E step computes

$$Q(\beta|\beta^c) = E[l_0(\beta)|y,z,\beta^c] , \quad (2.8)$$

where y,z represents the observations $(y_i,z_i)$, $i = 1,...,n$. The function Q is assumed to exist for all possible values of $(\beta,\beta^c,y,z)$. The M step finds $\beta^{c+1}$ to maximize $Q(\beta|\beta^c)$ over $\beta$. The two steps are iterated, with $\beta^{c+1}$ replacing $\beta^c$, until convergence to an estimate $\hat{\beta}$. Under mild regularity conditions $\hat{\beta}$ maximizes the loglikelihood $l(\beta)$ based on (2.4) [1,16,17].

The covariance matrix for $\hat{\beta}$ can be estimated as the inverse of the observed information matrix for $l(\beta)$, which can be computed using a method due to Louis [18]. Let $S(\beta)$ denote the vector of partials of $l(\beta)$ with respect to $\beta$, and let $-I(\beta)$ denote the matrix of second partials. Let $S_0(\beta)$ and $-I_0(\beta)$ denote the corresponding derivatives of $l_0(\beta)$. $I(\hat{\beta})$ can be computed from the latter according to the formula

$$I(\hat{\beta}) = E[I_0(\hat{\beta}) - S_0(\hat{\beta})S_0^T(\hat{\beta}) \mid (y_i,z_i),\ i=1,...,n,\ \hat{\beta}] ,$$

where the expectation is taken over the unobserved $x_i$, $i = 1,...,n$ [18].

The algorithm simplifies when $f_{Y|X}$ belongs to the regular exponential family. This means that, up to an additive data-dependent constant independent of $\beta$,

$$\log f_{Y|X}(y|x,\beta) = w^T(y)G(\beta,x) - A(\beta,x) . \quad (2.9)$$

Here w is a sufficient statistic for $\beta$. The term regular means that the range of the vector valued function G is restricted to a convex set $\Omega$ such that $f_{Y|X}$ defines a distribution for all $G(\beta,x)$ in $\Omega$. Substituting (2.9) into (2.5) and (2.5) into (2.8) gives

$$Q(\beta|\beta^c) = \sum \{w^T(y_i)E_i^c[G(\beta,x)] - E_i^c[A(\beta,x)]\} . \quad (2.10)$$

In (2.10) $E_i^c[G(\beta,x)]$ denotes expectation with respect to the conditional distribution of X given the data $(y_i,z_i)$ and the current parameter $\beta^c$:

$$E_i^c[G(\beta,x)] = \int G(\beta,x)f_{X|YZ}(x|y_i,z_i,\beta^c)dx .$$

Thus the E step computes for each distinct observation (y,z) the expected values of G and A with respect to the posterior distribution of X obtained from the prior $f_X$ and the data (y,z), with $\beta$ at its current value.

When response Y, conditional on X = x, is normally distributed about a linear function of x, then G and A are linear in x, and the E step computes only the expected values of X. In general, however, G and A are nonlinear in x, and computing Q requires numerical integrations for each distinct pair (y,z), and each trial value of $\beta$ examined in the following M step. Substantial computing time may be involved unless the data are grouped so that many observations have the same (y,z) values, or unless the needed expectations can be approximated.

An important exceptional case occurs when the sample space of X contains only finitely many values $c_1,\dots,c_K$ in $R^m$. Then one can linearize the E step as follows. Introduce the K-dimensional parameter vector $\xi$ with $k^{th}$ component $\xi_k = \beta^T c_k$, and let the K-dimensional random vector V = V(X) take value the $k^{th}$ unit vector in $R^K$ when X takes the value $c_k$, k = 1,...,K. Then $\beta^T x = \xi^T v$, and for any r-dimensional vector valued function G, $G(\beta^T x) = \Gamma(\beta)v$, where $\Gamma(\beta)$ is the rxK matrix whose $k^{th}$ column is $G(\beta,c_k)$, k = 1,...,K. Thus

$$E^c[G(\beta,x)]) = \Gamma(\beta)E^c[v(x)] \equiv \Gamma(\beta)\chi ,$$

and (2.10) becomes

$$Q(\beta|\beta^c) = \sum \{w^T(y_i)\Gamma(\beta)\chi_i - [\alpha(\beta)]^T\chi_i\} , \tag{2.11}$$

where $\alpha(\beta) = [A(\beta,c_1),\dots,A(\beta,c_K)]^T$. Hence the E step requires for each (y,z) only the multinomial probability vector $\chi = E^c[V(X)]$, whose $k^{th}$ component is the probability that X = $c_k$, conditional on (y,z) and $\beta^c$.

To determine the $\chi$'s, let z be an L dimensional column vector of indicators for one of L observed values, and specify $f_{X|Z}(x|z) = v^T\Theta z$, where $\Theta = (\theta_{kl})$ is a known KxL probability matrix. Then from Bayes' Theorem the $k^{th}$ component of $\chi$ is

$$\chi^{(k)} = \varepsilon_k\theta_{kl}(\varepsilon^T\Theta z)^{-1} , \tag{2.12a}$$

where $\varepsilon$ is a K-dimensional column vector with $k^{th}$ component

$$\varepsilon_k = \exp[w^T(y)G(\beta,c_k) - A(\beta,c_k)] . \tag{2.12b}$$

The likelihood equation needed for maximizing (2.11) in the M step is

$$\sum_i w^T(y_i)\,\nabla_\beta\Gamma(\beta)\chi_i = [\nabla_\beta\alpha(\beta)]^T \sum \chi_i . \tag{2.13}$$

Here $\nabla_\beta$ denotes the gradient vector of partial derivatives with respect to $\beta$. Solving (2.13) for $\beta$ may itself involve an iterative procedure, such as Newton-Raphson.

## EXAMPLES

We illustrate the preceding theory with examples from Section 1.

### Dysplasia and DES.

Here Y,X and Z are indicators for presence of dysplasia, DES exposure and a positive DES report, respectively. We parameterize $f_{Y|X}$ as

$$\text{logit } f_{Y|X}(1|x,\beta) = \beta_0 + \beta_1 x , \tag{3.1}$$

where logit p = p/(1−p). We also assume as known the probabilities $\theta_z$ of DES exposure, given recalled exposure Z = z, z = 1,0. The conditional probability of dysplasia status y given recall z is then the mixture

$$f_{Y|Z}(y|z,\beta) = \theta_z f_{Y|X}(y|1,\beta) + (1-\theta_z) f_{Y|X}(y|0,\beta) . \tag{3.2}$$

The observed data loglikelihood is

$$l(\beta) = \sum_i \log f_{Y|Z}(y_i|z_i,\beta) ,$$

where $f_{Y|Z}$ is given by (3.2). Several papers (e.g. [19-21] have shown that erroneously specifying no error (i.e. $\theta_z = z$) leads to maximum likelihood estimates for $\beta_1$ that are biased toward zero.

The corresponding complete data loglikelihood kernel $l_0(\beta)$ is the usual logistic loglikelihood, given by (2.9) with w = y, $G(\beta,x) = \beta_0 + \beta_1 x$, and $A(\beta,x) = \log[1 + \exp(\beta_0 + \beta_1 x)]$. Since x assumes K = 2 values $c_1 = 0$ and $c_2 = 1$, $\chi$ is the binomial probability vector $(1-\pi,\pi)^T$ where $\pi$ is the probability of DES exposure, conditional on disease and recall status, and on the current parameter estimate $\beta^c$. From (2.12),

$$\pi = \{1 + [(\theta_z)^{-1} - 1]\exp(-\beta_1^c y)[1 + \exp(\beta_0^c)]^{-1}[1 + \exp(\beta_0^c + \beta_1^c)]\}^{-1} .$$

The E step involves computing four $\pi$ values, corresponding to the four values assumed by the pair (y,z).

In this example,

$$\Gamma(\beta) = (\beta_0, \beta_0 + \beta_1) ,$$

and

$$\alpha(\beta) = \{\log[1+\exp(\beta_0)], \log[1+\exp(\beta_0 + \beta_1)]\}^T .$$

Therefore the M step likelihood equation (2.13) determines $(\beta_0^{c+1},\beta_1^{c+1})$ as the usual logistic estimator

$$\beta_0^{c+1} = \log [\sum_i y_i (1-\pi_i) / \sum (1-y_i)(1-\pi_i)]$$

$$\beta_1^{c+1} = \log\{[\sum_i y_i \pi_i][\sum_i (1-y_i)(1-\pi_i)]/[\sum_i (1-y_i)\pi_i][\sum_i y_i(1-\pi_i)]\} ,$$

with each woman's DES exposure indicator $x_i$ replaced by her probability $\pi_i$ of exposure, given her dysplasia and DES recall status.

## Colorectal Cancer and Diet.

Here Y is an indicator for case (vs. control) status, and X and Z represent actual and recalled average daily nutrient in the year before interview. For simplicity we consider an unmatched case-control study consisting of a random sample $z_{y1},....z_{yn}$ from each of the distributions $f_{X|Z}(z|y)$, $y = 0,1$. We make the standard discriminant analysis assumption that the joint distribution of X and Z, conditional on disease status y, is bivariate normal with mean

$$(\mu + \Delta y, \mu + \Delta y) ,\qquad\qquad (3.2a)$$

and covariance matrix $\Sigma$. Further we assume that

$$\Sigma = \begin{pmatrix} \sigma_x^2 & \sigma_x^2 \\ & \\ \sigma_x^2 & \sigma_x^2 + \tau \end{pmatrix} \qquad\qquad \sigma_x^2 > 0 , \quad \tau > 0 . \qquad (3.2b)$$

Interest centers on testing the null hypothesis that $\Delta = 0$ , and on estimating the standardized difference $\Delta/\sigma_x$.

Standard normal theory [22] verifies the basic assumption (2.0) of independence between Y and Z, conditional on the value x assumed by X. Indeed $f_{Z|X,Y} = f_{Z|X}$ is given by the normal distribution with mean x and variance $\tau$. The distribution $f_{Z|Y}$ governing the observed data is normal with mean $\mu + \Delta y$ and variance $\sigma_x^2 + \tau$. This variance is the sum of the between-person variance component $\sigma_x^2$, representing the population variance of actual nutrient intakes, and the within-person component $\tau$, representing the variance of recall errors. Thus in this special case of joint normality for X and Z, the observed data distribution is available in closed form, and the EM algorithm is not needed.

The usual estimate of $\Delta/\sigma_x$ is given by the difference $\bar{z}_1 - \bar{z}_0$ between case and control means, divided by the square root of the pooled variance estimate. This estimate converges in probability to $\Delta/(\sigma_x^2 + \tau)^{1/2}$. Therefore it underestimates $\Delta/\sigma_x$ by the factor $\rho^{1/2}$, where $\rho = \sigma_x^2/(\sigma_x^2 + \tau)$ is the intraclass correlation coefficient, i.e. the proportion of total variation in reported intakes due to population heterogeneity of actual intakes.

To see how this downward bias can apply to estimates for $\beta_1$ obtained from unconditional logistic analysis of case control studies, we invoke the normality assumptions (3.2) and Bayes Theorem to obtain the logistic distribution (3.1) for $f_{Y|X}$ with $\beta_1 = \Delta/\sigma_x^2$ [23]. The same arguments give $f_{Y|Z}$ as logistic with $\beta_1$ replaced by $\beta_1^* = \Delta/(\sigma_x^2 + \tau)$. Anderson [24] and Prentice and Pyke [25] have shown that one obtains consistent estimates for $\beta_1$ from complete data $x_{yi}$, $i = 1,....,n$, $y = 0,1$, by maximizing the likelihood based on $f_{Y|X}$ as if the data were obtained from a prospective or cross-sectional study. When recalled intakes $z_{yi}$ replace the actual $x_{yi}$, these estimates converge in probability to the deflated coefficient $\beta_1^* = \beta_1\rho$.

Wu *et al.* [26] estimated the variance components $\sigma_x^2$ and $\tau$ and the intraclass correlation coefficient $\rho$ for several nutrients by administering repeat dietary history questionnaires to the same healthy white middle-aged U.S. subjects. The estimates for $\rho$ ranged from 83% to 21%, depending on the nutrient. They showed that these values lead to substantial power loss for the moderate to small odds-ratios expected of dietary-chronic-disease associations. The results suggest that case-control studies of diet be restricted to populations with larger dietary heterogeneity (i.e. larger $\sigma_x^2$) than typically found in U.S. populations, since reduction of the recall error variance $\tau$ by averaging repeated dietary assessments is infeasible.

The normality assumptions in this example make it special in two ways: i) the observed data loglikelihood is easily maximized without special numerical algorithms; ii) covariate errors lead to estimates for the regression coefficients that are deflated toward zero. These properties do not hold in general.

Breast Cancer Survival and Extent of Disease.

We shall use the EM algorithm to investigate the effects of covariate misclassification and grouping on the relationship between survival time and disease stage for 112 women aged 45-49 diagnosed with breast cancer in the San Francisco Bay Area during the period 1972 to 1977. To simplify the presentation, we suppose first that each woman's time to death is uncensored by loss-to-followup or study termination. Then her data consist of a pair (y,z), with y representing her time to death, and z representing an L-dimensional stage indicator vector that may be incomplete.

We assume that a woman's correct complete stage indicator $x^T = (x^{(1)},...,x^{(K)})$ and her observed indicator $z^T = (z^{(1)},...,z^{(L)})$ are related by

$$f_{X|Z}(x|z) = x^T\Theta z \quad (3.3)$$

Here $\Theta$ is a known KxL matrix of classification probabilities, with $\theta_{kl}$ denoting the probability that a woman observed in stage l is truly in stage k. (In general, the matrix could vary from woman to woman.)

We also assume that the death times y arise independently from an exponential density whose hazard rate depends on the corresponding stage indicators x via the form $\exp(\beta^T x)$. Thus

$$\log f_{Y|X}(y|x,\beta) = \beta^T x - y\exp(\beta^T x)\,, \quad (3.4)$$

and the exponential family form (2.9) holds with $w(y) = y$, $G(\beta,x) = -\exp(\beta^T x)$, and $A(\beta,x) = -\beta^T x$. Moreover $v = x$, $\xi = \beta$, $\Gamma(\beta) = [-\exp(\beta_1),...,-\exp(\beta_K)]^T$, and $\alpha(\beta) = -\beta$. Substituting these values into (2.11) gives the expected complete data loglikelihood

$$Q(\beta|\beta^c) = \beta^T\sum \chi_i - \sum y_i \sum_k \chi_i^{(k)}\exp(\beta_k)\,,$$

where $\chi_i^{(k)}$ is the probability that the $i^{th}$ woman was in stage k at diagnosis, given her death time y, her observed stage l, and the current parameter $\beta^c$. From (2.12) and (3.3), this probablility is

$$\chi_i^{(k)} = \exp[\beta_k^c - y\exp(\beta_k^c)]\theta_{kl}\left\{\sum_j \exp[\beta_j^c - y\exp(\beta_j^c)]\theta_{jl}\right\}^{-1}. \tag{3.5}$$

The M-step likelihood equation (2.13) is

$$\sum \chi_i - \sum y_i \sum_k \chi_i(k)\exp(\beta_k),$$

with solution

$$(\exp(\beta_k^{c+1}) = \sum_i \chi_i^{(k)} / \sum_i \chi_i^{(k)} y_i. \tag{3.6}$$

Equation (3.6) shows that the updated death rate $\exp(\beta_k^{c+1})$ is the reciprocal of a weighted average time in stage k, with the $i^{th}$ woman's contribution weighted by the proportion $\chi_i^{(k)}$, $0 \leq \chi_i^{(k)} \leq 1$, $k = 1,...,K$. In the absence of misclassification or grouping, the $\chi_i = x_i$ are the multinomial indicators for stage at diagnosis, and the estimated death rate $\exp(\hat{\beta}_k)$ is the usual reciprocal of average woman-months of survival time for stage k.

When a woman's death time U can be censored by a random variable C, we observe for her a triple $(t,\delta,z)$, where $t = \min(u,c)$ and $\delta$ is an indicator for the event that $t = u$. Both response $y = (t,\delta)^T$ and covariate z are incomplete. We assume that the complete observations $(u_i,c_i,x_i,z_i)$ are a random sample of size n from a distribution function that satisfies

$$f_{UCXZ}(u,c,x,z) = f_{U|X}(u|x,\beta)f_{X|Z}(x|z)f_{C|Z}(c|z)f_Z(z). \tag{3.7}$$

The factorization (3.7) implies that censoring times are stochastically independent of death times, given x and z. This assumption is basic to regression analysis of censored data. The form (3.7) also implies that, conditional on a woman's observed stage, her censoring time is independent of her true stage vector x. This second assumption, which may hold only approximately in practice, assures that the expected values of X obtained at each E step do not depend on the censoring mechanism.

We infer $\beta$ from the loglikelihood $l(\beta)$ of (2.4). The $i^{th}$ summand of (2.4) is $\log f_{Y|Z}(y_i|z_i,\beta)$, where $f_{Y|Z}(y|z,\beta)$ is obtained by integrating the first three terms of (3.7) over all values of x and over the space S(y) of pairs (u,c) corresponding to y:

$$f_{Y|Z}(y|z,\beta) = \int f_{X|Z}(x|z)\left[\int_{S(y)} f_{U|X}(u|x,\beta)f_{C|Z}(c|z)du\,dc\right]dx. \tag{3.8}$$

The integral in square brackets equals

$$[f_{U|X}(t|x,\beta)F_{C|Z}(t|z)]^{\delta}[F_{U|X}(t|x,\beta)f_{C|Z}(t|z)]^{1-\delta}, \tag{3.9}$$

where $F(t) = \int_t^{\infty} f(s)ds$ is the survivor function. Substitution of (3.9) into (3.8) and (3.8) into (2.4) gives, up to an additive term,

$$l(\beta) = \sum \log \int f_{X|Z}(x|z_i)[f_{U|X}(t_i|x,\beta)^{\delta_i} F_{U|X}(t_i|,x,\beta)^{1-\delta_i}]dx . \tag{3.10}$$

The corresponding complete data loglikelihood is

$$l_0(\beta) = \sum \log f_{U|X}(t_i|x_i,\beta) - (1-\delta_i)\log[f_{U|X}(t_i|x_i,\beta)/F_{U|X}(t_i|x_i,\beta)] . \tag{3.11}$$

When $f_{U|X}$ is the exponential density (3.4), (3.11) reduces to (2.9) with $w = y = (t,\delta)^T$, $G(\beta,x) = (-\exp(\beta^T x),\beta^T x)^T$, and $A(\beta,x) = 0$. As in the uncensored case, $v = x$ and $\xi = \beta$. The 2 x K matrix $\Gamma(\beta)$ has $k^{th}$ column $[-\exp(\beta_k),\beta_k]^T$. From (2.11)

$$Q(\beta|\beta^c) = \beta^T \sum_i \delta_i \chi_i - \sum_i t_i \sum_k \chi_i^{(k)}\exp(\beta_k),$$

with likelihood equation

$$\sum_i \delta_i \chi_i^{(k)} = \sum_i t_i \chi_i^{(k)}\exp(\beta_k), \quad k = 1,...,K .$$

Thus $\beta^{c+1}$ satisfies

$$\exp(\beta_k^{c+1}) = \sum \delta_i \chi_i^{(k)} / \sum t_i \chi_i^{(k)} . \tag{3.12}$$

The updated death rates (3.12), which generalize the uncensored ones (3.6), represent the number of deaths in stage k divided by the total time in the stage, with each woman contributing a fractional part $\chi^{(k)}$ of her time (and death) to the stage. From (2.12)

$$\chi^{(k)} = \theta_{kl} \exp(\delta\beta_k^c - t \exp \beta_k^c) \; / \; \sum_j \theta_{jl} \exp(\delta\beta_j^c - t \exp \beta_j^c) ,$$

a generalization of (3.5).

Table 1 shows numbers of women, person-months of survival time, and deaths in each of five stages. Stages 1-4 are defined by tumor size and number of involved lymph nodes (see [27] for details). Stage 5 consists of women diagnosed with metastatic disease. An additional "Stage" 2.5 consists of women known only to be in Stages 2 or 3. "Stage" 2.5 accounts for a large proportion of women, person-months and deaths. The death rates are virtually indistinguishable for Stages 1 and 2, and for Stages 2.5, 3 and 4. Those with metastatic disease exhibit substantially higher rates, with a rate-ratio of 32.5 relative to women diagnosed in Stage 1.

Table 2 shows the classification matrix $\Theta$ introduced in (3.3) and represented as a function of a parameter $\delta$, $0 \le \delta \le 1$. The value $\delta = 0$ corresponds to no misclassification for women observed in Stages 1-5, with those in Stage 2.5 having 67% probability of being in Stage 2. Positive values for $\delta$ indicate positive probabilities of understaging for women in Stages 1-4; it is assumed that no one was overstaged.

Table 1

Survival vs. Disease Stage for Women Aged 45-49 at Breast Cancer Diagnosis

| Stage | Number of Women | Number of Person-Months | Number of Deaths | Death rate (Deaths/$10^3$ Woman-Months) |
|---|---|---|---|---|
| 1 | 14 | 967 | 2 | 2.068 |
| 2 | 30 | 2314 | 5 | 2.161 |
| 2.5[a] | 46 | 3141 | 17 | 5.412 |
| 3 | 11 | 754 | 4 | 5.305 |
| 4 | 5 | 362 | 2 | 5.510 |
| 5 | 6 | 88 | 6 | 68.182 |
| Total | 112 | 7626 | 36 | 4.721 |

[a]Women in "Stage" 2.5 were known only to be in either Stage 2 or Stage 3.

Table 2

CLASSIFICATION MATRIX $\Theta$

| Actual Stage x | Observed Stage z: 1 | 2 | 2.5 | 3 | 4 | 5 |
|---|---|---|---|---|---|---|
| 1 | $1-\delta$ | 0 | 0 | 0 | 0 | 0 |
| 2 | $\delta/2$ | $1-\delta$ | $.67-\delta/4$ | 0 | 0 | 0 |
| 3 | $\delta/3$ | $\delta/2$ | $.33-\delta/4$ | $1-\delta$ | 0 | 0 |
| 4 | $\delta/6$ | $\delta/3$ | $\delta/4$ | $2\delta/3$ | $1-\delta$ | 0 |
| 5 | 0 | $\delta/6$ | $\delta/4$ | $\delta/3$ | $\delta$ | 1 |

Tables 3 and 4 show the values of $\beta^c$ and the maximized observed data loglikelihood for the first 12 iterations of the EM algorithm corresponding to $\delta = 0$ and $\delta = 0.10$, respectively. The initial values $\beta^0$ were taken to be the logs of the death rates in Table 1, ignoring the death rate for Stage 2.5. The maximized loglikelihood at the 12th iteration is higher for $\delta = 0$ than $\delta = 0.10$. Neither of them exceeds the maximized loglikelihood of -215.2398 for the model with one additional parameter obtained by fitting six separate death rates to the data of Table 1.

Table 3

Iterations of EM Algorithm for Data in Table 1 using Classification Matrix $\Theta$ of Table 2 with $\delta = 0$

| Iteration | $\beta_1$ | $\beta_2$ | $\beta_3$ | $\beta_4$ | $\beta_5$ | Observed Data loglikelihood |
|---|---|---|---|---|---|---|
| 0 | -6.181 | -6.137 | -5.239 | -5.198 | -2.686 | -217.3847 |
| 1 | -6.181 | -5.820 | -4.931 | -5.198 | -2.686 | -216.2042 |
| 2 | -6.181 | -5.816 | -4.915 | -5.198 | -2.686 | -216.2021 |
| 3 | -6.181 | -5.819 | -4.909 | -5.198 | -2.686 | -216.2019 |
| 4 | -6.181 | -5.825 | -4.911 | -5.198 | -2.686 | -216.2018 |
| 5 | -6.181 | -5.822 | -4.907 | -5.198 | -2.686 | -216.2017 |
| 6 | -6.181 | -5.823 | -4.906 | -5.198 | -2.686 | -216.2017 |
| 7 | -6.181 | -5.823 | -4.906 | -5.198 | -2.686 | -216.2017 |
| 8 | -6.181 | -5.824 | -4.906 | -5.198 | -2.686 | -216.2017 |
| 9 | -6.181 | -5.824 | -4.905 | -5.198 | -2.686 | -216.2017 |
| 10 | -6.181 | -5.824 | -4.905 | -5.198 | -2.686 | -216.2017 |
| 11 | -6.181 | -5.824 | -4.905 | -5.198 | -2.686 | -216.2017 |
| 12 | -6.181 | -5.824 | -4.905 | -5.198 | -2.686 | -216.2017 |
| Death Rate ($e^{\beta}x10^3$) | 2.068 | 2.956 | 7.409 | 5.528 | 68.153 | |

While the death rates in Table 3 are identical to the ones in Table 1 for Stages 1, 4 and 5, those in Stages 2 and 3 are elevated. The increase in Stage 2 reflects the fractional contribution of deaths and person-months from women in Stage 2.5, whose mortality experience was less favorable than that of women in Stage 2. The increase in Stage 3 reflects the contribution from those women in Stage 2.5 with shorter survival times, and puts women in Stage 3 at greater risk than those in Stage 4.

Comparison of the death rates in Tables 3 and 4 shows that taking account of a 10% probability of understaging has the surprising effect of lowering the rates in all stages. (This phenomenon has been dubbed "the Will Rogers effect", because of his remark that when the Okies moved from Oklahoma to California, they raised the average I.Q. in both states.) Rates in the lower stages are decreased due to loss to higher stages of part of the mortality experience of women who died early. Rates in the higher stages are decreased due to gain of experience from women observed in the lower stages, who apparently survived longer than did women observed in the higher recipient stage. If $\delta = 10\%$ were the correct model, misspecifying $\delta = 0$ can be shown to produce death rate estimates for Stage 5 that are biased toward zero. Therefore the elevated Stage 5 rates and elevated loglikelihood for the model $\delta = 0$, relative to the model $\delta = 10\%$, suggest that the latter fits poorly.

Table 4

Iterations of EM Algorithm for Data in Table 1 using Classification Matrix $\Theta$ of Table 2 with $\delta = 0.10$

| Iteration | $\beta_1$ | $\beta_2$ | $\beta_3$ | $\beta_4$ | $\beta_5$ | Observed Data loglikelihood |
|---|---|---|---|---|---|---|
| 0 | -6.181 | -6.137 | -5.239 | -5.198 | -2.686 | -218.2181 |
| 1 | -6.238 | -5.911 | -5.003 | -5.201 | -2.862 | -217.4241 |
| 2 | -6.268 | -5.899 | -4.972 | -5.281 | -2.894 | -217.3955 |
| 3 | -6.272 | -5.900 | -4.960 | -5.319 | -2.903 | -217.3907 |
| 4 | -6.272 | -5.903 | -4.953 | -5.336 | -2.906 | -217.3895 |
| 5 | -6.272 | -5.905 | -4.949 | -5.343 | -2.907 | -217.3892 |
| 6 | -6.272 | -5.907 | -4.946 | -5.346 | -2.908 | -217.3890 |
| 7 | -6.272 | -5.909 | -4.945 | -5.348 | -2.908 | -217.3889 |
| 8 | -6.272 | -5.910 | -4.944 | -5.349 | -2.908 | -217.3889 |
| 9 | -6.272 | -5.911 | -4.943 | -5.349 | -2.908 | -217.3889 |
| 10 | -6.272 | -5.911 | -4.942 | -5.349 | -2.908 | -217.3889 |
| 11 | -6.272 | -5.911 | -4.942 | -5.349 | -2.908 | -217.3889 |
| 12 | -6.272 | -5.911 | -4.942 | -5.349 | -2.908 | -217.3889 |
| Death Rate ($e^{\beta} x 10^3$) | 1.888 | 2.707 | 7.140 | 4.753 | 54.585 | |

## DISCUSSION

The preceding examples show that the EM algorithm provides a feasible and heuristically appealing procedure for estimating regression coefficients relating disease to true exposures by maximizing the likelihood of the observed, incomplete data. In these examples the updated estimates obtained at each M step were available in closed form. More generally, standard software packages such as GLIM-3 [28] can be embedded in the algorithm as subroutines. Usually the M step is less computer intensive than the E step. The latter is particularly time consuming when response y or observed covariates z are continuous, necessitating separate numerical integrations for each individual under study. Further work is needed to shorten computing time needed by the algorithm, and to compare its performance to that of alternative "one-pass-through-the-data" procedures [29].

It should be emphasized that there is no satisfactory substitute for complete or nearly complete data. The conditional independence assumption used for response and observed covariates may fail in practice, and the models assumed for true covariates given the observed ones may be difficult to verify. Nevertheless, the procedures described above allow one to test robustness of inferred associations against plausible departures from the simple assumptions typically used to deal with incomplete covariates, and to make alternative, more realistic assumptions when warranted. Therefore the procedures provide a useful tool for analyzing observational data.

## REFERENCES

[1] A. P. DEMPSTER, N. M. LAIRD, and D. B RUBIN. Maximum likelihood from incomplete data via the EM algorithm (with discussion). J. R. Statist. Soc. B, 39 (1977), pp. 1-38.

[2] R. GREENBERG, M. VESSEY, K. MCPHERSON, R. DOLL, and D. YEATES. Body size and survival in premenopausal breast cancer. Br. J. Ca., 51 (1985), pp. 691-697.

[3] A. S. WHITTEMORE, R. S. PAFFENBARGER, K. ANDERSON, and J. LEE. Early precursors of site-specific cancers in college men and women. J. National Cancer Inst., 74 (1985), pp. 43-51.

[4] M. G. KENDALL and A. STUART. The Advanced Theory of Statistics. Vol. 2, Fourth Edition, MacMillan (1979), New York.

[5] L. J. GLESER. Estimation in a multivariate "errors in variables" regression model: large sample results. Annals Statist., 9 (1981), 24-44.

[6] R. L. PRENTICE. Covariate measurement errors and parameter estimation in a failure time regression model. Biometrika, 69 (2) (1982), pp. 331-342.

[7] R. L. PRENTICE. Statistical issues arising in the analysis of A-bomb survival data. Environmental Epidemiology: Risk Assessment (1982). Prentice, R. L. and Whittemore, A. S., eds., SIAM, Philadelphia, pp. 22-28.

[8] R. L. PRENTICE. Covariate measurement errors in the analysis of cohort and case-control studies. Survival Analysis (1982). Crowley, J. and Johnson, R. A., eds., Inst. of Math. Statist. Lecture Notes, Monograph Series V2, pp. 137-151.

[9] M. GAIL, S. WIEAND, and S. PIANTADOSI. Biased estimates of treatment effect in randomized experiments with nonlinear regressions and omitted covariates. Biometrika, 71 (1984), pp. 431-444.

[10] D. B RUBIN. Inference and missing data. Biometrika, 63 (1983), pp. 581-592.

[11] D. R. COX and D. V. HINKLEY. Theoretical Statistics. Chapman and Hall (1974), London, New York.

[12] K.-Y. LIANG. On information and ancillarity in the presence of a nuisance parameter. Biometrika, 70 (1983), pp. 607-712.

[13] E. B. ANDERSEN. Asymptotic properties of conditional maximum likelihood estimators. J. R. Statist. Soc. B, 32 (1970), pp. 283-301.

[14] I. V. IBASAWA. Efficiency of conditional maximum likelihood estimators and confidence limits for mixtures of exponential families. Biometrika, 68 (1981), pp. 515-523.

[15] J. M. BEGUN, W. J. Hall, W.-M. HUANG, and J. A. WELLNER. Information and asymptotic efficiency in parametric-nonparametric models. Ann. Statist., 11 (1983), pp. 432-452.

[16] R. SUNDBERG. Maximum likelihood theory for incomplete data from an exponential family. Scand. J. Statist., 1 (1974), pp. 49-58.

[17] R. A. REDNER and H. F. WALKER. Mixture densities, maximum likelihood and the EM algorithm. SIAM Review, 26 (1984), pp. 195-240.

[18] T. A. LOUIS. Finding the observed information matrix when using the EM algorithm. J. Roy. Statist. Soc. B, (1982), pp. 226-233.

[19] I. BROSS. Misclassification in 2x2 tables. Biometrics, 10 (1954), pp. 474-486.

[20] G. G. KOCH. The effect of nonsampling errors on measures of association in 2x2 contingency tables. J. Amer. Statist. Assn., (1969), pp. 851-864.

[21] E. ROGOT. A note on measurement errors and detecting real differences. J. Amer. Statist. Assn., 56 (1961), pp. 314-319.

[22] T. W. ANDERSON. An Introduction to Multivariate Statistical Analysis. John Wiley and Sons (1958), New York.

[23] A. A. AFIFI and S. P. AZEN. Statistical Analysis: A Computer-Oriented Approach. Academic Press (1979), New York.

[24] J. ANDERSON. Separate sample logistic discrimination. Biometrika, 59 (1972), pp. 19-35.

[25] R. L. PRENTICE and R. PYKE. Logistic disease incidence models and case control studies. Biometrika, 66 (1979), pp. 403-411.

[26] M. L. WU, A. S. WHITTEMORE, and D. JUNG. Errors in reported dietary intakes: A. Short-term recall. Am. J. Epid., (in press).

[27] J. MOHLE, S. GROSSER, M. MALEC, J. KAMPERT, A. S. WHITTEMORE, and R. S. PAFFENBARGER. Hormonal factors as determinants of breast cancer survival (in preparation).

[28] R. J. BAKER and J. A. NELDER. The GLIM system, Release 3. Numerical Algorithms Group (1978), Oxford.

[29] D. M. TITTERINGTON. Recursive parameter estimation using incomplete data. J. Roy. Statist. Soc. B, 46 (1984), pp. 257-267.

# Partial and Marginal Matching in Case-Control Studies

*Sander Greenland**

Abstract. A common problem in epidemiologic studies is the inability to match all study subjects on all potential matching factors. I examined the effects of partial matching relative to full matching and no matching on the efficiency of case-control designs. For the case of two binary matching covariates, I compared five types of design: unmatched, matched on only one of the two factors, fully matched on both factors, partially matched on both factors, and a design matched on the marginal distribution of both factors. I further compared the unmatched, partially matched, and fully matched designs using a matching factor with five interval-scaled categories.

Marginal matching always gave an efficiency nearly equal to full matching. Although the efficiency of partial matching often fell between that of unmatched and fully matched designs, partial matching could sometimes be more or less efficient than the extremes of no matching or full matching, as could matching on a nonconfounding correlate of an unmatched confounder. Furthermore, even when partial matching was not the most efficient of the designs it often came close to the best efficiency among the designs when only 60% of the subjects were matched. These results indicate that, in practice, complete matching is unnecessary to produce most of the efficiency benefits (or penalties) of matching.

I also compared various analysis options for the study designs, including the option of controlling the matching factor by entering it directly into an unconditional analysis. The results indicate that the latter strategy may be particularly worthwhile for partially matched designs involving small sample sizes.

1. Introduction. Over the past five years or so many authors have considered the statistical properties of matched versus unmatched designs in case-control research [1-11]. Most of these investigations compared the extremes of a completely unmatched design and a design in which matched controls are successfully recruited for all cases. Those

---

*Division of Epidemiology, UCLA School of Public Health, Los Angeles, California 90024.

studies that attempted to take account of the difficulty of finding a matched control did so by assuming that in the matched study one would have to exclude cases for whom no perfectly matched control could be found, thus reducing the sample size of the study. The latter approach is often unnecessary, however, and will be inefficient whenever a method of employing unmatched case information exists. A logical alternative to excluding imperfectly matched cases would be a "partially matched" design: one would perfectly match as many cases as practical, and collect unmatched or partially matched controls for the remaining cases.

My initial reasons for investigating partial matching were practical. Since the decision to match on a covariate is at least partly based on the difficulty of finding a match, a partially matched design might be a compromise design option for situations in which the investigator felt a strong desire to match on a covariate but was doubtful about the prospects of successfully (or perfectly) matching all cases when the covariate was included as a matching factor. A partially matched design might also serve as a viable option when the number of covariates for which matching was felt desirable was so large as to make it unlikely that all cases could be successfully matched on all such covariates.

This paper presents the results from a preliminary investigation of the conditions under which partial matching is a viable alternative, focusing especially on the efficiency of various degrees of matching relative to unmatched and fully matched designs for estimating main effects. In the course of this research I was led to review analytic methods for partially matched designs, and I briefly examine these methods and their attendant problems.

2. Preliminaries. This section describes the concepts, terms, and notation I will employ in presenting the results.

On an individual level, one can distinguish two elementary types of imperfect matching: one applying to all types of matching variables, in which imperfect matching involves employing subjects that are unmatched on one or more of the matching variables; and one applying only to continuous matching variables, in which the imperfection of matching refers to residual case-control differences in the matching variables. Although real situations may involve both types of imperfection, in this paper partial matching will refer only to the first type.

Full matching (perfect matching) insures that the joint distribution of matching factors will be the same among cases and controls. If, in the design of subject recruitment phase of a study, one has accepted the inevitability of partial matching, one may still attempt to recruit subjects in a sequential fashion such that the sample marginal distribution of each matching factor is the same among the cases and the controls, without regard to the joint distribution of the factors or the quality of the individual matches. Such a strategy may be termed a "marginal matching," and may be viewed as a kind of frequency matching.

In this paper, matched design and analysis strategies will be evaluated in terms of the reduction or inflation in variance they yield relative to the unmatched design. This evaluation is particularly illuminating for those situations in which a perfectly matched study is less efficient than an unmatched one. Because of the large number of possible combinations of parameter values, combinations were selected by varying parameters one or two at a time from a few "baseline" population models; the baseline models were chosen to represent some realistic situations.

3. Case of Two Binary Matching Factors. Consider a case-control study of the effect of a single binary exposure variable x on incidence of a disease d, and in which two binary covariates y and z are to be considered for matching (all variables taking the values 0,1). Suppose that in the population under study

$$\mathrm{Prob}(y = 1) = P_y \ , \ \mathrm{Prob}(z = 1) = P_z \ ,$$

$$\mathrm{Prob}(y = 1|z) = [1 + \exp(-\alpha_0 - \alpha_1 z)]^{-1} \ ,$$

$$\mathrm{Prob}(x = 1|y,z) = [1 + \exp(-\theta_0 - \theta_1 y - \theta_2 z)]^{-1} \ ,$$

$$\mathrm{Prob}(d = 1|x,y,z) = [1 + \exp(-\beta_0 - \beta_1 x - \beta_2 y - \beta_3 z)]^{-1} \ ,$$

If we define $EO_0 = \exp(\theta_0)$, $OR_{dx} = \exp(\beta_1)$, $OR_{dy} = \exp(\beta_2)$, $OR_{dz} = \exp(\beta_3)$, $OR_{xy} = \exp(\theta_1)$, $OR_{xz} = \exp(\theta_2)$, and $OR_{yz} = \exp(\alpha_1)$, then $EO_0$ will be the odds of exposure when y and z are absent; $OR_{dx}$, $OR_{dy}$, and $OR_{dz}$ will be the odds ratios for the association of x, y, and z with disease, each conditional on the remaining two factors; $OR_{xy}$ and $OR_{xz}$ will be the odds ratios for the associations of x with y and x with z, each conditional on the remaining factor; and $OR_{yz}$ will be the crude odds ratio for the association of y and z.

All the results assume a 1:1 case-control ratio. Other case-control ratios were also examined, but increasing the number of controls per case did not alter the relationships observed other than to attenuate the efficiency differences between the designs. Because the variance for the marginally matched strategy never deviated more than 2% from the variance for the fully matched strategy, results for the marginal matched design are not presented.

In the case of a binary exposure factor x and categorical covariates y and z, all the designs may be analyzed by stratifying on the covariates and applying an appropriate method for testing and estimation of a common odds ratio. Thus, analysis of partially matched data simply involves pooling all the subjects (unmatched and matched) in the same stratum followed by the application of standard stratified procedures.

The variance ratios presented in Tables 1, 2, 3, 4, and 5 were computed from the asymptotic variance of the unconditional maximum-likelihood estimator of the log common odds ratio. For each design, this variance was computed from the multiway cross-classification of the data (cell counts) expected under the design, using the δ-method formula for the variance [12, sec. 14.6] (which yields the same formula as derived from the inverse of the expected information [12, sec. 14.8]): in the above notation, $\mathrm{var}(\hat{\beta}_1) = (\Sigma_{jk} V_{jk}^{-1})^{-1}$, where $V_{jk} = \Sigma_{hi} N_{hijk}^{-1}$ and $N_{hijk}$ is the expected number of subjects at level h of d, i of x, j of y, and k of z. (Note that in a fully matched design, $\Sigma_i N_{0ijk}$ is constrained to equal $\Sigma_i N_{1ijk}$ for all j,k, whereas in a marginally matched design, $\Sigma_{ij} N_{0ijk}$ and $\Sigma_{ik} N_{0ijk}$ are separately constrained to equal $\Sigma_{ij} N_{1ijk}$ for all k and $\Sigma_{ik} N_{1ijk}$ for all j, respectively; in a partially matched design, $N_{0ijk}$ is a combination of matched and unmatched subjects, and no constraints are imposed on cell counts). Application of this formula to the partially matched design assumes that the probability of finding a match is independent of x conditional on the remaining factors, but does not require that the final proportion matched is fixed. Valid application of the formula does, however, assume a large-stratum limiting model, and so the findings given below may not generalize to small-sample or sparse-data situations.

Table 1 gives the baseline model (model A) used for the presentations in Tables 2 and 3, as well as some illustrations of the influence of $P_m$, the expected proportion of subjects matched, on the large-sample variance of the common odds ratio estimator. Under model A, matching clearly reduces variance, but most of the reduction achieved by matching is achieved by the time 60% of the subjects have been

TABLE 1

Examples of the effect of varying the proportion matched on the asymptotic variance of the common odds ratio estimator obtained from a partially matched design, relative to unmatched and fully matched designs. Case of one binary exposure and two binary matching covariates.*

Model A: $P_y = P_z = 0.4$, $OR_{dx} = 2$, $OR_{dy} = 4$, $OR_{dz} = 8$, $EO_o = ¼$, $OR_{xy} = OR_{xz} = 4$, $OR_{yz} = 1$ (see text for definitions of these symbols).

| | Proportion matched ($P_m$): | | | | |
|---|---|---|---|---|---|
| | 0.2 | 0.4 | 0.6 | 0.8 | 1.0 |
| $V_p/V_o$ | 0.92 | 0.87 | 0.84 | 0.83 | 0.84 |
| $V_p/V_f$ | 1.09 | 1.03 | 1.00 | 0.99 | 1.00 |

Model B: Same as A except $OR_{xy} = OR_{xz} = ¼$

| | Proportion matched ($P_m$): | | | | |
|---|---|---|---|---|---|
| | 0.2 | 0.4 | 0.6 | 0.8 | 1.00 |
| $V_p/V_o$ | 0.99 | 0.99 | 1.00 | 1.03 | 1.13 |
| $V_p/V_f$ | 0.88 | 0.87 | 0.88 | 0.92 | 1.00 |

*$V_p$ = variance under partial matching, $V_o$ = variance under no matching, $V_f$ = variance under fully matched design, P = proportion matched on y and z.

matched on y and z. Furthermore, the dependence of variance on the proportion matched is not monotonic: 80% matching yields a slightly smaller variance than perfect matching. In other words, 80% matching is closer to the optimal design than 100% matching. Under model B in Table 1, matching clearly inflates variance, but most of the inflation occurs after 60% of the subjects have been matched. Thus, in the categorical case, the extent of matching ($P_m$) bears no simple relationship to the degree of variance change.

Table 2 explores the effects of varying the population parameters on the variances of designs matched on y only, z only, 60% matched on y and z, and perfectly matched on y and z, all relative to the variance of the unmatched design. Designs 20, 40, and 80% matched on y and z were also examined but are omitted for the sake of brevity. The most important features to note about these comparisons are that, as in the baseline models, when matching reduces variance, most of the reduction

TABLE 2

Examples of the effect of varying $P_z$, $OR_{dx}$, $OR_{dy}$, $OR_{dz}$, $EO_o$, $OR_{xy}$, and $OR_{xz}$ on the asymptotic variance obtained under various matching strategies, relative to no matching (assuming all analyses involved stratification on both y and z). All parameter variations are done using Model A of Table 1 as baseline.

| | Matching on y only | Matching on z only | 60% Matched on both y and z | Fully matched on both y and z |
|---|---|---|---|---|
| Baseline | 0.99 | 0.87 | 0.84† | 0.84† |
| $P_z$ = 0.1 | 0.92 | 0.91 | 0.83† | 0.84 |
| $OR_{dy}$ = 1/5 | 0.94 | 0.82 | 0.80 | 0.75† |
| $OR_{dx}$ = 1 | 0.96 | 0.84 | 0.82 | 0.79† |
| $OR_{dy}$ = 1 | 1.01 | 0.81† | 0.84 | 0.82 |
| $OR_{dy}$ = 1, taking variances relative to an unmatched design with analysis stratified on z only: | | | | |
| | 1.11 | 0.89(0.82*)† | 0.93 | 0.90 |
| $OR_{dz}$ = 1/8 | 0.87 | 0.84 | 0.78 | 0.73† |
| $OR_{dy}=OR_{dz}=1$ | 1.00 | 1.00 | 1.00 | 1.01 |
| $OR_{dy}=OR_{dz}=1$, taking variances relative to an unmatched design with unstratified analysis: | | | | |
| | 1.22(1.10*) | 1.22(1.10*) | 1.22 | 1.22 |
| $EO_o$ = 1/16 | 0.85 | 0.75 | 0.70 | 0.64† |
| $EO_o$ = 3/2 | 1.05 | 0.96 | 0.94† | 0.99 |
| $OR_{xy}$ = 1 | 0.90 | 0.78 | 0.74 | 0.70† |
| $OR_{xy}$ = 1, using an analysis stratified on z only for all five designs: | | | | |
| | 1.00 | 0.77† | 0.81 | 0.77† |
| $OR_{xy}=OR_{xz}=1$ | 0.91 | 0.81 | 0.77 | 0.72† |
| (If $OR_{xy}=OR_{xz}=1$, all five designs will be unbiased and have equal variances using an unstratified analysis) | | | | |
| $OR_{xy}$ = 1/4 | 0.97 | 0.74 | 0.75 | 0.69† |
| $OR_{xy}=OR_{xz}=1/4$ | 1.08 | 1.01 | 1.00 | 1.13 |

* Using analysis stratified on matching variable only.

†Minimum variance of the five designs (no dagger appears in row if unmatched design has minimum variance).

is achieved by the time 60% of the subjects are matched; in a few instances, 60% matching yields a lower variance than any of the other designs; and 60% matching generally yields a lower variance than perfectly matching only one of the two variables whenever both the covariates are associated with both the exposure and the disease (and so would be confounders).

In Tables 1 and 2 the covariates y and z were assumed to be unconditionally independent of one another. If covariates are highly correlated, however, it would seem intuitively reasonable to suppose that matching on a subset of them might produce most of the benefit (or harm) achievable by matching on all of them. Table 3 presents some investigations of the influence of $OR_{yz}$, the covariate association, on the relative variances of the designs. As expected from intuitive arguments, the presence of a y-z association appears to bring the results of matching on one covariate closer to the results of matching on both, although not dramatically or consistently so. The net impact of the y-z association on the variances of the designs relative to the unmatched design follows no simple pattern, but as before, partial matching does well relative to the other designs.

Lines 4 and 5 of Table 3 illustrate a situation in which y is a non-risk factor associated with a strong risk factor z, and in which matching on z alone is beneficial. In such a situation, one might intuitively expect that matching on y as a proxy for z would also be beneficial; nevertheless, matching on y is harmful in this case.

TABLE 3

Examples of the effect of varying $OR_{yz}$ on the asymptotic variance obtained under various matching strategies, relative to no matching (assuming all analyses involve stratification on both y and z). All parameter variations are done using Model A of Table 1 as baseline.

| Model | Matching on y only | Matching on z only | 60% Matched on both y and z | Fully matched on both y and z |
|---|---|---|---|---|
| $OR_{yz} = 1/5$ | 1.02 | 0.92 | 0.89† | 0.89† |
| $OR_{yz} = 1$ (Baseline) | 0.99 | 0.87 | 0.84† | 0.84† |
| $OR_{yz} = 5$ | 0.89 | 0.82 | 0.80 | 0.79† |
| $OR_{yz} = 5$, $OR_{dy} = 1$ | 1.02 | 0.83† | 0.85 | 0.84 |
| $OR_{yz} = 5$, $OR_{dy} = 1$, taking variances relative to an unmatched design with analysis stratified on z only: | | | | |
| | 1.08 | 0.90(0.82*)† | 0.92 | 0.91 |
| $OR_{xy} = OR_{xz} = 1/4$, with: | | | | |
| $OR_{yz} = 1/5$ | 1.03 | 0.98† | 1.00 | 1.07 |
| $OR_{yz} = 1$ | 1.08 | 1.01 | 1.00 | 1.13 |
| $OR_{yz} = 5$ | 1.10 | 1.03 | 0.97† | 1.14 |

*Using analysis stratified on matching variable only.

†Minimum variance of the five designs (no dagger appears in row if unmatched design has minimum variance).

4. Case of One Interval-Scaled Matching Factor. For this case, we will assume that, in the population at risk,

$$\mathrm{Prob}(d = 1|x,y) = [1 + \exp(-\alpha - \beta x - \gamma y)]^{-1} \quad .$$

This leads to an analysis of unmatched case-control data using the unconditional logistic model

$$\mathrm{Prob}(\mathrm{case}|x,y) = [1 + \exp(-\alpha^* - \beta x - \gamma y)]^{-1} \quad , \qquad [1]$$

where $\alpha^*$ is a nuisance parameter (and is estimated). For case-control data pair-matched on y, this leads to an analysis using conditional methods to estimate $\beta$ in the logistic model

$$\mathrm{Prob}(\mathrm{case}|x,y) = (1 + \exp[-\alpha(y) - \beta x])^{-1} \quad , \qquad [2]$$

where $\alpha(y)$ is an unknown nuisance function (and is not estimated). Suppose the study successfully matches only a proportion $P_m$ of the cases, and selects unmatched controls for the remainder. Several analysis methods are then available.

One possibility would be to analyze the matched and unmatched subjects separately and then pool the results. The matched subjects can be analyzed conditionally to yield an estimate $\hat{\beta}_m$ of $\beta$ with estimated variance $\hat{V}_m$, and the unmatched subjects can be analyzed unconditionally to yield an estimate $\hat{\beta}_u$ of $\beta$ with estimated variance $\hat{V}_u$. A pooled estimate $\hat{\beta}_p$ of $\beta$ can then be obtained by inverse-variance weighting of the two estimates,

$$\hat{\beta}_p = \frac{\hat{\beta}_m/\hat{V}_m + \hat{\beta}_u/\hat{V}_u}{1/\hat{V}_m + 1/\hat{V}_u} \qquad [3]$$

which will have large-sample variance $V_p = (1/V_m + 1/V_u)^{-1}$. $V_p$ is a monotonic function of the proportion matched. (In fact, in the middle ranges of $P_m$ the overall dependence of the variance on the proportion matched is linear to a rough approximation.) Thus in all cases a lower variance is yielded by either the unmatched or fully matched design, with variance in direct proportion to the proportion matched.

The preceding approach has a number of drawbacks. Because the unmatched cases will tend to be highly discrepant from the unmatched controls on the matching-factor values, the unmatched portion of the results (represented by $\hat{\beta}_u$ and $\hat{V}_u$) will be highly vulnerable to bias due to misspecification of the analysis model. Furthermore, if some of the matching factors are unquantified, one would have to attempt to control such factors among the unmatched subjects by entering quantified correlates of them into the unconditional model (model 1). Finally, as will be shown below, a more efficient analysis of the partially matched design may be obtained by breaking the matching and directly entering the matching factors into the analysis model.

One alternative (suggested by James Robins) to the pooling method just discussed would be to perform two analyses of the data: one a conditional analysis of the matched sets, the other an unconditional analysis of all cases and the unmatched controls. The results of the two analyses would then be pooled in a fashion that would take account of the covariance of their results (this covariance of results arises from the "double use" of all the cases). As before, all the matching factors would have to be entered into the unconditional model (at least this would be necessary in principle).

Another approach to partially matched data would be to break the matching and enter all the quantified matching factors into an unconditional model; this approach can be used to pool unmatched and matched subjects, as well as deal with "loose" matching. Some problems with this approach are discussed by Breslow et al. [13], though not in the context of partial matching. The chief drawback to breaking the matching is that asymptotic bias can occur if one of the matching factors (e.g., neighborhood) cannot be adequately quantified and entered into the model. Such bias may be minimized, however, if some quantified variables are available that account for most of the association of the study exposure with the unquantified factors. For example, a study of dietary factors might adequately deal with effects of neighborhood matching by including variables for ethnicity, income, and education in the unmatched analysis. It should be noted, however, that the use of modelling to control such factors depends on the correctness of a more restrictive model than that used in the matched analysis, and so is more vulnerable to specification bias [13]. In addition, the act of matching will distort the sample regression relative to the population regression; in particular, a continuous matching factor cannot be expected to exhibit a simple dose-response relationship to disease (even if one existed in the population) after the matching is broken, and as a result adequate control of such a factor may require that it be discretized and entered as several indicator variables. Finally, the number of regressors required after the matching is broken may be too large to allow simultaneous entry of all variables into the model.

If the study is focused on a single binary exposure factor, another analysis option is to break the matching and enter all the quantified matching factors into a logistic regression of exposure status on disease status, as described by Prentice [14]. This approach can entail the same bias problems as discussed above in the disease regression case. But if one wishes to break the matching, the justification for exposure regression is much more straightforward than for disease regression. When viewing the exposure as the dependent variable, matching amounts to nothing more than manipulation of the design matrix of the regressors, and if the model is correctly specified no distortion of the sample regression relative to the population regression will result. Thus, one might reasonably expect that only linear or possibly quadratic terms would be required to control continuous matching factors using an exposure regression. Nevertheless, an analysis based on exposure regression has only limited capacity to investigate the form of exposure interaction with the covariates; in contrast, the methods based on disease regression models can employ general relative risk models (such as those given by Thomas [15]).

To get some idea of the relative merits of the preceding strategies, I investigated the case of one binary study factor x and one potential matching factor y with five discrete but interval-scaled values (0, 1, 2, 3, 4). A 1:1 matching ratio was assumed; the distributions of y, x, and disease were specified as

$$\text{Prob}(y = n) = \alpha_0 + \alpha_1 n \text{ (where } \alpha_0 + \alpha_1 n > 0,\ 5\alpha_0 + 10\alpha_1 = 1),$$

$$\text{Prob}(x = 1 | y) = [1 + \exp(-\theta_0 - \theta_1 y)]^{-1}, \text{ and}$$

$$\text{Prob}(d = 1 | x,y) = [1 + \exp(-\beta_0 - \beta_1 x - \beta_2 y)]^{-1} \quad .$$

For comparison to Table 1-3, let $EO_0 = \exp(\theta_0)$, $OR_{xy} = \exp(\theta_1)$, $OR_{dx} = \exp(\beta_1)$, and $OR_{dy} = \exp(\beta_2)$. Table 4 presents some results of comparing unmatched, 60% matched, and fully matched designs, and for the matched designs comparing analyses based on pooling, breaking the matching and

TABLE 4

Comparison of variances obtained under different design-analysis combinations. Each tabulated value is the asymptotic variance of the logistic coefficient estimator for the combination, relative to unmatched design with categorical analysis, times 100. All parameter variations are done using the following model as baseline: $EO_o = 1/4$, $OR_{xy} = OR_{dx} = OR_{dy} = 5/2$, $\text{Prob}(y = n) = 0.32 - 0.06n$ (see text for definition of symbols).

| | | Model | | | | | | |
|---|---|---|---|---|---|---|---|---|
| Percent matched | Analysis* | Base | $EO_o = 2$ | $OR_{xy} = 2/5$ | $OR_{dx} = 2/5$ | $OR_{dy} = 2/5$ | $OR_{xy} = 1/2$, $OR_{dy} = 1/2$ | † |
| Zero % | D, int | 99 | 99 | 97 | 99 | 99 | 100 | 99 |
| | X, int | 100 | 99 | 100 | 99 | 99 | 100 | 99 |
| 60% | D, cat | 90 | 98 | 109 | 84 | 87 | 82 | 95 |
| | D, com | 97 | 105 | 117 | 86 | 88 | 84 | 99 |
| | D, int | 89 | 96 | 101 | 83 | 87 | 82 | 94 |
| | X, int | 90 | 98 | 108 | 83 | 87 | 82 | 95 |
| 100% | D, cat | 95 | 110 | 135 | 79 | 82 | 76 | 99 |
| | D, int | 93 | 108 | 132 | 78 | 82 | 76 | 98 |
| | X, int | 95 | 110 | 135 | 79 | 82 | 76 | 99 |

*D = disease used as outcome; X = exposure used as outcome; cat = covariate treated as categorical (i.e., y entered as 4 indicator variables); int = covariate treated as interval-scaled; com = unmatched subjects analyzed with interval model, matched subjects analyzed with categorical model, results then combined. Notes: The combination "X, cat" has the same variance as the "D, cat" combination; "D, int" is biased under the matched designs, and therefore the tabulated variance is understated [16].

†Using $\text{Prob}(y = n) = 0.08 + 0.06n$.

employing disease regression, and breaking the matching and employing exposure regression. Results are presented in terms of the large-sample variance of the logistic coefficient estimator for x, relative to this variance under an unmatched design treating y as a categorical variable (i.e., entering y as four indicator variables). Variances were derived from the expected information matrix, and thus the tabulated values somewhat misstate the actual large-sample variances in the misspecified models [16]. Note that for this "large-stratum" setup, an analysis treating y as categorical yields the same large-sample variance as a conditional logistic analysis. The parameter values used in the exploration in Table 4 were chosen to yield expected data in a typical range, rather than to represent extreme situations. Other explorations were conducted using various baseline models, and these yielded qualitatively similar results.

Unsurprisingly, design appears to be a much more important determinant of variance than the analysis method. No design-analysis combination is consistently best or worst, although within designs the analysis using disease as outcome and the covariate y as continuous nearly always yields the smallest computed variance. With one exception, in practical terms there appears to be little difference between the variances associated with the different analysis methods. The one exception is that the analysis method for partially matched designs based on separate analysis of the matched and unmatched subjects, followed by pooling of results, has consistently higher variance than the other analysis options. It appears that, much like the binary case considered before, when matching is beneficial 60% matching captures most of the variance benefit of matching, while when matching is detrimental 60% matching retains most of the precision of the unmatched design. Thus, under the models considered here, partial matching does not deviate as far from optimality as the other two designs.

While the analysis based on interval scaling for y yields a lower computed variance than the categorical analysis, in the partial and fully matched designs the interval-scaled analysis with disease as outcome yields a biased coefficient for x. (This arises because the matched-sample conditional distribution of disease given x and y does not follow a first-order logistic model with y interval-scaled.) Table 5 exhibits the large-sample bias (computed by the multivariate $\delta$-method [12, sec. 14.6]) associated with the two biased design-analysis combinations. This exhibits a sharp difference between the partially matched and fully matched designs: the bias induced by treating y as interval-scaled is consistently very small in the fully matched situations. This observation is readily explained by the fact that in the fully matched case, the residual y-disease association is very small (the crude y-disease association having been removed by matching) and misspecification of its form can thus have little impact; in contrast, considerable residual y-disease association can remain in the partially matched design.

The residual bias of the estimators in the two combinations in Table 5 leads naturally to consideration of their mean-squared error relative to analysis of the same design treating y categorically (which yields an asymptotically unbiased estimator of the x coefficient). Table 5 displays the large-sample mean-squared errors of the biased analyses (relative to the categorical analyses) for several sample sizes; mean-squared errors were computed as the sum of variance and the square of bias. At the small sample size (100 cases and 100 controls) the large-sample bias appears to be of little importance, in that the interval-scaled analysis never does worse than the categorical analysis and often retains the smaller computed mean-squared error. At the large sample size (900 cases and 900 controls), however, the disadvantage resulting from large bias becomes apparent. Furthermore, because the variance portions of the mean-squared errors were computed without regard to specification error, the values in Table 5 understate the disadvantage. In the fully matched situation the choice of analalysis method appears unimportant.

5. Discussion. The partial-matching pattern used to obtain the results given above is unrealistic, in that it assumes the probability of finding a match is unrelated to the matching factors. The reason for using this pattern was to avoid adding extra free parameters to the presentation; also, limited investigations of the impact of such a dependency indicated that introducing it would yield practical observations little different from those made here. For example, I experimented with allowing the probability of finding a match to equal Pr(y,z)/Pr(y´,z´), where Pr(y,z) is the joint distribution of y and z,

TABLE 5

Asymptotic bias and mean-squared error (MSE) of biased design-analysis combinations, relative to mean-squared error of same design with categorical analysis, times 100. N = size of case sample = size of control sample. In all models, absolute value of true coefficient is log(5/2) = 0.916.

| | Model | | | | | | |
|---|---|---|---|---|---|---|---|
| Design/Analysis* | Base | $EO_o = 2$ | $OR_{xy} = 2/5$ | $OR_{dx} = 2/5$ | $OR_{dy} = 2/5$ | $OR_{xy} = 1/2$, $OR_{dy} = 1/2$ | † |
| 60%, D, int — | | | | | | | |
| % bias in coefficient | 5 | 8 | -10 | 0 | 1 | -1 | 3 |
| Relative MSE: | | | | | | | |
| at N = 100 | 100 | 98 | 95 | 99 | 100 | 100 | 96 |
| at N = 300 | 102 | 100 | 99 | 99 | 100 | 100 | 96 |
| at N = 900 | 109 | 106 | 113 | 99 | 101 | 100 | 98 |
| 100%, D, int — | | | | | | | |
| % bias in coefficient | 1 | 2 | -2 | 0 | 0 | 0 | -1 |
| Relative MSE: | | | | | | | |
| at N = 100 | 98 | 98 | 98 | 100 | 100 | 100 | 99 |
| at N = 300 | 98 | 98 | 98 | 100 | 100 | 100 | 99 |
| at N = 900 | 99 | 98 | 98 | 100 | 100 | 100 | 99 |

*Percent matched, followed by analysis code; see footnote on Table 4.

†Using Prob(y = n) = 0.08 + 0.06n.

and $(y',z')$ is the most frequent combination of matching-factor values. For Model A of Table 1, this yielded an overall proportion matched $P_m$ of 0.48, with only 40% of cases matched when $y = z = 1$. Yet the variance ratio for partial matching relative to full matching under this setup was only 1.02 (virtually the same as under the simpler partial-matching scheme with a 48% proportion matched). Thus, in this situation, even variable partial matching captures most of the efficiency benefit of matching (which, as apparent from Table 1, is non-negligible).

This paper has treated imperfect matching as failure to find a match. When the matching factors are continuous, partial matching may represent "loose" matching, with some degree of matching present for all subjects, rather than complete failure to match some subjects. One approach to this problem would be to extend Rubin's [17] method for continuous outcomes to the logistic model: assuming the logistic population model given earlier, the analysis of case-control data imperfectly pair-matched on y could proceed by letting $\Delta x$ and $\Delta y$ be the pairwise case-control difference in x and y, and fitting the logistic model

$$\Pr(\text{success}|\Delta x,\Delta y) = (1 + \exp[\beta(\Delta x) + \gamma(\Delta y)])^{-1}$$

obtained by treating each pair as a binomial trial with outcome one ("success") and regressors $\Delta x$ and $\Delta y$. Note that in this formulation x, y, $\beta$, and $\gamma$ may be vectors, and that the matching may involve variables (not included in y) for which a perfect match was obtained; in particular, the pairs may be matched on unquantified factors such as neighborhood. More general matched designs might be dealt with by defining (for each matched subject) $\Delta y$ to equal the deviation of the subject's y-value from the mean of y in the subject's matched set; $\Delta y$ could then be entered as a covariate in a conditional logistic model. It would be of interest to compare this approach (or some refinement of it) to approaches that break the matching and control the covariate via modelling only.

Studies of epidemiologic designs (including the present one) have been hampered by the need to consider a large number of free parameters and the general lack of simple relationships between these parameters and relative efficiency. Conclusions will necessarily depend on the region of the joint parameter space that is explored, and subjective judgments about whether observed relationships are of practical importance or not; counter-examples to some earlier conclusions continue to be found [11], and recommendations have not been consistent (e.g., contrast Kupper et al [3] to Howe and Choi [6,7]). The current paper has examined a somewhat more complex situation than those in earlier studies, but the pattern of efficiency of matching relative to no matching appears consistent with those found in most earlier studies; that is, no consistently superior design strategy emerges. Nevertheless, I would interpret the results in Tables 1-5 as supportive of earlier recommendations [5] that one should limit matching to strong risk factors.

Even with this constraint, one may still have too many good matching candidates to perfectly match on them all. Nearly all the previous literature has talked as if the choice then is to pick only a small subset and attempt perfect matching on these, when in fact partial matching on a larger subset would have been a viable alternative. Since partial matching often occurs involuntarily anyway (due to failure to find perfect matches), a study of its properties seemed overdue.

Now the number of free parameters in a study of partial matching is even larger than in studies of simply matching versus not matching (especially when one considers the enormous variety of possible partial-matching patterns), and my explorations of the parameter space should be regarded as quite preliminary. With this caveat in mind, I offer the following tentative observations:

A) For all practical purposes, marginal matching appears to have about the same impact on efficiency as full matching, and so one should be quite content if marginal matching can be attained.

B) Even if relatively large proportions (perhaps up to a third) of subjects remain unmatched on one or more factors, as long as optimal analytic methods are used the efficiency of the study will rarely deviate much further from optimality than the fully matched design.

C) In practice, partially matched data can be efficiently and validly analyzed by breaking the matching and entering the matching factors in the analysis model; consequently, one need never discard unmatched subjects as unanalyzable. One should, however, be wary of the specification bias that can occur when modelling partially matched interval-scaled covariates in their interval-scaled form.

D) The efficiency loss engendered by treating an interval-scaled covariate as categorical appears very small. (Note that this comment does <u>not</u> apply to the study exposure.)

Of course, all the preceding observations apply only to the investigation of main effects. The impact of matching in the study of interactions is quite different [9, 10] and is not addressed here.

With regard to observation C, the results in Table 5 reflect a general rule that the importance of bias relative to variance is directly proportional to the sample size. This is fortunate for the situation at hand, for it is precisely in the small-sample case that one would be tempted to economize on parameters in an unconditional ("unmatched") analysis by entering y as an interval-scaled variable rather than as a categorical variable.

Objections are often raised to including unmatched cases in a study on the grounds that their failure to be matched reflects a property of these cases that would bias the analysis, were they to be included. In fact, the only distinguishing property of unmatched cases is the rarity of their matching-factor pattern in the control source population. In this case, adequate control of the matching factors should prevent bias from use of unmatched cases. One caution does apply, however, if some of the factors are to be controlled as interval-scaled covariates in a model: the unmatched cases may represent extreme values of the factors and thus may unduly influence the regression results. Regression diagnostics would hopefully reveal such a situation, but this problem (along with the specification-bias problem seen in Table 5) suggests that regression results of partially matched studies will be especially sensitive to dose-response specifications.

The conclusions presented here (especially the last paragraph) have assumed throughout that both the matched and unmatched cases arise from the same population at risk. Failure to match may, however, be a consequence of the unmatched cases arising from a different population than the matched cases (one possibly different in its distribution of uncontrolled covariates conditional on controlled covariates). If so, it may be essential for validity that the random-sample controls obtained for the unmatched cases be obtained from the population generating those cases, and that an indicator for population of origin be entered in any analysis of the combined data. This should include analysis of possible exposure-population interactions; if numbers permit, I would also recommend one perform and compare separate analyses of each population, in case of extensive heterogeneity of effects across populations.

In closing, I would again emphasize that the conclusions presented here are tentative, and I would like to encourage further research on the efficiency and analysis of partially matched designs. Particularly valuable would be examinations of more realistic partial-matching patterns than those used here, and more detailed study of analytic methods for dealing with interval-scaled matching factors in a partially matched study.

ACKNOWLEDGEMENTS:

I wish to thank Edward Lustbader, Suresh Moolgavkar, and James Robins for their helpful comments. I also thank Virginia Hansen for her help in preparing the manuscript.

## REFERENCES

[1] M.L. SAMUELS, Matching and design efficiency in epidemiological studies. Biometrika, 68 (1981), pp. 577-588.

[2] P.G. SMITH and N.E. DAY, Matching and confounding in the design and analysis of epidemiological case-control studies, in Perspectives in Medical Statistics, J.F. Bithell and R. Coppi (eds.), Academic Press, New York, 1981.

[3] L.L. KUPPER, J. M. KARON, D.G. KLEINBAUM, H. MORGENSTERN, and D.K. LEWIS, Matching in epidemiologic studies: validity and efficiency considerations. Biometrics, 37 (1981), pp. 271-291.

[4] W.D. THOMPSON, J.L. KELSEY, and S.D. WALTER, Cost and efficiency in the choice of matched and unmatched case-control study designs. Am. J. Epidemiol., 116 (1982), pp. 840-851.

[5] D.C. THOMAS and S. GREENLAND, The relative efficiencies of matched and independent sample designs for case-control studies. J Chronic Dis., 36 (1983), pp. 685-697.

[6] G. R. HOWE and B.C.K. CHOI, Methodological issues in case-control studies: validity and power of various design/analysis strategies. Int. J. Epidemiol., 12 (1983), pp. 238-245.

[7] B.C.K. CHOI and G.R. HOWE, Methodological issues in case-control studies: II. Test statistics as measures of efficiency. Int. J. Epidemiol., 13 (1984), pp. 229-234.

[8] B.C.K. CHOI, Unnecessary stratification/pairing can never increase efficiency – a mathematical proof. Int. J. Epidemiol., 13 (1984), pp. 116-117 (Letter to the Editor).

[9] P.G. SMITH and N.E. DAY, The design of case-control studies: the influence of confounding and interaction effects. Int. J. Epidemiol., 13 (1984), pp. 356-365.

[10] D.C. THOMAS and S. GREENLAND, The efficiency of matching in case-control studies of risk-factor interactions. J Chronic Dis., 38 (1985), in press.

[11] L.A. KALISH, Matching on a non-risk factor in case-control studies does not always result in an efficiency loss. Am. J. Epidemiol. (1986), in press.

[12] Y.M.M. BISHOP, S.E. FIENBERG, and P.W. HOLLAND, Discrete Multivariate Analysis: Theory and Practice, MIT Press, Cambridge, MA, 1975.

[13] N.E. BRESLOW, N.E. DAY, K.T. HALVORSEN, R.L. PRENTICE, and C. SABAI, Estimation of multiple relative risk functions in matched case-control studies. Am. J. Epidemiol., 108 (1978), pp. 299-307.

[14] R.L. PRENTICE, Use of the logistic model in retrospective studies. Biometrics, 32 (1976), pp. 599-606.

[15] D.C. THOMAS, General relative-risk models for survival time and matched case-control analysis. Biometrics, 37 (1981), pp. 673-686.

[16] H. WHITE, Maximum Likelihood Estimation of Misspecified Models, Discussion Paper 80-32, Dept. of Economics, Univ. of California, San Diego, CA, 1980.

[17] D.B. RUBIN, The use of matched sampling and regression adjustment to remove bias in observational studies, Biometrics, 29 (1973), pp. 185-203.

# Design Options for Sampling Within a Cohort

*Ross L. Prentice*, Steven G. Self*, and Mark W. Mason**

Abstract. Designs are considered which permit efficient relative risk regression estimation without requiring the assembly of covariate histories on all members of a defined cohort. A standard 'case-control within cohort' design is described along with a more structured time-matched design in which a subject can serve as a control in at most one risk set. The latter design is expected to typically give rise to some small efficiency improvement, but at the expense of more complex variance estimation. A case-cohort design is described as an alternative to case-control sampling. This design involves the selection of a (stratified) random subcohort of the entire cohort which then provides the comparison group for all cases, regardless of whether such cases arise within or outside of the selected subcohort. This design is expected to typically give noteworthy efficiency gains relative to the case-control designs. Simulation results permit comparison among these designs in selected circumstances.

## INTRODUCTION

Epidemiologic cohort studies frequently involve the periodic acquisition of extensive raw materials. Such raw materials are used to construct individual 'covariate' histories, which may then be related to subsequent failure (disease) occurrence. For example, the raw materials may include detailed occupational exposure records, dietary intake records, blood samples or cells. The processing of such raw materials to obtain the desired covariate histories can be time-consuming and expensive. For example, such processing may involve abstraction from and interpretation of industrial exposure records, hand coding of individual diet records to obtain nutrient intake estimates, biochemical analysis of blood sera for micronutrient and trace metal levels, or examination of individual cells for chromosomal aberrations or for the presence of viral fragments. Very often the temporal relationship between covariate histories that are evolving over time and failure rate is of particular interest. In such

---

*Division of Public Health Sciences, Fred Hutchinson Cancer Research Center, 1124 Columbia Street, Seattle, WA., 98104. This work partially supported by NIH grants GM-24472, GM-28314, CA-38526 and CA-34847.

circumstances it is natural to take the instantaneous failure rate or hazard function as the primary target of estimation. The ratio of such failure rates for a general covariate history to that for a standard history will often provide an insightful summary of the relationship between failure rate and covariates. This relative risk function, or relative risk process, can be efficiently estimated under a variety of sampling schemes that can reduce, to a fraction of the cohort, the set of subjects for whom covariate data need be assembled.

Before describing these sampling procedures let us introduce necessary notation and briefly review full-cohort relative risk estimation procedures. Let $Z(t)$ denote a covariate measurement for a subject at time t. Let $\lambda\{t;Z(u),0 \leq u < t\}$ denote the instantaneous failure rate at time t for a subject with covariate history $\{Z(u),0 \leq u < t\}$ prior to time t. A relative risk regression model (e.g., Cox [1]; Kalbfleisch and Prentice [ 2 ]) may be defined by

$$\lambda\{t;Z(u),0 \leq u < t\} = \lambda_0(t)\; r\{X(t)\beta\} \quad , \tag{1}$$

where the modeled regression vector $X(t) = \{X_1(t),\cdots,X_p(t)\}$ consists of functions of $\{Z(u);0 \leq u < t\}$ or products of such functions with time, $\beta$ is a corresponding column p-vector of regression parameters to be estimated, $r(\cdot)$ is a fixed function, usually $r(\cdot) = \exp(\cdot)$ or $r(\cdot) = 1+(\cdot)$, standardized so that $r(0) = 1$, and $\lambda_0(\cdot)$ is a baseline failure rate function corresponding to a standard covariate history for which $X(t) \equiv 0$. Consider a cohort of size n and let $\{N_i(u),Y_i(u),0 \leq u \leq t\}$ denote failure time counting and censoring processes up to time t for the $i^{th}$ subject. Thus $N_i$, with right continuous sample paths, takes value zero prior to an observed failure on subject i and value one thereafter, while $Y_i$ with left continuous sample paths takes value one at times at which the $i^{th}$ subject is 'at risk' for failure and value zero otherwise. The sample paths for $X_i$ are assumed to be left continuous with right hand limits.

If counting, censoring and covariate data are available on all subjects in the cohort then estimation of the relative risk regression parameter $\beta$ can be based on the partial likelihood (Cox [ 3 ]) function

$$L(\beta) = \prod_{i=1}^{n} \{r_{ii} / \sum_{\ell=1}^{n} r_{\ell i}\}^{\delta_i} \quad , \tag{2}$$

where the observed failure or censoring time for the $i^{th}$ subject is given by $t_i = \inf\{t|Y_i(u) = 0,\text{ all } u > t\}$, the corresponding censoring indicator is defined by $\delta_i = 1$ if $N_i(t_i) \neq N_i(t_i^-)$ and $\delta_i = 0$ otherwise, and $r_{\ell i} = Y_\ell(t_i)\; r\{X_\ell(t_i)\beta\}$. That (2) possess a partial likelihood interpretation can be seen by defining the $\sigma$-algebras

$$F(t) = \sigma\{N_i(u),Y_i(u),Z_i(u);0 \leq u < t\}$$

and noting that, under standard independent failure time and censorship assumptions,

$$\mathrm{pr}\{N_i(t)\neq N_i(t^-)\,|\,\mathcal{F}(t), N(t)\neq N(t^-)\} = Y_i(t)r\{X_i(t)\beta\}/\sum_{\ell=1}^{n} Y_\ell(t)r\{X_\ell(t)\beta\}, \quad (3)$$

where $N(t) = \{N_1(t),\cdots,N_n(t)\}$. $L(\beta)$ can be manipulated as if it were an ordinary likelihood function in respect to asymptotic likelihood inference on $\beta$ (Andersen and Gill [4]; Prentice and Self [5]).

Synthetic Case-Control Designs. In order to reduce the number of subjects for whom covariate data need be assembled, and in order to reduce computations in maximizing (2), a number of authors (e.g., Liddell et al, [6], Breslow and Patton [7], Whittemore [8], Thomas [9], Oakes [10], Whittemore and McMillan [11], Breslow et al, [12], Lubin and Gail [13]) have suggested that at each observed failure ($\delta_i=1$) the denominator summation in (2) be replaced by a sum over i and a random sample of all other subjects $\{j\neq i\}$. Typically random sampling at a particular failure time $t_i$ would continue until a specified number of 'at risk' $\{Y_\ell(t_i)=1\}$ 'controls' had been sampled. If the random sampling at each failure time takes place without replacement, while the random samplings at distinct failure times are independent (hereafter referred to as case-control design A) then the resulting function

$$L(\beta) = \prod_{i=1}^{n} \{r_{ii} / \sum_{\ell\in\tilde{R}(t_i)} r_{\ell i}\}^{\delta_i} \quad (4)$$

again has a partial likelihood interpretation (Oakes [10]), where $\tilde{R}(t_i)$ includes the failing subject at $t_i$ along with its time-matched controls. That (4) is a partial likelihood can be seen by defining

$$\mathcal{F}(t) = \sigma[\{N_i(u), Y_i(u), Z_i(u), 0\leq u < t, i\in K(t)\}; \tilde{R}(u), 0\leq u\leq t],$$

where $K(t)$ consists of all cases occurring at time t or earlier along with their matched controls and $\tilde{R}(u)$ is empty unless a failure occurs at t, and noting that under standard independent failure and censorship assumptions

$$\mathrm{pr}\{N_i(t)\neq N_i(t^-)\,|\,\mathcal{F}(t), N(t)\neq N(t^-)\} = Y_i(t)r\{X_i(t)\beta\} / \sum_{\ell\in\tilde{R}(t)} Y_\ell(t)r\{X_\ell(t)\beta\}. \quad (5)$$

Expression (4) was also developed by Prentice and Breslow [14] under time-matched case-control sampling from a 'large', conceptually infinite, population in which the matched sets $\tilde{R}(t)$, could be assumed disjoint at distinct failure times, in which circumstance (4) is a conditional likelihood. In the context of case-control sampling within a cohort one could ask whether improved estimation properties would accrue if the sampling were restricted so that a subject, once selected as a control, is ineligible for control selection at all subsequent failure times (hereafter referred to as case-control design B). Such a sampling procedure is mentioned in Robins et al [15] and is examined in some detail in Prentice [16]. Expression (4) can again be used for relative risk parameter estimation with $\tilde{R}(t)$, at a failure time t, defined to consist of the failure and matched controls at risk at t as before. If, however, the failing subject was at risk and had been selected as a control at $t' < t$, $\tilde{R}(t)$ will consist only of the failing subject together with the matched controls that were also at risk at both t and $t'$. With this requirement expression (5) again holds with $\mathcal{F}(t)$ defined by

$$\mathcal{F}(t) = \sigma[\{N_i(u), Y_i(u), Z_i(u), 0 \le u < t, i \in K(t)\}, \tilde{R}(t), A(t,u), \Delta(t,u), 0 \le u < t],$$

where $K(t)$ is the union of $\tilde{R}(u)$ for all $u \le t$, $A(t,u) = \tilde{R}(t) \cup \tilde{R}(u)$, and $\Delta(t,u) = 1$ if a failure occurs at time t and the failing subject is in $\tilde{R}(u)$, and $\Delta(t,u) = 0$ otherwise. Case-control design B induces a typically negative correlation between the score statistic contributions at t and u if $\Delta(t,u) = 1$. Hence (4) is generally not a partial likelihood function. It can be referred to as a pseudolikelihood following Besag [17]. Correlations among distinct score statistic contributions are, however, readily estimated [16] and since they are typically negative the more structured case-control design B can be expected to have slightly better efficiency properties than does the corresponding design A.

Case-Cohort Designs. An opposite extreme to the disjoint control samples of case-control design B involves the selection of a random subset $C \subset \{1, 2, \cdots, n\}$ of the cohort and the specification $\tilde{R}(t) = D(t) \cup C$ in (4), where $D(t) = \{\ell \mid N_\ell(t) \ne N_\ell(t^-)\}$ is the set of subjects failing at t. Assuming absolutely continuous failure times $D(t)$ will include at most one subject. This design allows each selected 'control', that is each member of C, to contribute to the comparison group at every failure time at which that control is at risk. This design requires covariate data assembly on all failures (cases) and on all members of the subcohort C, and hence may be termed a case-cohort design. Such designs are discussed in Prentice [18]. Related designs with a binary response, rather than time-to-response, and binary covariate are considered by Kupper et al [19] and Miettinen [20].

A retrospective application of a case-cohort design may involve selection of a subcohort C with size that is a specified multiple of the number of observed failures in the cohort. Under extreme censorship it may be advisable to continue subcohort sampling until some minimum number of subjects in C are at risk at each observed failure time. A major advantage of the case-cohort design relative to the above case-control designs arises from the fact that the subcohort can be selected in advance and the corresponding covariate histories can be assembled and monitored during the course of cohort follow-up. This feature seems particularly valuable in the context of large scale prevention/intervention trials. Raw covariate data may be processed on an ongoing basis on a suitably selected subcohort in order to monitor the achievement of intervention goals and in order to monitor compliance on a groupwise basis. Covariate data necessary for the monitoring of individual safety or individual compliance would, of course, need to be processed on the entire trial cohort.

In order to be specific consider the so-called Women's Health Trial currently in a feasibility phase in this country. This trial hopes to randomize up to 15,000 women at increased risk for breast cancer to either their usual diet or to a diet in which fat constitutes only about 20% of calories, as compared to the customary level of approximately 40% in America. The achievement of dietary fat goals will be monitored primarily on the basis of hand-coded 4-day diet records obtained at baseline and periodically thereafter. Serum levels of micronutrients and hormones (estrogens) will play an important role in understanding and interpreting any difference in breast cancer occurrence between the two randomization groups during a follow-up period of 5-10 years. The cost of dietary data coding and biochemical analysis of blood sera on the entire cohort could run into the millions of dollars on a cohort of this size. Much of this cost could be averted if such analyses were restricted to a subcohort of perhaps 20-25% of the entire cohort along with the approximately 5% of the cohort expected to develop breast cancer during follow-up. Note that dietary records and blood sera need to be collected on the entire cohort, but processed only for the subcohort and for cases as they arise. Note also that attention needs to be paid to the stability of covariate values over time when such values are obtained from stored materials, and to the constancy over time in the means of processing such raw materials.

There are additional motivations for a case-cohort as opposed to a case-control within cohort design: the selected subcohort provides a natural comparison group for a variety of failure time endpoints in the case-cohort design, whereas the control selection in a case-control design focuses on a single endpoint definition. Also, a case-cohort analysis, like the corresponding full-cohort analysis, permits the estimation of the cumulative baseline disease rate in addition to the relative risk process. Perhaps most importantly, the case-cohort design appears capable of recovering a loss of efficiency that arises from the fact that a given subject contributes to the comparison set only at selected time points in the synthetic case-control approach. Whittemore and McMillan [11] note that the efficiency properties of the unmatched case-control design for odds ratio estimation are noticeably better ($\beta \neq 0$) than the corresponding efficiency properties for the time-matched case-control design for relative risk estimation. Simulation calculations, described below suggest that efficiency properties for the case-cohort design will agree closely with those for the corresponding unmatched case-control design in situations in which both designs can be applied (i.e., fixed covariates, common follow-up period, censorship only at end of follow-up period).

Estimation under a case-cohort design [18] will now be briefly outlined. Let $K(t) = \{i | N_i(t) = 1\}$ denote the set of subjects failing at or before time t. Covariate histories at time t will be assumed available for subjects in $M(t) = K(t) \cup C$. Denote $\tilde{R}(t) = D(t) \cup C$ as above and let $\Delta(t) = 1$ if $\tilde{R}(t) = C$ and $\Delta(t) = 0$ otherwise. Thus $\Delta(t) = 1$ only if a failure occurs at time t outside the subcohort C. Expression (4) generally is not a partial likelihood under this design and will again be referred to as a pseudolikelihood function. The maximum pseudo-likelihood estimate $\hat{\beta}$ is defined by $U(\hat{\beta}) = 0$ where

$$U(\beta) = \partial \log L(\beta)/\partial\beta = \sum_{i=1}^{n} U_i(\beta) = \sum_{i=1}^{n} \delta_i \{c_{ii} - \sum_{\ell \varepsilon \tilde{R}(t_i)} b_{\ell i} / \sum_{\ell \varepsilon \tilde{R}(t_i)} r_{\ell i}\} ,$$

and where $b_{\ell i} = Y_{\ell i}(t_i) X_\ell(t_i) r'\{X_\ell(t_i)\beta\}$, $c_{\ell i} = b_{\ell i} r^{-1}\{X_\ell(t_i)\beta\}$ and $r'(u) = dr(u)/du$.

Upon defining

$$F(t) = \sigma[\{N_i(u), Y_i(u), 0 \le u < t, i=1,\cdots,n\}, \{Z_i(u), 0 \le u < t, i \varepsilon M(t)\}, \tilde{R}(t), \Delta(t)]$$

one can readily show that (5) again holds. It follows easily that each $U_j(\beta)$ has mean zero conditional on $\{F(t_j), N(t_j) \neq N(t_j^-)\}$, and has conditional variance

$$v_{jj} = \sum_{i \varepsilon \tilde{R}(t_j)} c_{ij}' c_{ij} R_j^{-1} - B_j' B_j R_j^{-2} ,$$

where $R_j = \sum_{\ell \varepsilon \tilde{R}(t_j)} r_{\ell j}$, $B_j = \sum_{\ell \varepsilon \tilde{R}(t_j)} b_{\ell j}$ .

Furthermore, since at most one subject in $\tilde{R}(t_j)$ is not a member of $R(t_k)$ for $t_k < t_j$ one can readily calculate, if $\delta_k = \delta_j = 1$, that

$$E\{U_k(\beta)U_j(\beta)\,|\,\mathcal{F}(t_j),N(t_j)\neq N(t_j^-)\} = -\Delta(t_j)\sum_{i\in\tilde{R}(t_j)}\left\{\frac{B_k+b_{jk}-b_{ik}}{R_k+r_{jk}-r_{ik}}\right\}\left\{c_{ij}-\frac{B_j}{R_j}\right\}r_{ij}R_j^{-1}$$

$$= \Delta(t_j)\,v_{kj} \quad .$$

Hence $U(\beta)$ has mean zero and variance estimated by

$$V(\beta) = \sum_{j=1}^{n}\delta_j[v_{jj} + 2\Delta(t_j)\sum_{\{k|t_k<t_j\}}\delta_k v_{kj}] \quad .$$

Under regularity and stability conditions one then expects $n^{\frac{1}{2}}(\hat{\beta}-\beta)$ to converge weakly to a normal variate with mean zero and with variance consistently estimated by $n\,I(\hat{\beta})^{-1}\,V(\hat{\beta})\,I(\hat{\beta})^{-1}$ where $I(\beta) = -\partial^2\log L(\beta)/\partial\beta^2$. Though flexible sufficient conditions for the convergence just mentioned are still under development, the asymptotic normality of the standardized score statistic $n^{\frac{1}{2}}U(\beta)$ can be shown under the conditions of [4] and [5], along with additional conditions relating to (a) the convergence of $m\,n^{-1}$ to a positive constant where m is the subcohort size, (b) the asymptotic stability of processes appearing in the first and second derivatives of the logarithm of (4), (c) the 'tightness' of the difference between certain full-cohort and subcohort sample averages appearing in the derivatives just mentioned, and (d) additional Lindeberg assumptions. These conditions, along with a representation of $n^{-\frac{1}{2}}U(\beta)$ as a sum of a martingale and an asymptotically uncorrelated term to which finite population convergence results apply, yield the desired asymptotic normality and give a variance expression that is the sum of the full-cohort score statistic asymptotic variance and a term involving covariances among the difference between certain subcohort and full-cohort sample averages. The details of this work will be presented elsewhere.

A natural 'estimator' of the cumulative baseline failure rate $\Lambda_0(t) = \int_0^t \lambda_0(u)du$ is given by

$$\hat{\Lambda}_0(t) = m\,n^{-1}\int_0^t [\sum_{\ell\varepsilon C} Y_i(w)\,r\{X_\ell(w)\beta\}]^{-1}\, d\,\bar{N}(w) \quad ,$$

where m is the size of the selected subcohort and $\bar{N} = N_1+\cdots+N_n$.

Simulation Results. A small simulation was conducted in order to compare the properties of $\hat{\beta}$ and related quantities under full-cohort partial likelihood estimation (2), under case-control designs A and B with estimation based on (4), and under a case-cohort design with estimation based on (4). Most results of this simulation have previously been reported in [16] and [18].

A cohort of size n=500 was selected and exponentially distributed failure times, censored at unity, were generated corresponding to a binary covariate that took each of values zero and one for 250 cohort members. The exponential failure rate parameter was selected to give 50 expected failures for each sample. One hundred samples were generated at each of relative risks one and two for the binary covariate. An exponential form relative risk model, $r(\cdot) = \exp(\cdot)$, was used throughout. Case-control designs A and B were applied both with one and with five controls per case. Such analyses will involve covariate data on an expected 100 and 300 subjects, respectively. Subcohorts of size 55 and 275 were selected for the case-cohort design in order to also yield an expected 100 and 300 subjects, respectively, for which covariate data is required. All calculations took place on an HP3000 minicomputer.

Table 1 gives summary statistics for these analyses. Convergence of a Newton-Raphson iterative procedure was achieved for each estimation method for every sample. The upper half of Table 1 suggests rather similar properties at $\beta=0$ for the two case-control designs and the case-cohort design, both with 100 and 300 subjects requiring covariate data. The sample mean of $\hat{\beta}$ values differs from zero by more than one estimated standard error only for case-control design A and one case per control. Sample standard errors for $\hat{\beta}$ and the average of estimated standard errors for $\hat{\beta}$ are slightly larger for case-control design A than for the other designs. There is also a suggestion of anticonservatism with case-control design A for a test of $\beta=0$ based on $\hat{\beta}$ divided by its standard error (i.e., a suggestion that actual significance levels exceed nominal levels). This point merits further study. The sample standard errors for analyses involving an expected 300 subjects are within 10% of the full-cohort sample standard errors for all methods. Moreover, this would not likely change appreciably if the basic cohort size were 5,000 or 50,000 rather than 500. With only 100 samples there is considerable random variation in the sample standard errors for $\hat{\beta}$. Upon acknowledging this randomness one can note that sample standard errors are all in good agreement with the corresponding mean of standard error estimates with the exception of case-control design A with one case per control where the sample standard error (0.484) exceeds the corresponding mean (0.420) by about two standard errors.

The situation is rather different at a relative risk of two ($\beta=0.693$) as shown in the lower half of Table 1. The case-cohort sample standard errors are about midway between the full-cohort and the case-control sample standard errors, both at 100 and 300 expected subjects. This

TABLE 1

Simulation summary statistics for various methods of estimating the logarithm of the relative risk (β)

| Estimation Procedure | Full-Cohort | Case-Control Design A | Case-Control Design B | Case-Cohort | Case-Control Design A | Case-Control Design B | Case-Cohort |
|---|---|---|---|---|---|---|---|
| Expected subjects requiring covariate data | 500 | 100 | 100 | 100 | 300 | 300 | 300 |
| Relative Risk = 1 ($\beta$ = 0) | | | | | | | |
| Sample mean ($\hat{\beta}$) | -0.031 | -0.064 | -0.037 | -0.006 | -0.034 | -0.027 | -0.021 |
| Mean of Std. Error Ests. | 0.286 | 0.420(47)* | 0.404(40) | 0.389(36) | 0.312(9) | 0.298(4) | 0.304(7) |
| Sample Std. Error ($\hat{\beta}$) | 0.335 | 0.484(44) | 0.411(23) | 0.412(23) | 0.364(9) | 0.337(1) | 0.348(4) |
| Est. Significance Level ($\alpha$ = 0.10) | 0.10 | 0.12 | 0.10 | 0.10 | 0.12 | 0.10 | 0.13 |
| Est. Significance Level ($\alpha$ = 0.05) | 0.08 | 0.10 | 0.04 | 0.06 | 0.09 | 0.05 | 0.08 |
| Relative Risk = 2 ($\beta$ =0.693) | | | | | | | |
| Sample mean ($\hat{\beta}$) | 0.731 | 0.748 | 0.721 | 0.676 | 0.729 | 0.729 | 0.728 |
| Mean of Std. Error Ests. | 0.303 | 0.444(47)* | 0.430(45) | 0.399(32) | 0.330(9) | 0.316(4) | 0.318(5) |
| Sample Std. Error ($\hat{\beta}$) | 0.258 | 0.417(62) | 0.461(79) | 0.337(31) | 0.282(9) | 0.280(9) | 0.269(4) |
| Est. Rejection Rate+ ($\alpha$ = 0.10) | 0.84 | 0.50 | 0.53 | 0.56 | 0.78 | 0.77 | 0.78 |
| Est. Rejection Rate ($\alpha$ = 0.05) | 0.72 | 0.39 | 0.38 | 0.33 | 0.63 | 0.68 | 0.63 |

* Percentage increase over full-cohort value given in parentheses.

\+ Fraction of samples in which $|\hat{\beta}$ / (Est. Std. Error $\hat{\beta})|$ exceeds 1.65 ($\alpha$ = 0.10) and 1.96 ($\alpha$ = 0.05)

reduction in sample standard error is practically important at 100 expected subjects, but with 300 expected subjects both case-cohort and case-control standard errors are within 10% of the full-cohort sample standard errors. Power estimates for the test of $\beta=0$ are similar under the three designs both at 100 and 300 expected subjects. Though not shown in Table 1 standard error estimates were stable (i.e., their own standard errors were small) for all estimators, somewhat moreso for the full-cohort and case-cohort estimators than for the case-control estimators.

Whittemore and McMillan [11], drawing on results reported in Whittemore [8] and in Breslow et al [12], noted that the asymptotic efficiency of a time-matched case-control design (design A) agreed with that of an unmatched case-control design at a relative risk of unity, but that the efficiency of the time-matched design compared poorly to that for the unmatched design if the relative risk departed substantially from unity. In fact, a comparison with unmatched case-control results, or equivalently, with unmatched case-cohort results gives additional insight into Table 1. Specifically, at a relative risk of unity asymptotic standard errors for the maximum likelihood estimate of the log-odds ratio are 0.298, 0.400 and 0.310 under full-cohort, case-cohort (100 expected) and case-cohort (300 expected), respectively. These numbers agree well with the corresponding standard error means in the upper part of Table 1. The corresponding asymptotic standard errors for the log-odds ratio estimator at a relative risk of two are 0.313, 0.411 and 0.324, respectively. Note that the percentage increase of the latter two compared to the first are 31% and 5%, respectively, virtually identical to the corresponding case-cohort to full-cohort standard error increments in Table 1. It then seems sensible to interpret Table 1 as indicating that the poor efficiency properties of the synthetic case-control design for the estimation of relative risks ($\neq 1$) as compared to the corresponding unmatched case-control design for odds ratio estimation are attributable to the use of a subject as a control only at failure times at which the subject is a member of the matched case-control set. It appears that this loss can be obviated by employing a case-cohort design in which a selected control contributes to the comparison group of all cases in that control's risk period. One might speculate further that efficiency results for case-cohort designs will parallel closely those for a corresponding unmatched case-control design in situations in which the latter design applies.

Discussion. Each of the designs described above are readily extended to a stratified relative risk model

$$\lambda\{t;Z(u),0\le u<t\} = \lambda_{0s}(t)\, r\{X(t)\beta_s\} ,$$

where the stratification $s = s\{t; Z(u), 0 \leq u < t\} \varepsilon \{1, \cdots, q\}$ may be time-dependent, where $\lambda_{0s}(\cdot)$ is a baseline failure rate function for stratum s, and where the relative risk parameters can be allowed to differ among strata. Partial and pseudolikelihood procedures generalize to products of terms (2) and (4) over strata. In the case-cohort approach the subcohort sampling rates may be allowed to vary among baseline-defined strata. The case-control designs would typically involve selection of a specified number of controls at risk in the same stratum as the case at each distinct failure time.

The above estimation procedures all generalize, in the manner of Peto [21] and Breslow [22] to accommodate a limited degree of failure time grouping.

The case-cohort approach may also be considered as an alternative to a case-control design in the presence of a population-based disease registry, since the above relative risk estimation procedures do not require a cohort roster. Efficiency gains relative to time (age)-matched case-control analyses can be anticipated, though recall bias would be as much an issue for the case-cohort design as for the case-control design in such a context.

The topic of efficiency relative to time-matched case-control studies merits additional study. Certainly one would expect better efficiency properties for the case-cohort approach in a broad range of circumstances. One can, however, imagine situations with detailed stratification and short individual risk periods in which the sub-cohort risk set may be small at some failure times or in which a small stratum-specific subcohort constitutes the comparison group for a large number of cases. In such circumstances reduced efficiency may arise relative to a case-control approach in which the size of the referent group is specified for each case. Even here, however, one can presumably define a subcohort that is appropriately related to the strata and failure times of the failing subjects in order to ensure an efficiency improvement relative to a matched case-control analysis. Specifically, one could choose to augment the subcohort at preselected follow-up times with minimal change in the above procedures.

## REFERENCES

[1] D.R. Cox. Regression models and life tables (with discussion). J.R. Statist. Soc. B, 34, (1972), pp. 187-220.

[2] J.D. Kalbflesich and R.L. PRENTICE. The Statistical Analysis of Failure Time Data. Wiley, New York, (1980).

[3] D.R. COX. Partial likelihood. Biometrika, 62, (1975), pp. 269-276.

[4] P.K. ANDERSEN and R.D. Gill. Cox's regression model for counting processes: a large sample study. Ann. Statist, 10, (1982), pp. 1100-1120.

[5] R.L. PRENTICE and S.G. SELF. Asymptotic distribution theory for Cox-type regression models with general relative risk form. Ann. Statist., 11, (1983), pp. 804-813.

[6] F.D.K. LIDDELL, J.C. MCDONALD, D.C. THOMAS. Methods for cohort analysis: appraisal by application to asbestos mining. J.R. Statist, Soc. A., 140, (1977), pp. 469-490.

[7] N.E. BRESLOW and J. PATTON. Case-Control Analysis of Cohort Studies. IN Energy and Health, (1979), Breslow, N.E. and Whittemore, A.S., Eds., pp. 226-242.

[8] A.S. WHITTEMORE. The efficiency of synthetic retrospective studies. Biom. J., 23, (1981), pp. 73-78.

[9] D.C. THOMAS. General relative risk models for survival time and matched case-control analysis. Biometrics 37, (1981), pp. 673-686.

[10] D. OAKES. Survival times: aspects of partial likelihood. Int. Statist. Review, 49, (1981), pp. 235-264.

[11] A.S. WHITTEMORE and A. MCMILLAN. Analyzing Occupational Cohort Data: Application to U.S. Uranium Miners. IN Environmental Epidemiology: Risk Assessment, (1982), Prentice, R.L. and Whittemore, A.S., Eds., SIAM, Philadelphia, pp. 65-81.

[12] N.E. BRESLOW, J.H. LUBIN, P. MAREK, B. LANGHOLTZ. Multiplicative models and cohort analysis. J. Amer. Statist. Assoc., 78, (1983), pp. 1-12.

[13] J.H. LUBIN and M.H. GAIL. Biased selection of controls for case-control analyses of cohort studies. Biometrics, 40, (1984), pp. 63-75.

[14] R.L. PRENTICE and N.E. BRESLOW. Retrospective studies and failure time models. Biometrika, 65, (1978), pp. 153-158.

[15] J.M. ROBINS, M.H. GAIL, J.H. LUBIN. More on 'biased selection of controls for case-control analyses of cohort studies'. Submitted for publication (1985).

[16] R.L. PRENTICE. On the design of synthetic case-control studies. Submitted for publication (1985).

[17] J.E. BESAG. Efficiency of pseudolikelihood estimation for simple Gaussian fields. Biometrika, 64, (1977), pp. 616-618.

[18] R.L. PRENTICE. A case-cohort design for epidemiologic cohort studies and disease prevention trials. In press, Biometrika, (1985).

[19] L.L. KUPPER, A.J. MCMICHAEL, R. SPIRTAS. A hybrid epidemiologic study design useful in estimating relative risk. J. Amer. Statist. Assoc., 70, (1975), pp. 524-528.

[20] O.S. MIETTINEN. Design options in epidemiologic research: an update. Scand. J. Work Environ. Health 8, Suppl 1, (1982), pp. 7-14.

[21] R. PETO. Contribution to discussion of 'Regression models and life tables'by D.R. Cox. J.R. Statist. Soc. B, 34, (1972), pp. 205-207.

[22] N.E. BRESLOW. Covariance analysis of censored survival data. Biometrics, 30, (1974), pp. 89-99.

# SECTION 2
## Topics in Relative Risk Regression Analysis of Epidemiologic Data

As mentioned in the general introduction, relative risk regression methods are coming to occupy a prominent unifying place in the analysis of epidemiologic data. Various aspects of the use of such methods were examined by conference speakers. A relative risk analysis requires the specification of a time to response endpoint, of a covariate history (for each subject) that will include both the primary covariates and control covariates, and of a relative risk form. Elja Arjas considers the choice of time variable. He argues for the use of chronological time, both from the viewpoint of ease of interpretation and for reasons of clarity of the relationships among the stochastic processes that are evolving over time. Per Andersen discusses the uses, and potential abuses, of the inclusion of time-dependent covariates in a relative risk model. He notes particularly that the interpretation of key regression parameters may be much affected by the inclusion of 'responsive' covariates, and that the relative risk analysis may be usefully supplemented by the modelling and analyses of the stochastic covariates themselves.

Relative risk forms other than the usual exponential form have been used in a number of epidemiologic applications. The paper by Moolgavkar and Venzon illustrates the poor quality of asymptotic distributional approximations for relative risk parameters when linear and certain mixture model forms are employed. These authors then describe a geometric approach to the production of parameter transformations that lead to much improved asymptotic approximations.

Ed Lustbader describes diagnostic procedures for relative risk regression. These procedures are designed to identify in a computationally simple manner, data points (e.g., subjects) that might exert substantial influence on the regression analysis. Such analyses may identify faulty data and, more generally, provide insight into the stability of analytic results.

Davis, Hyde, Bangdiwala and Nelson consider another aspect of data analysis stability. They argue, in the context of a specific data set, that correlation among predictor variables have adversely affected the ability to draw meaningful inferences in a logistic regression analysis. Methods for identifying dependencies among predictor variables are proposed and compared.

Relative risk regression methods are also discussed and extended in other sections of these proceedings.

# Stanford Heart Transplantation Data Revisited: A Real-Time Approach

*Elja Arjas**

Abstract. A form of the discrete time logistic regression model is considered as a means to analyze complicated failure time data. A characteristic property of this approach is that the events recorded in the data are always treated in the model in the order in which they occurred in real time, without first aligning them according to some particular "basic time measurement". Parametric modelling is used throughout. The technique is illustrated by a detailed analysis of the Stanford Heart Transplantation Data. Computational aspects are discussed briefly.

## INTRODUCTION

In recent years, the dominant role among regression models of hazard has been played by the semiparametric model of Cox [14] and its extensions (see Andersen and Gill [5] and Andersen and Borgan [4]). An unspecified time-dependent baseline hazard, common to all individuals, is assumed to act multiplicatively on a relative risk function, which is a function of the parameters of interest. Estimation of parameters is based on considering relative risks within risk sets, formed by aligning individuals according to some particular measurement of time, such as age or time since diagnosis. A drawback of such alignment is that it usually changes the natural sequencing of events in real time. In particular, it can destroy the natural martingale structure of the real time counting process models (cf. Sellke and Siegmund [22] and Arjas [6]).

The idea of a multiplicative baseline factor is also present in most fully parametric models of hazard (see Borgan [10] for a general model, Thompson [23], Laird and Olivier [20], Aitkin, Laird and Francis [2] or Tibshirani and Ciampi [24] for piecewise exponential models, and

*Department of Applied Mathematics and Statistics, University of Oulu, Oulu, Finland. This work was completed while the author was visiting the Fred Hutchinson Cancer Research Center in Seattle. It was supported in part by the National Institutes of Health Grant 5R01 GM-28314 and by the Finnish Academy.

Aitkin and Clayton [1] for models having log-linear structure).

We have, in Arjas and Haara [7] and Arjas [6], advocated what might be called a real-time approach to hazard regression, arguing that if a hazard model uses time-dependent covariates, all dependence on time-related quantities can actually be accommodated into such covariates. Then, instead of postulating the existence of a common unspecified multiplicative baseline hazard, a function of some particular measurement of time, one attempts to model how an individual's hazard at a certain (real) time t depends on "the currently prevailing conditions for survival". Frequently, some such conditions are best expressed in terms of conveniently chosen time readings, such as age, time from diagnosis, time from treatment, or indeed, calendar time. Several time readings may be needed simultaneously for a realistic description. Some suitably chosen functions of these readings can then be listed as covariates, among other factors that are thought to be relevant to the individual's survival.

Arjas and Haara [7] showed that, under general conditions, the real time approach leads to likelihood expressions of a common form. This approach has intuitive appeal in that the histories, representing the past and used in the conditioning of the hazards, are always compatible with the actual experiment in the sense of having the events sequenced in the correct order. This makes the results easy to interpret.

On the other hand, the general likelihood formula in [7] has too little structure for immediate statistical application such as parameter estimation. The purpose of this paper is to suggest a concrete way to fill this gap.

In trying to fill the gap, we have incorporated two features that have practical, rather than conceptual or theoretical motivation. First a discrete time parameter is used, which, together with a natural conditional independence assumption, removes all difficulties concerning tied failure times. Second, a logistic regression model with binomial response is the primary statistical tool. This allows us to work within the log-linear family of distributions, and leads to an elegant asymptotic theory and unproblematic numerical routines in ordinary ML-estimation.

In the next section we set up our statistical model. The exact derivation of the corresponding likelihood function and the asymptotic normality of the regression coefficient estimates are deferred respectively to Appendices 1 and 2. We then illustrate the method by considering the well-known Stanford Heart Transplant data. Finally, we make some remarks concerning computation.

## THE STATISTICAL MODEL

Choosing some convenient point in real time as the origin, we split the time axis into the unit intervals $(t-1,t]$, $t \geq 1$. As an approximation, we then think that individuals at risk at the beginning of an interval remain so to the end of it. Consequently, deaths occurring during (t-1,t] are thought of as occurring at t. Similarly, we think of the covariates as remaining fixed during each time interval, with the possible new value always being determined at the beginning of the interval. When the time unit is small, the approximations are unlikely to influence statistical inference a great deal.

The individuals included in the study are indexed by j, $j \geq 1$. We define the risk indicators $Y_j(t-1)$, $j,t \geq 1$, by

$$Y_j(t-1) = \begin{cases} 1 & \text{if individual } j \text{ is at risk during } (t-1,t] \\ 0 & \text{otherwise} \end{cases} \tag{2.1}$$

and the failure indicators $\Delta N_j(t)$, $j,t \geq 1$, by

$$\Delta N_j(t) = \begin{cases} 1 & \text{if individual } j \text{ at risk during } (t-1,t] \\ & \text{fails during this period} \\ 0 & \text{otherwise} \end{cases} \tag{2.2}$$

Denote by $R(t-1) = \{j \geq 1 : Y_j(t-1) = 1\}$ the risk set during (t-1,t]. The size of the risk set, card $R(t-1) = \sum_{j\geq 1} Y_j(t-1)$, is assumed to be finite for all $t \geq 1$.

We do not assume that all individuals are present at time 0; they may enter and leave the risk set many times, and they may also "fail" many times.

Suppose then that, for every individual j and time interval (t-1,t] such that $Y_j(t-1) = 1$, the investigator knows the value of a p-vector $\underset{\sim}{Z}_j(t-1) = (Z_{j1}(t-1),\cdots,Z_{jp}(t-1))$ of the relevant covariates. We shall view the value of $\Delta N_j(t)$ as the outcome of a Bernoulli experiment, where the probability of the event $\{\Delta N_j(t) = 1\}$ depends on $\underset{\sim}{Z}_j(t-1)$. For convenience, we may assume that $\underset{\sim}{Z}_j(t-1) = \underset{\sim}{0}$ whenever $Y_j(t-1) = 0$.

We then assume that the likelihood function corresponding to data up to time t can be expressed as the product

$$L_t^{\beta} = \prod_{s \leq t} \prod_{j \in R(s-1)} P^{\underset{\sim}{\beta}}(\Delta N_j(s) = \Delta n_j(s) \mid \underset{\sim}{Z}_j(s-1); Y_j(s-1) = 1) \quad , \tag{2.3}$$

where $\{\Delta n_j(s);\ j \in R(s-1),\ s \leq t\}$ are the observed values of the indicators (2.2). Moreover, we assume that

$$\log \frac{P^{\underset{\sim}{\beta}}(\Delta N_j(s) = 1 \mid \underset{\sim}{Z}_j(s-1);\ Y_j(s-1) = 1)}{P^{\underset{\sim}{\beta}}(\Delta N_j(s) = 0 \mid \underset{\sim}{Z}_j(s-1);\ Y_j(s-1) = 1)} = \underset{\sim}{\beta}'\underset{\sim}{Z}_j(s-1) \quad . \tag{2.4}$$

The precise sequence of assumptions leading to this logistic regression model for binary data is discussed in Appendix 1. Note the formal similarity of this model and the discrete time model in Cox [14] if one in the latter sets $\lambda_0(t) = 1$. However, setting $\lambda_0(t) = 1$ is a way of specifying the baseline hazard completely. Here we use a different likelihood than in [14], one that does not suppress $\lambda_0(t)$ by only considering the relative risks of individuals in a risk set, and only at times of failure. Thus (2.3) uses information from all time intervals, whether any failures occur in them or not.

The score function is easily seen to be

$$\frac{\partial}{\partial \beta_i} \log L_t^{\underset{\sim}{\beta}} = \sum_{s \leq t} \sum_j Z_{ji}(s-1)[\Delta N_j(s) - P^{\underset{\sim}{\beta}}(\Delta N_j(s) = 1 | \underset{\sim}{Z}_j(s-1), Y_j(s-1))] \quad , \tag{2.5}$$

$1 \leq i \leq p$. The equations $\frac{\partial}{\partial \beta_i} \log L_{t_{max}}^{\underset{\sim}{\beta}} = 0$, $1 \leq i \leq p$, with $t_{max}$ = calendar time of the latest observation, can then be used in the standard way to obtain the ML-estimate $\hat{\underset{\sim}{\beta}}_{t_{max}}$ of the "true" parameter $\underset{\sim}{\beta}_0$. The asymptotic normality of $\hat{\underset{\sim}{\beta}}_t$ as $t \to \infty$ is briefly considered in Appendix 2.

## AN EXAMPLE: STANFORD HEART TRANSPLANT DATA REVISITED

The Model. We now apply the above logistic regression model to the Stanford Heart Transplant Data. This famous data set, originally introduced in Clark et al [12], has been since considered and analyzed many times. (See Crowley and Hu [16], Kalbfleisch and Prentice [19]; Section 5.5, and Aitkin, Laird and Francis [2], with discussion, for results and for more references.) Our motive for choosing this data set was that it is widely known from previous analyses, and that the transplantation introduces a set of random and/or time-dependent covariates whose treatment illustrates well our real time approach.

We emphasize that our goal is only to demonstrate the use of a particular statistical technique. Thus, this section should not be taken as one more reanalysis of the Stanford data. Extreme caution should be used in the interpretation of the results, see in particular Gail [18].

We use the data exactly as reported in Crowley and Hu [16]. The follow-up covers 99 patients between September 13, 1967 and March 23, 1974 (4 being deselected because of missing information). The information available about all patients is (j is again the index used to identify the patient):

(1) $T_{BIRTH(j)}$, the date of birth

(2) $T_{ACC(j)}$, the date of acceptance into the program

(3) Previous open heart surgery (1=yes, 0=no)

(4) $T_{EXIT(j)}$, the date last seen

(5) Status on the last day (1=dead, 0=alive)

About transplanted patients there is additionally information about:

(6) $T_{TRANS(j)}$, the date of the transplantation

(7) MM(j), mismatch score, indicating the degree to which donor and recipient are mismatched for tissue type

Crowley and Hu [16] and Kalbfleisch and Prentice [19] applied the semiparametric Cox [14] model on the data, using a single model to accommodate both pretransplant and posttransplant survival. Aitkin, Laird and Francis [2] chose a fully parametric approach and they modelled pretransplant and posttransplant survivals separately.

We follow Aitkin, Laird and Francis in choosing a fully parametric approach, but Crowley and Hu, or Kalbfleisch and Prentice, in that we work with a single model covering both pretransplant and posttransplant survival.

Write for simplicity $T_0$ for the date September 12, 1967 (the beginning of the follow-up). The variable t always refers to a day in calendar time. We then define the following covariates, some with two alternatives (with and without taking logarithms). A code for each covariate is given in parentheses:

$$Z_{j1}(t-1) = 1$$

$$Z_{j2}(t-1) = \log(t-T_{ACC(j)}+1)$$ ("TIME FROM ACC")

$$Z_{j3}(t-1) = T_{ACC(j)} - T_0$$ ("ACC MONTH")

<u>or</u> $\log(T_{ACC(j)} - T_0 + 1)$

$$Z_{j4}(t-1) = T_{ACC(j)} - T_{BIRTH(j)}$$ ("ACC AGE")

<u>or</u> $\log(T_{ACC(j)} - T_{BIRTH(j)})$

$Z_{j5}(t-1)$ = 1(patient j has had a previous open heart surgery) ("SURGERY")

$$Z_{j6}(t-1) = 1(T_{TRANS(j)} \le t \le T_{TRANS(j)} + 70)$$ ("PHASE 1")

$$Z_{j7}(t-1) = Z_{j6}(t-1) \cdot \log(t-T_{TRANS(j)}+1)$$ ("TIME FROM TRANS")

$$Z_{j8}(t-1) = 1(T_{TRANS(j)} + 70 \le t \le T_{TRANS(j)} + 365)$$ ("PHASE 2")

$$Z_{j9}(t-1) = 1(T_{TRANS(j)} + 365 < t)$$ ("PHASE 3")

$$Z_{j10}(t-1) = 1(T_{TRANS(j)} \leq t) \cdot (T_{TRANS(j)} - T_{ACC(j)} + 1) \qquad (\text{"WAIT"})$$

$$\underline{\text{or}} \quad 1(T_{TRANS(j)} \leq t) \cdot \log(T_{TRANS(j)} - T_{ACC(j)} + 1)$$

$$Z_{j11}(t-1) = 1(T_{TRANS(j)} \leq t) \cdot MM(j) \qquad (\text{"MISMATCH"})$$

$$Z_{j12}(t-1) = 1(T_{TRANS(j)} \leq t) \cdot (T_{TRANS(j)} - T_0 + 1), \qquad (\text{"TRANSMONTH"})$$

$$\underline{\text{or}} \quad 1(T_{TRANS(j)} \leq t) \cdot \log(T_{TRANS(j)} - T_0 + 1)$$

$$Z_{j13}(t-1) = 1(T_{TRANS(j)} \leq t) \cdot (T_{TRANS(j)} - T_{BIRTH(j)} + 1) \qquad (\text{"TRANSAGE"})$$

$$\underline{\text{or}} \quad 1(T_{TRANS(j)} \leq t) \cdot \log(T_{TRANS(j)} - T_{BIRTH(j)} + 1)$$

$$Z_{j14}(t-1) = 1(T_{TRANS(j)} \leq t) \cdot Z_{j5}(t-1) \qquad (\text{"TRANSSURGERY"})$$

Here $1(\cdot)$ is the indicator of the event inside the parenthesis. Thus covariates $Z_{j6}, \cdots, Z_{j14}$ are only non-zero when $t \geq T_{TRANS(j)}$. In covariates $Z_{j4}$ and $Z_{j13}$ time is expressed in years, in $Z_{j3}$ and $Z_{j12}$ in months (in the latter rounded to the nearest full month). These choices were made purely for convenience.

According to the logistic regression model (2.3) and (2.4), we then assume that, for the $j^{th}$ individual during the $t^{th}$ day (calendar time), the odds ratio between death probability and survival probability is given by

$$\frac{P^{\beta}_{\sim}(j \text{ dies during the } t^{th} \text{ day} \mid \underset{\sim}{Z}_j(t-1);\ Y_j(t-1) = 1)}{P^{\beta}_{\sim}(j \text{ survives the } t^{th} \text{ day} \mid \underset{\sim}{Z}_j(t-1);\ Y_j(t-1) = 1)} \tag{3.1}$$

$$\begin{aligned} &= e^{\beta_1} \cdot (\text{TIME FROM ACC})^{\beta_2} \\ &\cdot \exp\{\beta_3 \cdot (\text{ACCMONTH}) + \beta_4 \cdot (\text{ACCAGE}) + \beta_5 \cdot (\text{SURGERY})\} \\ &\cdot f_j(t; \beta_6, \beta_7, \beta_8, \beta_9) \\ &\cdot \exp\{\beta_{10} \cdot (\text{WAIT}) + \beta_{11} \cdot (\text{MISMATCH}) + \beta_{12} \cdot (\text{TRANSMONTH}) \\ &\quad + \beta_{13} \cdot (\text{TRANSAGE}) + \beta_{14} \cdot (\text{TRANSSURGERY})\} \quad , \end{aligned}$$

where

$$f_j(t; \beta_6, \beta_7, \beta_8, \beta_9)$$

$$= \begin{cases} 1 \quad , & \text{if } t < T_{TRANS(j)} \\ e^{\beta_6} \ (\text{TIME FROM TRANS})^{\beta_7}, & \text{if } T_{TRANS(j)} \leq t \leq T_{TRANS(j)} + 70 \\ e^{\beta_8} \quad , & \text{if } T_{TRANS(j)} + 70 < t \leq T_{TRANS(j)} + 365 \\ e^{\beta_9} \quad , & \text{if } T_{TRANS(j)} + 365 < t \quad . \end{cases}$$

We call this the INITIAL MODEL. Note that, in practice, the denominator $P^{\underset{\sim}{\beta}}$(j survives the $t^{th}$ day$|\underset{\sim}{Z}_j(t-1)$; $Y_j(t-1) = 1$) is very close to one. Therefore the right hand side in (3.1) is "almost" an expression of discrete time hazard.

We then comment on how the time variable t comes up in the model. Consider first the pretransplant survival. Figure 1 describes cumulative hazard from the date of acceptance to the program. (Transplantation itself is treated as a censoring mechanism).

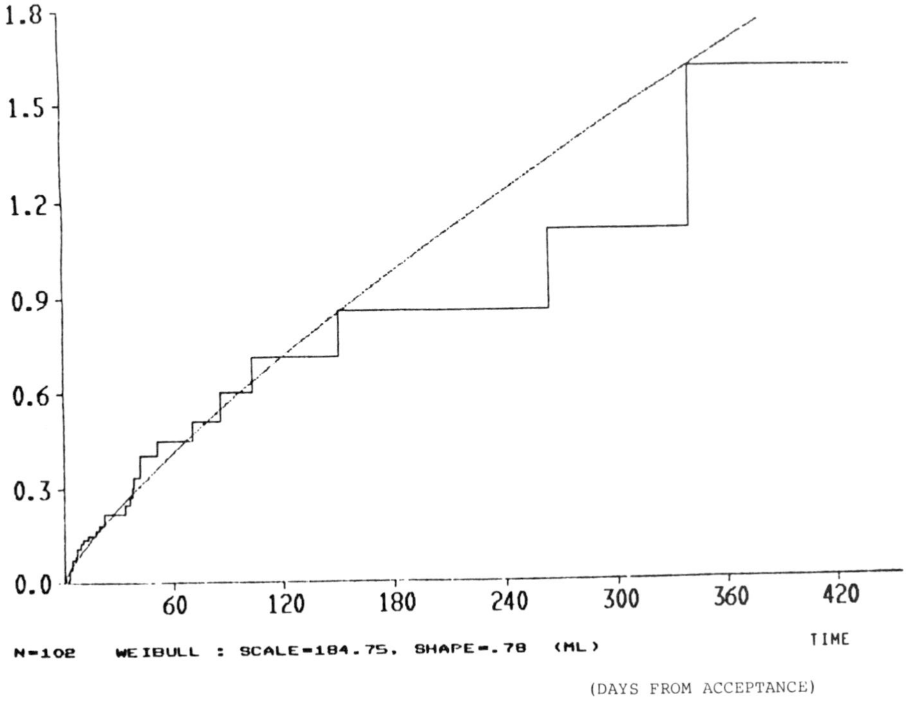


Figure 1. Nelson plot for pretransplant survival times and the fitted Weibull cumulative hazard function.

It is clear from Figure 1 that individuals who have survived long without transplantation, face a smaller risk than those who have only recently been accepted to the program. (This is probably because some of the incoming patients are healthier than others, and survival acts as a selection mechanism, with the healthier patients surviving longer.) Consequently, any reasonable functional expression for hazard should depend on the time from acceptance. We model this dependence by including the term $\beta_2 Z_{j2}(t-1)$ in the linear expression for the log-odds of dying during the $t^{th}$ day. Then the (discrete time) hazard becomes approximately proportional to a power of time from acceptance, in agreement with the Weibull hazard form (cf. Aitkin, Laird, and Francis [2]).

On the other hand, for transplanted individuals, the hazard depends crucially on the time since the transplantation. This is clear from Figure 2, which describes cumulative hazard after the transplantation.

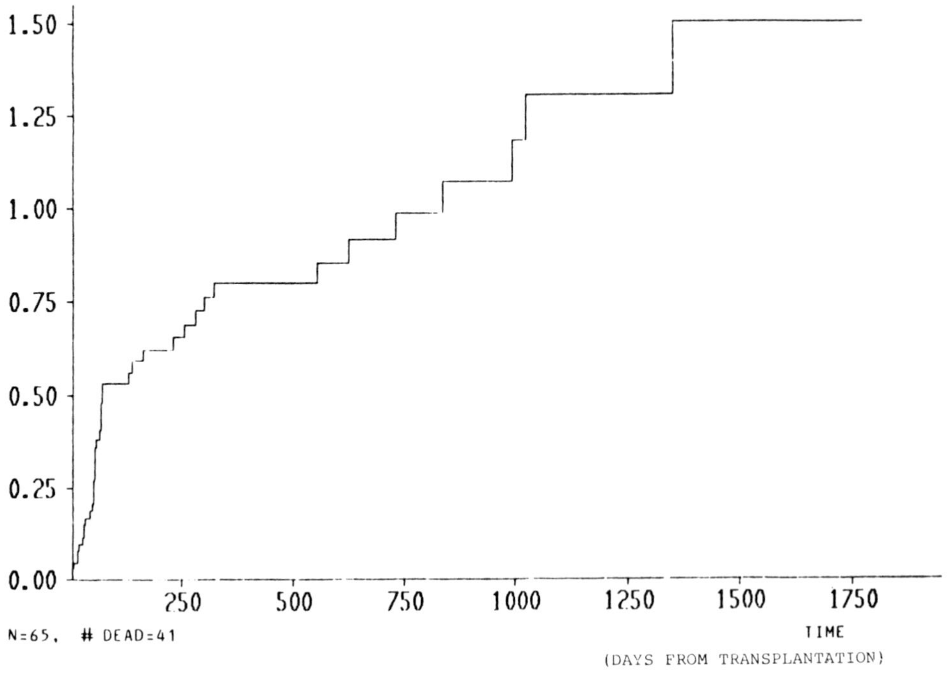


Figure 2. Nelson plot for posttransplant survival times.

There appears to be a very critical period of approximately 70 days after the transplantation ("PHASE 1") after which the hazard abruptly decreases (cf., again, Aitkin, Laird and Francis). In the INITIAL MODEL, we use a Weibull-type hazard model over the 70 day period, and thereafter two intervals of constant hazard ("PHASE 2" and "PHASE 3").

We want the model to describe the potential effect which the transplantation may have on survival. Therefore, it is natural to build it in such a way that, for a patient who is at risk during the $t^{th}$ day and who has been transplanted, the model would also give a value of the hazard corresponding to the alternative where the patient had not been transplanted. But then, by the above argument, it becomes necessary to express the hazard of a transplanted patient as a function which depends on both $(t-T_{ACC(j)})^+$ = time from acceptance and $(t-T_{TRANS(j)})^+$ = time from transplantation. (Compare this with the discussion in Crowley and Storer [17] and Aitkin, Laird and Francis [2]; rejoinder.) By mimicking the behavior found in Figures 1 and 2 by smooth functions, we describe this dependence by including in our model (3.1) the factor $((t-T_{ACC(j)}+1)^+)^{\beta_2}\ f_j(t;\beta_6,\beta_7,\beta_8,\beta_9)$. Later we are able to simplify this to some extent (see REDUCED MODELS below).

Thus there is some trade-off between our parametric and Cox's semi-parametric approach: We must try to find a reasonable parametric description of the various ways in which "time" influences hazard. But then we are not forced to work with a common baseline hazard, depending on a single time reading, and there is no need to artifically align the observations. We also get a "fuller" form of likelihood to work with (see Appendix 1), and obtain, by a straightforward ML-procedure, estimates for the absolute (instead of only relative) hazard.

We remark that we could have taken the real time approach even further, by employing more calendar time-dependent covariates. For example, we could have used $t-T_{BIRTH(j)}$ instead of $T_{ACC(j)}-T_{BIRTH(j)}$ as an age variable, and $t-T_0$ instead of $T_{ACC(j)}-T_0$ as a variable describing a time trend during the study. On the other hand, the method we use does not require any of the covariates to be a time reading.

Commenting finally on the fixed covariates we see that $\beta_3 Z_{j3}(t-1) + \beta_4 Z_{j4}(t-1) + \beta_5 Z_{j5}(t-1)$ is a patient dependent modification of the pre-transplant log-odds $\beta_1 + \beta_2 Z_{j2}(t-1)$ for survival. Recall that the transplantation effect $\beta_6 Z_{j6}(t-1) + \cdots + \beta_{14} Z_{j14}(t-1)$ is zero for $t < T_{TRANS(j)}$. Note also that information which is used in the fixed covariates to describe pretransplant survival, can come up again in a different role, now as part of the transplantation effect.

<u>Empirical Results</u>. We fitted INITIAL MODEL (3.1), trying the covariates $Z_{j2}$, $Z_{j3}$, $Z_{j10}$, $Z_{j12}$ and $Z_{j13}$ both in the logarithmic and non-logarithmic form. We also tried several simpler alternatives, which were obtained from the INITIAL MODEL by dropping some covariates, or replacing covariates by others. Numerical estimates of the regression coefficients, calculated from four different models, are given in Table 1. In REDUCED MODELS, covariates $Z_{j6}$, $Z_{j8}$ and $Z_{j9}$ corresponding to PHASE 1, PHASE 2 and PHASE 3 were replaced by the single covariate $1(T_{TRANS(j)} \leq t)$. Also, covariates $Z_{j5}$, $Z_{j10}$, $Z_{j12}$, $Z_{j13}$ and $Z_{j14}$ were eliminated.

In order to judge the goodness-of-fit of our models, we used both deviance and a graphical method based on total hazards (generalized residuals). Lack of space does not permit us to consider the graphical method here.

In line with our earlier comment that this section should not be viewed as a reanalysis of the Stanford data, we leave it to the reader to look for similarities and dissimilarities between our results and some earlier analyses. Neither do we comment on the values and significance levels of the regression coefficients in the four models reported. The numerical values of the regression coefficients were very stable from model to model provided that the corresponding covariate remained the same.

TABLE 1.

Parameter estimates from four models (standard errors in parentheses)

| PARAMETER | NON-LOGARITHMIC INITIAL MODEL | NON-LOGARITHMIC REDUCED MODEL*) | LOGARITHMIC INITIAL MODEL | LOGARITHMIC REDUCED MODEL*) |
|---|---|---|---|---|
| | *Pretransplant survival (all patients):* | | | |
| $\beta_1$ INTERCEPT | -4.7395 (.9532) | -4.5576 (.8205) | -3.4796 (1.0240) | -3.1965 (.9139) |
| $\beta_2$ TIME FROM ACC | - .3397 (.1147) | - .3634 (.0973) | - .2853 (.1185) | - .3394 (.0976) |
| $\beta_3$ ACCMONTH | - .0207 (.0090) | - .0172 (.0059) | - .6714 (.2229) | - .6267 (.1615) |
| $\beta_4$ ACCAGE | .0356 (.0174) | .0301 (.0141) | .0376 (.0189) | .0313 (.0141) |
| $\beta_5$ SURGERY | - .0703 (.6348) | --- | .0094 (.6363) | --- |
| | *Transplantation effect on survival (only transplanted patients):* | | | |
| $\beta$ TIME FROM TRANS | .4376 (.2559) | .4663 (.0997) | .4609 (.2600) | .4727 (.0998) |
| $\beta$ PHASE 1 | -1.4866 (1.2679) | | -1.2083 (1.4137) | |
| $\beta_8$ PHASE 2 | -1.5259 (.9593) | -1.7538 (.5170) (Combined estimate) | -1.2149 (1.1974) | -1.7612 (.5181) (Combined estimate) |
| $\beta_9$ PHASE 3 | -1.6182 (.9734) | | -1.3559 (1.2098) | |
| $\beta_{10}$ WAIT | $1.95 \times 10^{-5}$ (.0053) | --- | - .4543 (.3413) | --- |
| $\beta_{11}$ MISMATCH | .4052 (.2989) | .4739 (.2767) | .4779 (.3102) | .4732 (.2772) |
| $\beta_{12}$ TRANSMONTH | .0094 (.0121) | --- | .3463 (.7326) | --- |
| $\beta_{13}$ TRANSAGE | - .0083 (.0197) | --- | - .0102 (.0229) | --- |
| $\beta_{14}$ TRANSSURGERY | - .6164 (.8056) | --- | - .5556 (.8093) | --- |
| | Deviance = 892.42 | Deviance = 895.11 | Deviance = 886.93 | Deviance = 890.32 |

1) In the logarithmic models covariates $Z_{j3}$, $Z_{j10}$ and $Z_{j12}$ are logarithmic

We now consider survival prognoses that can be obtained from the estimated models. Taking a fictitious patient with given characteristics, we estimate survival distributions corresponding to different waiting times between acceptance and transplantation. In order to do this, we need to consider the time at which a donor heart becomes available as known at the time of acceptance, with no effect on the patient's pretransplant survival.

To take a concrete case, we consider two patients with similar characteristics as in Aitkin, Laird and Francis [2]:

| | Patient I | Patient II |
|---|---|---|
| ACCMONTH | 12 | 50 |
| ACCAGE | 42 | 55 |
| SURGERY | 0 | 0 |
| MISMATCH | .5 | 1.5 |

The options for waiting time are:

(1) transplantation at the time of acceptance (WAIT = 0)

(2) transplantation 50 days after the time of acceptance, if still alive (WAIT = 50)

(3) transplantation 200 days after the time of acceptance, if still alive (WAIT = 200)

(4) no transplantation (WAIT = ∞)

Survival curves were determined on the basis of the fitted models. The curves corresponding to NONLOGARITHMIC INITIAL MODEL are displayed in

Figures 3(a), (b).

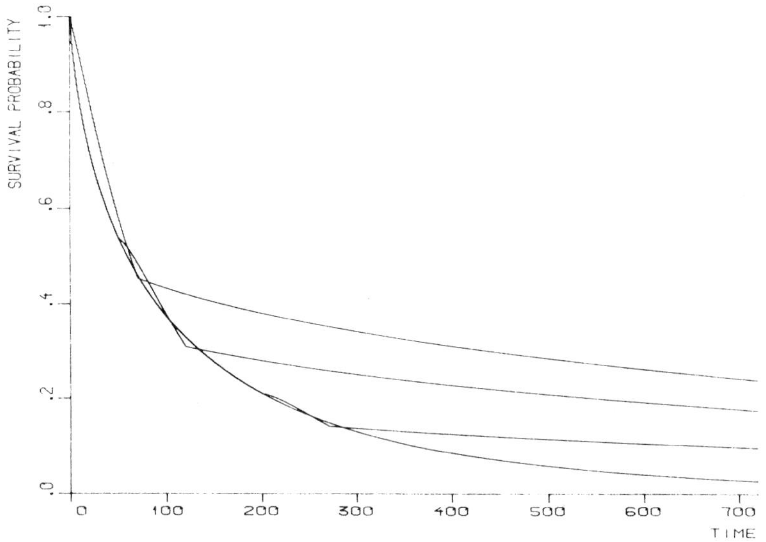


Figure 3(a). Estimated survival probabilities for Patient I (NON-LOGARITHMIC INITIAL MODEL).

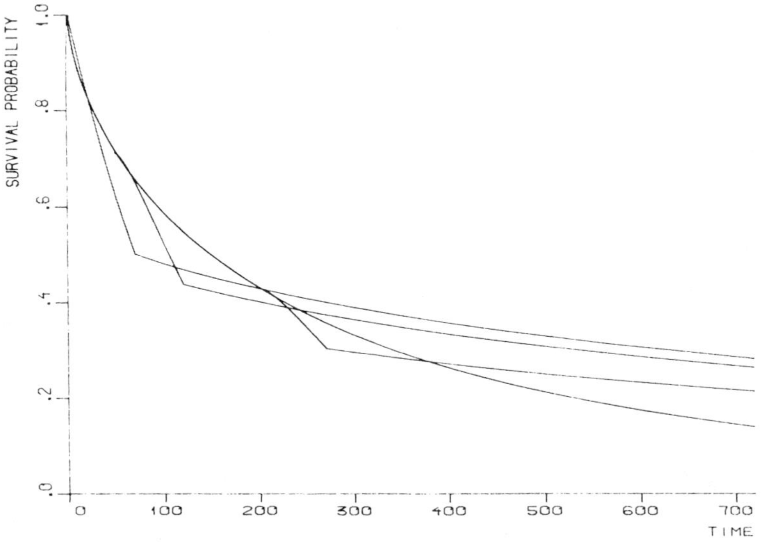


Figure 3(b). Estimated survival probabilities for Patient II (NON-LOGARITHMIC INITIAL MODEL).

For Patient I, all models indicate that transplantation would be beneficial (almost) uniformly over time as compared to no transplantation. The benefit is the bigger the earlier the transplantation. For Patient II, transplantation improves only long-term survival probabilities and the improvements are slight.

For either patient, there was relatively little variation between the prognoses obtained from different models.

## NOTES ON COMPUTATION

In a purely technical sense, we have considered a multiple logistic regression model for binary data. In principle, therefore, the parameter estimation could be done by using some well-known statistical package (such as GLIM or BMDP), which includes programs for handling logistic regression. However, there is a practical problem: The data matrix contains the values of $\underset{\sim}{Z}_j(t-1)$ and $\Delta N_j(t)$ for each $(j,t)$-pair such that $Y_j(t-1) = 1$. If the time unit is short (as it preferably should be in order to avoid serious discretization errors), the size of the data matrix becomes prohibitively large. For Stanford data the number of patient days exceeded 30,000. Such a data matrix cannot be stored conveniently into a core of a computer.

A computer program was devised to solve the problem. The key idea in the program is that, instead of computing the covariate values once and for all to be stored in a file, the covariate vectors $\underset{\sim}{Z}_j(t-1)$ are determined directly from the data every time they are needed in the iterations. A valuable computational aspect of our approach is that each $(j,t)$-pair can be treated separately, then only adding a term to the logarithmic likelihood expression. Thus there is no need to form, as in Cox's model, risk sets consisting of individuals with matching baseline hazards, also keeping track on their time-dependent covariates. Finally, as we have remarked earlier, no tie-breaking procedures are required.

A more detailed description of the program, together with examples and experiences about computing, will be reported later.

Acknowledgements. The programming and computing in this work was done by Risto Bloigu and Pekka Kangas. Without their skill and dedication to work, it would have been impossible to apply the method to any reasonable sized problem. My sincerest thanks to them. I am also grateful to Pentti Haara, Suresh Moolgavkar and John Crowley for useful discussions.

## APPENDIX I: DETAILS OF THE STATISTICAL MODEL

Let $(\Omega, \mathcal{F})$ be a measurable space in which the variables $Y_j(t-1)$, $\underset{\sim}{Z}_j(t-1)$ and $\Delta N_j(t)$ are defined. Let $\mathcal{F}_0$ be the $\sigma$-field representing "initial information"; usually $\mathcal{F}_0$ is the trivial field. Then the $\sigma$-fields $\mathcal{F}_t$ and $\mathcal{G}_{t-1}$, $t \geq 1$, defined inductively by

$$\mathcal{G}_{t-1} = \mathcal{F}_{t-1} \vee \sigma\{R(t-1), \{\underset{\sim}{Z}_j(t-1);\ j \in R(t-1)\}\} \quad ,$$

$$\mathcal{F}_t = \mathcal{G}_{t-1} \vee \sigma\{\Delta N_j(t);\ j \in R(t-1)\} \quad ,$$

represent the experimental history registered up to time t, $\mathcal{F}_t$ including and $\mathcal{G}_{t-1}$ excluding the failures during (t-1,t].

Consider a statistical model $\{P^\theta; \theta \in \Theta\}$ for the observation process $(R(s-1), \{\Delta N_j(s), \underset{\sim}{Z}_j(s-1);\ j \in R(s-1)\})_{s \geq 1}$ and a $P^\theta$-likelihood which corresponds to data collected up to time t, $t \geq 1$.

Suppose that the parameter $\theta$ can be represented in the form $\theta = (\theta_1, \theta_2)$, where $\theta_1$ is the parameter of interest and $\theta_2$ is a nuisance parameter. Typically, we think of $\theta_1$ as parametrizing the conditional distribution of the variables $\Delta N_j(s)$, conditioned on $\mathcal{G}_{s-1}$, and of $\theta_2$ as the parameter associated with the conditional law of the variables $R(s)$ and $\underset{\sim}{Z}_j(s)(j \in R(s))$, given $\mathcal{F}_{s-1}$. The full likelihood corresponding to the observed values $\{r(s-1), \{\Delta n_j(s), \underset{\sim}{z}_j(s-1);\ j \in r(s-1)\};\ s \leq t\}$ can then be expressed as the product of two terms, viz., as

$$\prod_{s \leq t} P^\theta(R(s-1) = r(s-1), \underset{\sim}{Z}_j(s-1) = \underset{\sim}{z}_j(s-1);\ j \in r(s-1) \,|\, \mathcal{F}_{s-1}) \cdot \prod_{s \leq t} P^\theta(\Delta N_j(s) = \Delta n_j(s);\ j \in r(s-1) \,|\, \mathcal{G}_{s-1}) \quad . \tag{A.1}$$

Following Cox [15], the second factor can be called a partial likelihood. Ordinary ML-estimation of $\theta_1$, the parameter of interest, can be done by considering that factor alone provided that the following condition holds:

<u>Assumption 1.</u> (i) For each $s \geq 1$, the conditional $P^\theta$-distribution of $\{R(s-1), \{\underset{\sim}{Z}_j(s-1);\ j \in R(s-1)\}\}$, given $\mathcal{F}_{s-1}$, does not depend on $\theta_1$; and (ii) For each $s \geq 1$, the conditional $P^\theta$-distribution of $\{\Delta N_j(s);\ j \in R(s-1)\}$, given $\mathcal{G}_{s-1}$, does not depend on $\theta_2$.

Of course, the validity of Assumption 1 depends on the model $\{P^\theta;\ \theta \in \Theta\}$. Actual verification of this assumption would require that the model were fully specified, including the probability law of the censoring mechanism and possible random covariates. This is usually not done explicitly. However, part (ii) of Assumption 1 becomes obvious if the censoring times and the covariates are fixed, or random but $\mathcal{F}_0$-measurable. More generally, we can consider (ii) to be valid if the censoring is non-informative about $\theta_1$ and the covariates are external (cf. Kalbfleisch and Prentice [19]). For internal covariates more caution is needed: If (i) is not met, also the first factor in (A.1) can depend on $\theta_1$, and then using only the second factor in the maximization is a potential source of bias. Finally, it seems that part (ii) in Assumption 1 can always be met in practice by making a convenient choice for $\theta_1$, the parameter of interest.

For a continuous time version of Assumption 1, see Arjas and Haara [7].

Our next assumption imposes an independence condition between the individuals and simplifies, in particular, the handling of ties.

Assumption 2. For each $s \geq 1$, and $\theta \in \Theta$, the random variables $\{\Delta N_j(s);\ j \geq 1\}$ are conditionally $P^\theta$-independent given $G_{s-1}$.

This assumption is likely to hold in practice if there are no multiple failures of common cause, or if such failures can occur but the background variable causing the failure can be included as a covariate.

Under Assumptions 1 and 2, the likelihood function (A.1) depends on $\theta_1$ only through the factor

$$\prod_{s \leq t} \prod_{j \in r(s-1)} P^\theta(\Delta N_j(s) = \Delta n_j(s) \mid G_{s-1}) \quad . \tag{A.2}$$

On the other hand, because of Assumption 1 (ii), this expression does not depend on $\theta_2$.

It remains to specify the conditional probabilities in (A.2). Our next assumption guarantees that all relevant information in $G_{s-1}$, when used as a condition for the probability of $\{\Delta N_j(s) = \Delta n_j(s)\}$, is actually contained in the p-vector $\underset{\sim}{Z}_j(s-1)$ and the indicator $Y_j(s-1)$.

Assumption 3. For all $s$, $j \geq 1$, and $\theta \in \Theta$, $\Delta N_j(s)$ and $G_{s-1}$ are conditionally $P^\theta$-independent given $Y_j(s-1)$ and $\underset{\sim}{Z}_j(s-1)$.

As a last step, we specify the conditional probabilities according to the logistic regression model for binomial response (see e.g., Bock [9], Cox [13], Thompson [23] and Plackett [21]). We also change the notation of the parameter, writing $\underset{\sim}{\beta} = (\beta_1, \cdots, \beta_p)'$ instead of $\theta_1$ and $P^{\underset{\sim}{\beta}}$ instead of $P^\theta$.

Assumption 4. For all $t \geq 1$,

$$P^{\underset{\sim}{\beta}}(\Delta N_j(s) = 1 \mid G_{s-1}) = Y_j(s-1)\ L(\underset{\sim}{\beta}'\underset{\sim}{Z}_j(s-1)) \quad , \tag{A.3}$$

where $L(x) = (1 + \exp(-x))^{-1}$.

As is well-known, an alternative way to (A.3) is to use "log-odds": For $(j,t)$ such that $j \in R(s-1)$,

$$\log \frac{P^{\underset{\sim}{\beta}}(\Delta N_j(s) = 1 \mid G_{s-1})}{P^{\underset{\sim}{\beta}}(\Delta N_j(s) = 0 \mid G_{s-1})} = \underset{\sim}{\beta}'\underset{\sim}{Z}_j(s-1) \quad .$$

## APPENDIX 2: ASYMPTOTIC NORMALITY

Apart from trivial cases, the exact distribution of the ML-estimate for $\underset{\sim}{\beta}$ is not known. Therefore, asymptotic results are needed to approximate this distribution. Here we only mention the key asymptotic theorem and a corollary. The exact regularity conditions and the proof of these results can be found in Arjas and Haara [8].

Let $\underset{\sim}{\beta}_0$ be the fixed "true value" of the parameter and let $\hat{\underset{\sim}{\beta}}_t$ be the ML-estimate corresponding to the data on the time interval $[0,t]$. For simplicity we write P in place of $P^{\underset{\sim}{\beta}_0}$. Denote $\underset{\sim}{I}_t(\beta) = -\frac{\partial^2}{\partial \underset{\sim}{\beta}^2} \log L_t^{\underset{\sim}{\beta}}$ .

Theorem (Asymptotic normality of $\hat{\underset{\sim}{\beta}}_t$). Suppose that there exists a sequence $(a_t)$ of constants such that

$$\frac{1}{a_t} \underset{\sim}{I}_t(\beta_0) \underset{P}{\to} \underset{\sim}{\Sigma} \text{ as } t \to \infty \quad ,$$

where $\underset{\sim}{\Sigma}$ is positive definite. Then, under further regularity conditions,

$$a_t \, (\hat{\underset{\sim}{\beta}}_t - \underset{\sim}{\beta}_0) \underset{D}{\to} N(0, \underset{\sim}{\Sigma}^{-1}) \quad \text{as } t \to \infty \quad ,$$

where "D" means convergence in distribution with respect to P.

Corollary. Under the conditions of the Theorem,

$$2(\log L_t^{\hat{\underset{\sim}{\beta}}_t} - \log L_t^{\underset{\sim}{\beta}_0}) \underset{D}{\to} \chi_p^2 \quad \text{as } t \to \infty \quad .$$

## REFERENCES


[1] M. AITKIN and D. CLAYTON. The fitting of exponential, Weibull and extreme value distributions to complex censored survival data using GLIM. Applied Statistics, 29, (1980), pp. 156-163.

[2] M. AITKIN, N.M. LAIRD and B. FRANCIS. Reanalysis of the Stanford heart transplant data. (With discussion), J. Am. Statist. Assoc., 78, (1983), pp. 264-292.

[3] A. ALBERT and J.A. ANDERSON. On the existence of maximum likelihood estimates in logistic regression models. Biometrika, 71, (1984), pp. 1-10.

[4] P.K. ANDERSEN and Ø. BORGAN. Counting process models for life history data: a review. (To appear), Scandinavian J. of Statist., (1985).

[5] P.K. ANDERSEN and R.D. GILL. Cox's regression model for counting processes: a large sample study. The Annals of Statist., 10, (1982), pp. 1100-1120.

[6] E. ARJAS. Contribution to the discussion on the paper by Andersen and Borgan. (To appear), Scandinavian J. of Statist., (1985).

[7] E. ARJAS and P. HAARA. A marked point process approach to censored failure data ith complicated covariates. Scandinavian J. of Statist., 11, (1984), pp. 193-209.

[8] E. ARJAS and P. HAARA. A logistic regression model for hazard: asymptotic theory. Manuscript in preparation, (1985).

[9] R.D. BOCK. Estimating multinomial response relations. In: Essays in Probability and Statistics (Ed. R.C. Bose et al). University of North Carolina Press, Chapel Hill, (1968).

[10] Ø. BORGAN. Maximum likelihood estimation in parametric counting process models. Scandinavian J. of Statist., 11, (1984), pp. 1-16.

[11] N. BRESLOW. Covariance analysis of censored survival data. Biometrics, 30, (1974), pp. 89-99.

[12] D.A. CLARK, E.B. STINSON, R B. GRIEPP, J.S. SCHOREDER, N.E. SHUMWAY and D.C. HARRISON. Cardiac transplantation in man, VI. Prognosis of patients selected for cardiac transplantation. Annals of Internal Medicine, 75, (1971), pp. 15-21.

[13] D.R. COX. The Analysis of Binary Data. Chapman and Hall, London, (1970).

[14] D.R. COX. Regression models and life tables. (With discussion), J. of the Royal Statist. Society, Ser. B, 74, (1972), pp. 187-220.

[15] D.R. COX. Partial likelihood. Biometrika, 62, (1975), pp. 269-276.

[16] J. CROWLEY and M. HU. Covariance analysis of heart transplant survival data. J. of the Am. Statist. Assoc., 72, (1977), pp. 27-36.

[17] J. CROWLEY and B.E. STORER. Comment on the paper by Aitkin, Laird and Francis. J. of the Am. Statist. Assoc., 78, (1983), pp. 277-281.

[18] M.H. GAIL. Comment on the paper by Aitkin, Laird and Francis. J. of the Am. Statist. Assoc., 78, (1983), pp. 275-277.

[19] J.D. KALBFLEISCH and R.L. PRENTICE. The Statistical Analysis of Failure Time Data. Wiley, New York, (1980).

[20] N.M. LAIRD and D. OLIVIER. Covariance analysis of censored survival data using log-linear analysis techniques. J. of the Am. Statist. Assoc., 75, (1981), pp. 231-240.

[21] R.L. PLACKETT. The Analysis of Categorical Data. Griffin, London, (1981).

[22] T. SELLKE and D. SIEGMUND. Sequential analysis of the proportional hazards model. Biometrika, 70, (1983), pp. 315-326.

[23] W.A. THOMPSON JR. On the treatment of grouped observations in life studies. Biometrics, 35, (1977), pp. 463-470.

[24] R.J. TIBSHIRANI and A. CIAMPI. A family of proportional- and additive-hazards models for survival data. Biometrics, 39, (1983), pp. 141-147.

# Time-Dependent Covariates and Markov Processes

*Per Kragh Andersen**

Abstract. Problems in connection with the Cox regression model with time-dependent covariates are studied including possible masking of treatment effects, prognostic measures and model evaluation. Possible ways of attacking these problems by means of multivariate counting processes, in particular Markov processes, are discussed. A study of survival with liver cirrhosis is used for illustration.

## INTRODUCTION

The semi-parametric regression model for censored survival data of Cox (1972) specifies the hazard rate function $\alpha(t)$ for the distribution of the time T to some event (in the following denoted the survival time or life time) for an individual with covariates $z(t) = (z_1(t),\cdots,z_p(t))$ at time t to be

$$\alpha(t) = \alpha_0(t)\exp(\beta' z(t)), \qquad t > 0. \tag{1}$$

Here $\beta$ is a vector of unknown regression coefficients and $\alpha_0(t)$ is an unknown and unspecified hazard rate function for individuals with covariate history $(Z(u),\ 0 \leq u \leq t)$ up to time t.

The possibility of allowing the covariates z to vary with time was introduced in the original paper by Cox (1972) rather as a convenient way to examining departures from the assumption of proportional hazards which is in the model (1) when the covariates do not depend on time than as a way of achieving more flexibility when building statistical models for survival data. The model (1) has become a very popular tool when analyzing data from randomized clinical trials where one wants to evaluate treatment effects on survival after adjusting for the effect of other covariates and also in other clinical and epidemiological follow-up studies. In this connection it seems obvious that taking into account time-dependent

*Statistical Research Unit, University of Copenhagen
Blegdamsvej 3, DK-2200 Copenhagen N, Denmark

measurements in an individual of some quantity when assessing the prognosis for that individual will allow one to give a more reliable forecast than is possible if only measurements taken at the time of entry into the study are considered. Examples of published analyses with time-dependent covariates are the Stanford heart transplant program (Crowley and Hu, [19]), a study of survival with leukemia after bone marrow transplantation (Farewell, [21]), a study of the short-term prognosis after acute myocardial infarction (Hougaard and Madsen, [22]), and a study of survival in infantile hydrocephalus, (Jansen and Jørgensen, [23]). In this report a clinical trial on the effect of prednisone treatment versus placebo on the survival with liver cirrhosis (Christensen et al, [13]) is used for illustration. Some details on this trial (called CSL1) are given in the next section.

The introduction of time-dependent covariates in the model (1) has, however, led to a series of new problems. We shall mention the theoretical statistical difficulties arising when inference is to be drawn from the model (1); can one find a suitable likelihood to use when estimating the parameters $\beta$ and $\alpha_0(t)$, and which large sample properties do the estimators have? These issues have been discussed in the statistical literature in the last decade and satisfactory solutions have now been obtained (Cox, [18]; Andersen and Gill, [5]).

The main problem arises when <u>interpreting</u> results from an analysis evaluating treatment effects when time-dependent covariates are taken into account. Oakes [25] mentioned a possible example concerning the effect of smoking on the risk of getting a stroke; if in such an analysis blood pressure is included as a time-dependent covariate then the effect of smoking may be masked since it might be so that smoking mainly influences the risk of stroke by increasing the blood pressure. A similar example was given by Kalbfleisch and Prentice ([24], Chapter 5). In Section 4 this problem of covariates acting both as treatment responses and as prognostic factors will be discussed in connection with the CSL 1 data and we shall suggest a way of approaching it. It will be demonstrated how the notion of a multivariate counting process, especially a Markov process, may be useful when discrete covariates are considered.

When a model of the form (1) including only time-independent covariates has been analyzed it is possible to estimate the survival probability and hence also the median survival time for a new patient with given covariates. If time-dependent covariates are included in the model then more care has to be taken since the further development of these should be taken into account in the estimation of such prognostic measures. We shall comment upon this in Section 5 where we also discuss the problem of <u>validating</u> a Cox regression model with time-dependent covariates.

## 2. THE CSL1 STUDY

CSL1 was the first study conducted by The Copenhagen Study Group for Liver Diseases. It was a double blind multicenter randomized clinical trial with the purpose of studying the effect of prednisone treatment versus placebo on the survival with liver cirrhosis (Copenhagen Study Group for Liver Diseases, [16]). During the accrual period 1962-69, 532 patients with histologically verified liver cirrhosis were included in the trial and the patients were followed from the date of entry into the trial to death or the closing date of the study: 1 September, 1974. Few patients were censored before that date. At entry, three, six and twelve months after start of treatment and thereafter once a year a number of clinical and biochemical variables were registered. Liver biopsies were taken at entry, and were scheduled to be taken every year after start of treatment but they were taken less frequently in some cases. In 488 patients the initial biopsy could later be re-evaluated and for these patients the effect on survival of variables recorded at entry into the trial was analyzed by Schlichting et al [27], and Christensen et al [14], using a Cox regression model with time-independent variables. The effect on survival of follow-up variables was analyzed by Christensen et al [13] using a Cox regression model of the form (1) with time-dependent covariates. In the latter study two variables: ascites (degree of oedema in the abdomen) and concentration of prothrombin (a substance which is produced in the liver) were found to interact with the treatment, i.e., their effects on the death intensity were significantly different in patients receiving prednisone treatment and in patients receiving placebo. These variables are studied in greater detail in the present paper. The variables in the final Cox regression model with time-dependent covariates and their scoring are shown in Table 1. Age was included as a time-independent covariate, i.e., as age at randomization. However, as the scoring of age was linear (age at randomization minus sixty years) the same estimated regression coefficient would have been obtained if age were included as current age minus sixty years. In this case the estimated integrated underlying hazard function $\hat{A}_0(t)$ (Breslow, [10]) would have been lower than the actual estimate shown in Figure 1. Except for the first three variables in Table 1 all covariates were time-dependent, $z_i(t)$ being defined as the recording of $z_i$ at the last follow-up preceding time t.

The curve in Figure 1 appears almost linear indicating a constant underlying intensity $\alpha_0(t) = \alpha_0$.

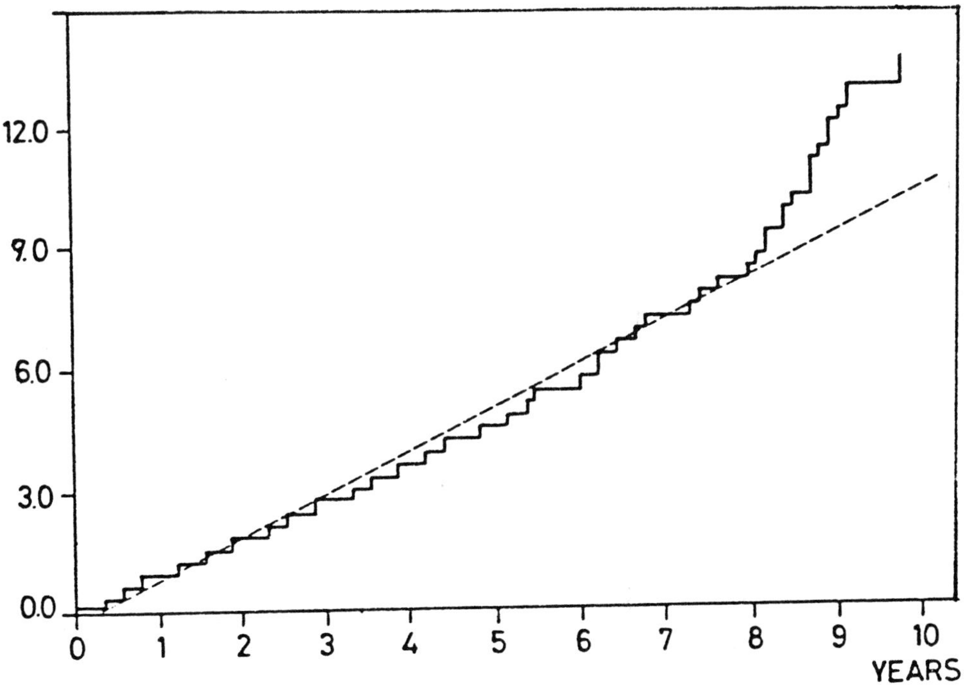


Figure 1. Estimated integrated underlying death intensity $\hat{A}_0(t)$ in final Cox regression model for the CSL1 study.

TABLE 1

Final Cox regression model with time-dependent covariates for the CSL 1 data.

| Variable | Scoring | | $\hat{\beta}$ | $\widehat{SE}(\hat{\beta})$ |
|---|---|---|---|---|
| Treatment (time-independent) | prednisone:<br>placebo: | 0<br>1 | -0.13 | 0.19 |
| Age (years) at randomization | age - 60 | | 0.052 | 0.0085 |
| Inflammation in liver connective tissue in biopsy at entry. | none or slight:<br>otherwise: | 0<br>1 | -0.56 | 0.14 |
| Prothrombin index (% of normal) | log(value) -4 | | pred -1.58<br>plac -0.83 | 0.22<br>0.19 |
| Ascites, slight | present:<br>absent: | 1<br>0 | pred 0.96<br>plac 0.34 | 0.25<br>0.27 |
| Ascites, moderate or marked | present:<br>absent: | 1<br>0 | pred 1.66<br>plac 1.17 | 0.25<br>0.23 |
| Gastrointestinal bleeding, marked | present:<br>absent: | 1<br>0 | 1.41 | 0.18 |
| Alcohol consumption (daily) | none:<br>10 - 50 g:<br>> 50g: | 0<br>3<br>9 | 0.14 | 0.024 |
| Bilirubin ($\mu$moles/$\ell$) | < 70:<br>$\geq$ 70: | 0<br>1 | 0.94 | 0.18 |
| Albumin (g/$\ell$) | log(value) -4 | | -1.20 | 0.27 |
| Alkaline phosphatase (KA units) | log(value) -4 | | 0.36 | 0.11 |
| Nutritional status | meagre or cachectic:<br>otherwise: | 1<br>0 | 0.56 | 0.16 |

## 3. A MULTISTATE MODEL FOR EACH INDIVIDUAL

The Cox regression model (1) with time-dependent covariates can be considered a special case of the simple two-state model for survival data displayed in Figure 2, namely a model where the state "alive" corresponds to the state space $\mathcal{Z}$ of the vector of covariate processes $(Z_1(t),\cdots,Z_p(t))$ and where the transition intensity to the state "dead" is

$$\alpha(t) = \alpha_0(t)\exp(\beta_1 z_1+\cdots+\beta_p z_p)$$

whenever

$$(Z_1(t),\cdots,Z_p(t)) = (z_1,\cdots,z_p) \; .$$

(As mentioned in the Introduction the covariates at time t may depend on the entire history of covariates up to time t.)

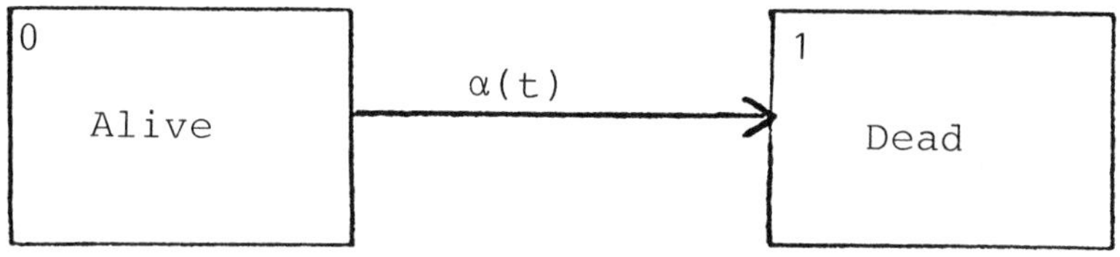


Figure 2. A two-state model for survival data.

Internal transitions within the state "alive" are not modelled in the Cox model (1) and thus only a small part of a complicated structure is modelled.

Let $N_i(\cdot)$ be the stochastic process counting 1 at t if and only if individual i is observed to die at t. Then (1) specifies only the conditional probability of observing a jump for the counting process $N_i$ at t given that i is at risk at time t and given the covariate history up to time t. One of the aims of this paper is to show how a small step towards a more detailed modelling of the entire process $(N_i(t), Z_{i1}(t), \cdots, Z_{ip}(t))$ may give more insight into the clinical or epidemiological problem at hand. Thus we model the development in time of Z(t) as occurrences of events which may change the death intensity $\alpha(t)$. This means that attention is restricted to discrete covariates and that continuous covariates have to be discretized in order to fit into the framework. Let us consider some examples.

In a study of survival in stage I cancer the occurrence of metastases is likely to increase the death intensity and one way of modelling this would be by means of a time-dependent covariate taking the value 1 at time t if metastases have occurred before time t and 0 otherwise. This corresponds to proportional death intensities $\alpha_{02}(t)$ and $\alpha_{12}(t)$ in Figure 3.

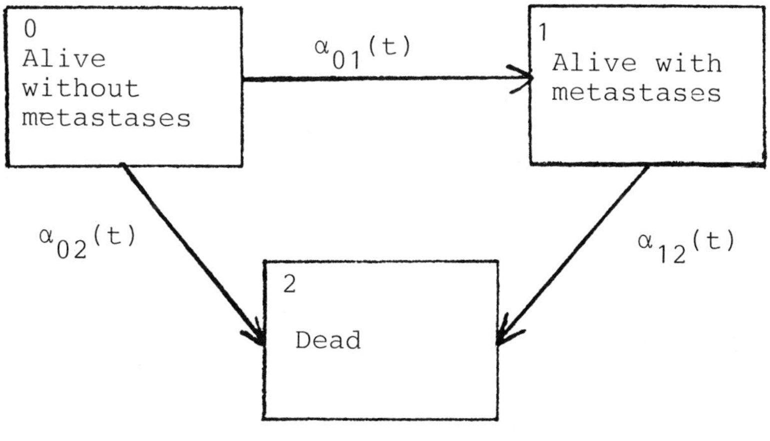


Figure 3. A model for cancer progression.

In this model $\alpha_{01}(t)$ is the relapse rate which is not specified in the Cox model for the survival time T. In the case where $\alpha_{12}(\cdot)$ only depends on t and not on the time since occurrence of metastases, the three state model for each individual is a Markov process and the transition probabilities are simple functions of $\alpha_{01}(\cdot)$, $\alpha_{02}(\cdot)$ and $\alpha_{12}(\cdot)$, (see Section 5); otherwise the process is semi-Markov.

Various extensions of the model in Figure 3 are possible, one possibility being the case where the event corresponding to the state 1 is a recurrent complication so transitions from state 1 to state 0 are also possible, see Figure 4.

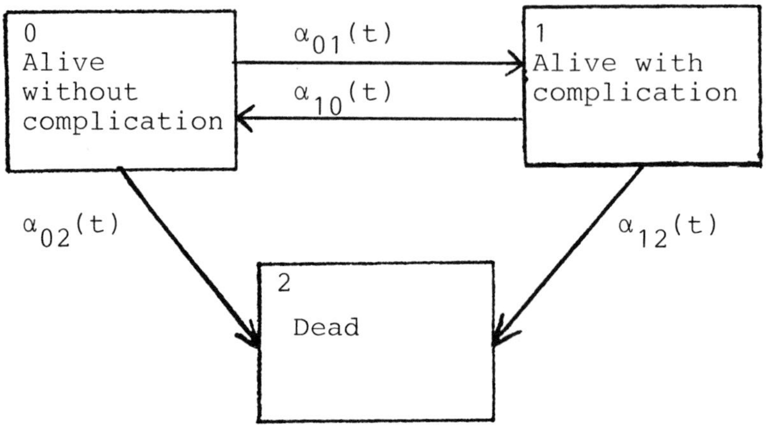


Figure 4. A model with a recurrent event.

A Cox regression model for survival time with information on the status of the complication included as a time-dependent indicator covariate taking the value 1 if the individual is alive at time t with the complication and 0 otherwise specifies the death intensities $\alpha_{02}(\cdot)$ and $\alpha_{12}(\cdot)$ to be proportional and it does not specify $\alpha_{01}(\cdot)$ and $\alpha_{10}(\cdot)$. An example of this type of model was used in two cases in the CSL1 study, where the complication was defined as either the presence of ascites or as an abnormal prothrombin index (defined as below 70% of normal). We return to these examples below.

A mathematical framework in which the models displayed in Figures 2-4 and similar models can be analyzed is multivariate counting processes. A multivariate counting process $N = \{(N_1(t), N_2(t), \cdots, N_k(t)); t \in [0,1]\}$ is a stochastic process with k components counting the occurrences, as time t proceeds, of k different types of events $N_h(t)$ being the number of type h events in the time interval $[0,t]$. Each component process $N_h$ has jumps of size +1, and no two component processes can jump simultaneously. Thus multiple events cannot occur. The events correspond to the transitions, for an individual or a group of individuals, between the various states of a stochastic process as exemplified in Figures 2-4. The development in time of a multivariate counting process N is governed by its (random) intensity process $\lambda = \{(\lambda_1(t),\cdots,\lambda_k(t));\ t\varepsilon[0,1]\}$, which is given as follows. Let $I_{dt}$ be a small time interval of length dt around time t, then $\lambda_h(t)dt$ is the conditional probability that $N_h$ jumps in $I_{dt}$ given all that has happened until just before time t. If we let $dN_h(t)$ denote the increment of $N_h$ over $I_{dt}$, and let $F_{t-}$ be the σ-algebra recording what has happened up to, but not including t, then we can write

$$\lambda_h(t)dt = \Pr[dN_h(t) = 1 \mid F_{t-}] .$$

Here $F_{t-}$ includes a complete specification of the path of N(u) on the interval [0,t) as well as all other events implicitly or explicitly included in the model which have happened before (but not at) time t. As a consequence we have that $F_s \subseteq F_t$, whenever $s < t$, reflecting the fact that as time proceeds more and more is learned about the process.

We consider models for the intensity process for the processes $N_{hi}$ counting the number of type h events for individual i of the form (cf. Andersen and Borgan, 1985)

$$\lambda_{hi}(t) = \alpha_{0h}(t)\exp(\beta' Z_{hi}(t))Y_{hi}(t) , \tag{2}$$

where $\alpha_{0h}(\cdot)$ is either left unspecified as in the Cox regression model or it is given a parametric specification $\alpha_{0h}(t,\Theta)$ with $\Theta\varepsilon R^q$. In either case $\alpha_{0h}(\cdot)$ is assumed to be locally integrable and left continuous. Other relative risk functions than the exponential can also be considered (Prentice and Self, [26]). The process $Y_{hi}(t)$ is a predictable indicator process taking the value 1 at time t if individual i is observed to be at risk just before time t for making a type h transition. Thus $Y_{hi}(\cdot)$ is also a function of possible censoring. One should notice that in the formulation of the model (2) it is assumed that we have the same vector of regression parameters $\beta = (\beta_1,\cdots,\beta_p)$ for all types h. This can always be obtained by introducing extra type specific covariates.

In the Cox regression model we estimate β by the solution $\hat{\beta}$ to the equation

$$\frac{\partial}{\partial\beta} C(\beta,1) = 0 ,$$

where

$$C(\beta,t) = \sum_{h=1}^{k} \Big[\sum_{i=1}^{n} \int_0^t \beta' Z_{hi}(s)dN_{hi}(s) - \tag{3}$$

$$\int_0^t \log\{\sum_{i=1}^{n} Y_{hi}(s)\exp(\beta' Z_{hi}(s))\}dN_h(s)\Big]$$

and $N_h = N_{h1}+\cdots+N_{hn}$. The integrated underlying intensities

$$A_{0h}(t) = \int_0^t \alpha_{0h}(s)ds, \quad h=1,\cdots,k$$

can be estimated by

$$\hat{A}_{0h}(t) = \int_0^t \sum_{i=1}^{n} \{Y_{hi}(s)\exp(\hat{\beta}'Z_{hi}(s))\}^{-1} dN_h(s) \tag{4}$$

and the asymptotic joint distribution (as $n\to\infty$) of $\hat{\beta}$ and the processes $\hat{A}_{01}(\cdot),\cdots,\hat{A}_{0k}(\cdot)$ can be derived using results for local square integrable martingales. It follows from (3) and the decomposition

$$N_{hi}(t) = \int_0^t \lambda_{hi}(s)ds + M_{hi}(t) ,$$

of $N_{hi}$ into the integrated intensity process and a local square integrable martingale $M_{hi}$, that the score statistics

$$U_j(\beta_0,t) = \frac{\partial}{\partial\beta_j} C(\beta,t)\Big|_{\beta=\beta_0} , \quad j=1,\cdots,p$$

evaluated at the true parameter value $\beta_0$ are also local square integrable martingales and so are the processes

$$V_h(t) = \int_0^t \{[\sum_{i=1}^{n} Y_{hi}(s)\exp(\beta_0'Z_{hi}(s))]^{-1} dN_h(s)$$

$$- I(Y_h(s) > 0)\alpha_{0h}(s)ds \} , \quad h=1,\cdots,k$$

where $Y_h = Y_{h1}+\cdots+Y_{hn}$. Furthermore any $U_j$ and $V_h$ are orthogonal. The conditions (including some regularity of the covariate processes) under which the asymptotic results hold can be found in Andersen and Borgan [4] and Andersen and Gill [5].

For the parametric regression model the estimation can be based on the joint likelihood function for $\Theta$ and $\beta$ given by

$$\log L(\Theta,\beta) = \sum_{h=1}^{k} \sum_{i=1}^{n} \Big[\int_0^\infty \{\log \alpha_{0h}(s,\Theta)+\beta'Z_{hi}(s)\}\, dN_{hi}(s) \tag{5}$$

$$- \int_0^\infty \alpha_{0h}(s,\Theta)\exp(\beta'Z_{hi}(s))Y_{hi}(s)ds\Big]$$

and results on the asymptotic distribution of $\hat{\theta}$ and $\hat{\beta}$ can again be derived using local martingale results (Borgan, [ 9], Andersen and Borgan, [ 4 ]).

## 4. EVALUATION OF TREATMENT EFFECTS IN THE MULTISTAGE MODEL

In the CSL1 study two time-dependent covariates: prothrombin index and ascites were found to interact with the treatment, cf. Table 1. Thus the death intensities given the levels of these variables were significantly different during prednisone treatment and during placebo treatment. To study how the development in time of these two covariates depended on the treatment a model as shown in Figure 4 was considered for each of the two treatments neglecting at the first stage in modelling the possible effect on the transition intensities of other covariates. As mentioned above the prothrombin index was dichotomized and the "complication" low prothrombin was defined as the prothrombin index being less than 70%. Since no other covariates than treatment were taken into account and since the transition intensities in the two treatment groups were assumed to vary freely the estimators (4) for the integrated transition intensities reduced to the ordinary Nelson-Aalen estimators (Aalen, [ 1 ]; Andersen and Borgan, [ 4 ]).

Figure 5 shows the estimated integrated death intensities for patients with low and normal prothrombin $\hat{A}_{12}(t)$ and $\hat{A}_{02}(t)$, respectively during prednisone and during placebo treatment. For both treatment groups the death intensity $\alpha_{12}(t)$ for patients with low prothrombin seems to be larger than the death intensity $\alpha_{02}(t)$ for patients with normal values. The relative increase in the death intensity $\alpha_{12}(t)/\alpha_{02}(t)$ when going from normal to low prothrombin seems to be larger in prednisone treated patients in accordance with the significantly different regression coefficients for log(prothrombin) for prednisone and placebo treated patients in Table 1.

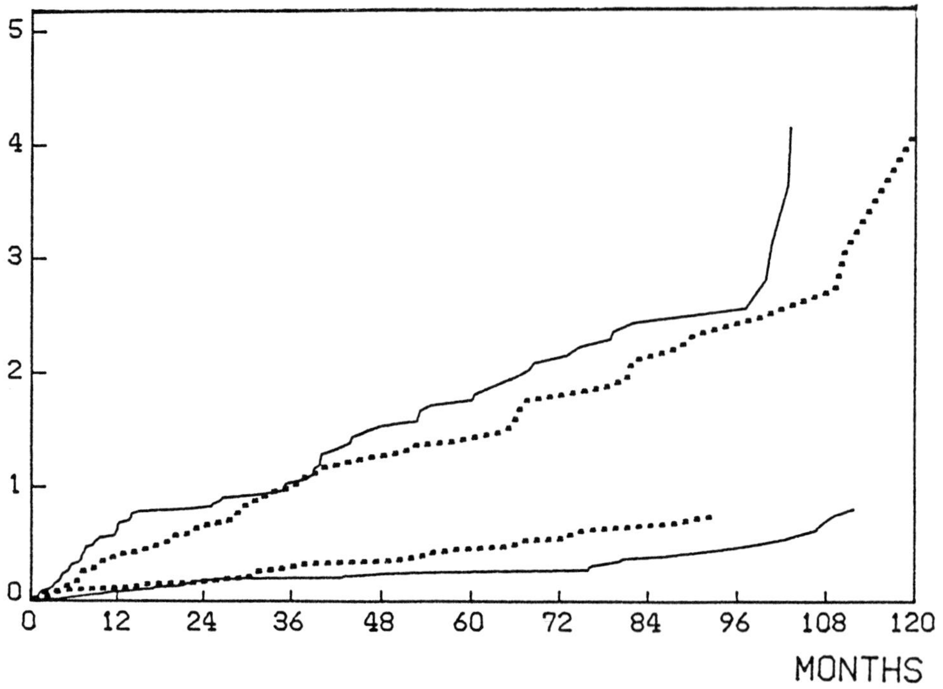


Figure 5. Estimated integrated death intensities in the CSL1 study: upper pair of curves ∿ low prothrombin, $\hat{A}_{12}(t)$, lower pair of curves ∿ normal prothrombin, $\hat{A}_{02}(t)$. Prednisone treatment: ——, placebo treatment: (••••).

Under the assumption of proportional death intensities within each treatment group the intensity ratios $\Theta_{pred}$ and $\Theta_{plac}$, say between patients with normal and low prothrombin can be estimated as described by Crowley et al [20], Begun and Reid [ 7 ], and Andersen [3]. The estimates (estimated standard errors) are $\hat{\Theta}_{pred} = 0.159$ (0.031) and $\hat{\Theta}_{plac} = 0.294$ (0.052) showing once more the interaction between treatment and prothrombin in that the hypothesis $\Theta_{pred} = \Theta_{plac}$ cannot be accepted, the standard normal deviate for the hypothesis being 2.23 ($P = 0.03$).

Since patients in the CSL1 trial were not monitored continuously the exact dates of transitions between low and normal prothrombin index were not observed. The convention was adopted that changes took place at the times of follow-up examination and for each time t the prothrombin value was defined as the value recorded at the last follow-up preceding t. An effect of this convention was a clustering of observed transition times around the scheduled follow-up examinations, cf. Figures 6 and 7. Figure 6 shows the estimated integrated transition intensities $\hat{A}_{10}(t)$ from low to normal prothrombin for both treatment groups and Figure 7 shows $\hat{A}_{01}(t)$ for both treatment groups. The intensity $\alpha_{10}(t)$ is significantly larger for prednisone treated patients, the estimated intensity ratio between the prednisone and the placebo group being $\hat{\theta} = 1.29$ corresponding to a logrank test statistic $X^2 = 4.37$ ($P = 0.04$). The intensity $\alpha_{01}(t)$ is significantly smaller for prednisone treated patients in that $\hat{\theta} = 0.72$, $X^2 = 9.98$, $P = 0.002$.

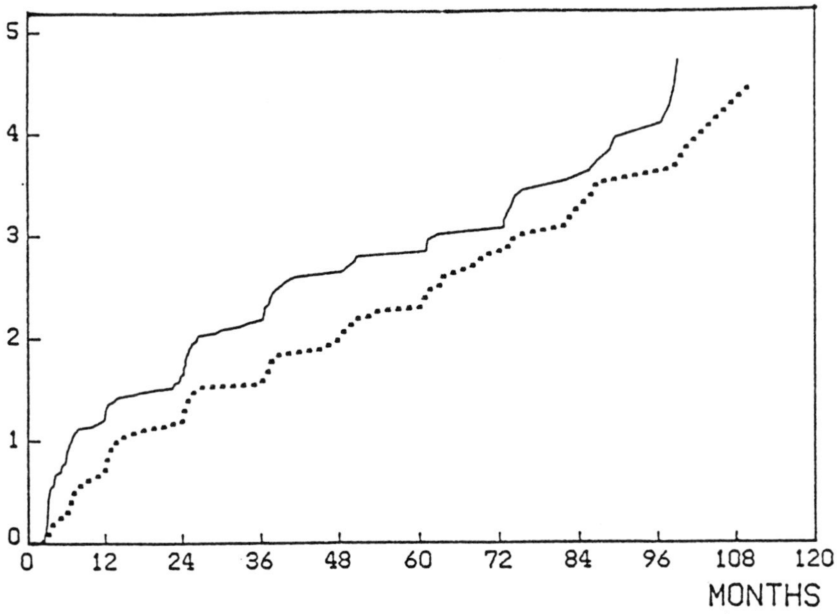


Figure 6. Estimated integrated transition intensities $\hat{A}_{10}(t)$ from low to normal prothrombin in the CSL1 study. (Prednisone treatment: ——, placebo treatment: ••••).

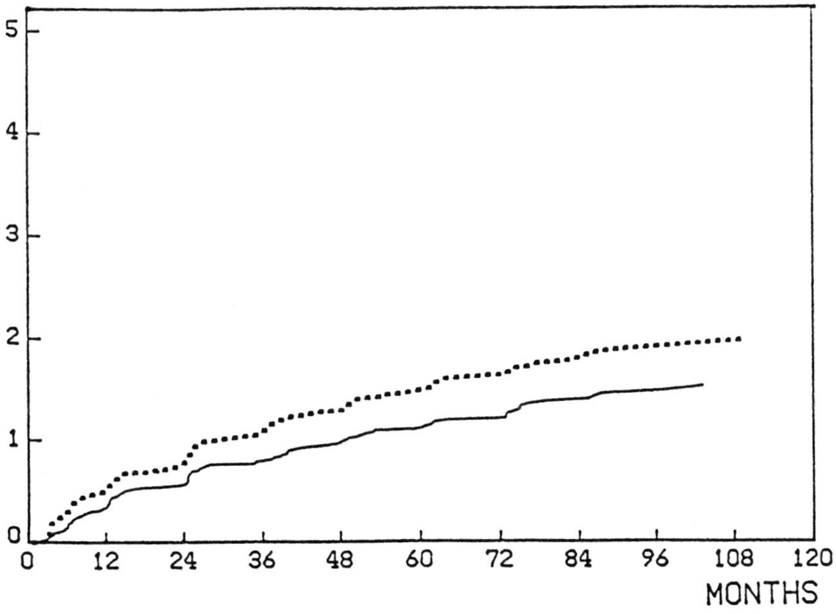


Figure 7. Estimated integrated transition intensities $\hat{A}_{01}(t)$ from normal to low prothrombin in the CSL1 study. (Prednisone treatment: ——, placebo treatment: ••••).

Thus in addition to the effect of treatment on the death intensities with low and normal prothrombin the transition intensities between the two "alive-states" are different during prednisone and placebo treatment. This means that it cannot be deduced directly from the estimates in Table 1 whether patients with high prothrombin index should be given prednisone and patients with a low index should not. To evaluate the treatment effects all four transition intensities must be taken into account. This can be done via the transition probabilities in the three-state Markov process displayed in Figure 4 which can be estimated non-parametrically as described by Aalen and Johansen [2] or under various parametric assumptions. In the following the transition probabilities are estimated under the assumption of constant transition intensities in which case the transition probabilities are simple explicit functions of the intensities (e.g., Chiang, [12]). In particular, the conditional probability of being alive at time t given that the initial state is j, j=0,1 is

$$S_j(t) = [(\alpha_{j2}+\gamma_2)e^{\gamma_1 t} - (\alpha_{j2}+\gamma_1)e^{\gamma_2 t}]/(\gamma_2-\gamma_1)$$

where

$$\gamma_1 = -[\alpha_0+\alpha_1+\{(\alpha_0-\alpha_1)^2+4\alpha_{01}\alpha_{10}\}^{\frac{1}{2}}]/2 \quad ,$$

$$\gamma_2 = -[\alpha_0+\alpha_1-\{(\alpha_0-\alpha_1)^2+4\alpha_{01}\alpha_{10}\}^{\frac{1}{2}}]/2$$

and $\alpha_0 = \alpha_{01}+\alpha_{02}$, $\alpha_1 = \alpha_{10}+\alpha_{12}$. The maximum likelihood estimates based on (5) for the transition intensities $\alpha_{hj}$ are ordinary occurrence/exposure rates and the estimates are shown in Table 2. The variance of log $\hat{\alpha}_{hj}$ can be estimated by the reciprocal of the observed number of transitions from h to j. The above mentioned differences between the two treatment groups are smaller judged from this model than from the non-parametric model above. This is partly due to the fact that the intensities are probably not quite constant.

TABLE 2

Estimates in model with constant transition intensities.

| Transition | Prednisone treatment<br>No. transitions | <br>Intensity per year | Placebo treatment<br>No. transitions | <br>Intensity per year |
|---|---|---|---|---|
| From low to normal | 164 | 0.69 | 159 | 0.53 |
| From normal to low | 137 | 0.20 | 150 | 0.26 |
| From low to dead | 95 | 0.40 | 99 | 0.33 |
| From normal to dead | 47 | 0.070 | 51 | 0.089 |

Christensen et al [15] noted that the changes in laboratory variables were larger during the first 6-12 months after start of treatment which is in accordance with Figures 6 and 7.

The estimated survival probabilities are shown in Figures 8 and 9. As expected the survival probability $\hat{S}_0(t)$ for patients with normal prothrombin is uniformly larger during prednisone treatment than during placebo treatment, whereas no clear tendency is seen in patients with low prothrombin. So, from these preliminary investigations the indication is that prednisone should be given only to patients with normal prothrombin.

For the other covariates in Table 1 which interacted with the treatment, ascites, similar analyses were performed restricting attention to absence or presence of ascites, i.e., without distinguishing between slight or moderate ascites. Again, the level of ascites at time t was defined as the value recorded at the last follow-up preceding t. The estimated ratios between the death intensities for patients with and for patients without ascites are

$$\hat{\phi}_{pred} = 8.91 \ (1.55)$$

and

$$\hat{\phi}_{plac} = 5.06 \ (0.86)$$

respectively confirming the interaction between ascites and treatment also seen in Table 1, the standard normal deviate for the hypothesis $\phi_{pred} = \phi_{plac}$ being 2.17 ($P = 0.03$). For both of the transition intensities between absence and presence of ascites we find insignificant tendencies to a smaller intensity during prednisone treatment than during placebo treatment. For transitions from ascites to no ascites the estimated intensity ratio is $\hat{\phi} = 0.81$ corresponding to a logrank statistic $X^2 = 1.56$ ($P = 0.21$). For transitions from no ascites to ascites $\hat{\phi} = 0.88$, $X^2 = 0.85$, $P = 0.36$. So, for this variable no further interaction with the treatment was found and the indication from Table 1 of not treating patients with ascites with prednisone is sustained and has been made even stronger in that the tendency of getting rid of ascites is (insignificantly) smaller for prednisone treated patients, the corresponding hazard ratio estimate $\hat{\phi}$ being smaller than unity.

It is interesting to compare the estimates $\hat{\phi}_{pred}$ and $\hat{\phi}_{plac}$ with those obtained from a Cox regression model stratified by treatment. For prednisone treated patients we find $\hat{\beta}_{pred} = 2.19 = \log 8.94$ (0.172) and for placebo treated patients $\hat{\beta}_{plac} = 1.60 = \log 4.95$ (0.167). The estimates are in close agreement with the $\hat{\phi}$ -values. It should be noticed that the estimated variances of the hazard ratios based on the Cox model are slightly smaller than those of $\hat{\phi}$ in agreement with

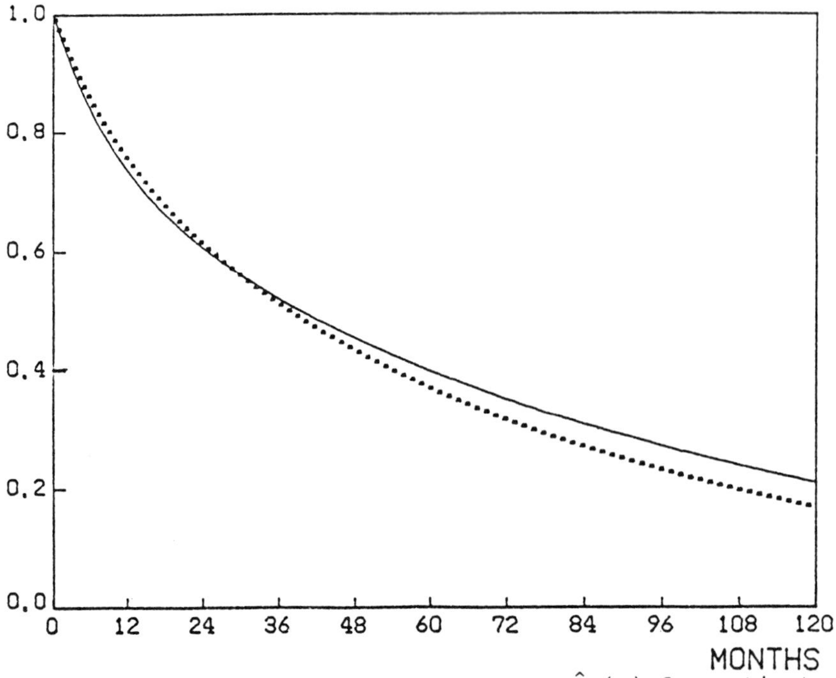


Figure 8. Estimated survival probabilities $\hat{S}_1(t)$ for patients with low prothrombin at time 0 assuming constant transition intensities. (Prednisone treatment: ——— , Placebo treatment: ···· .)

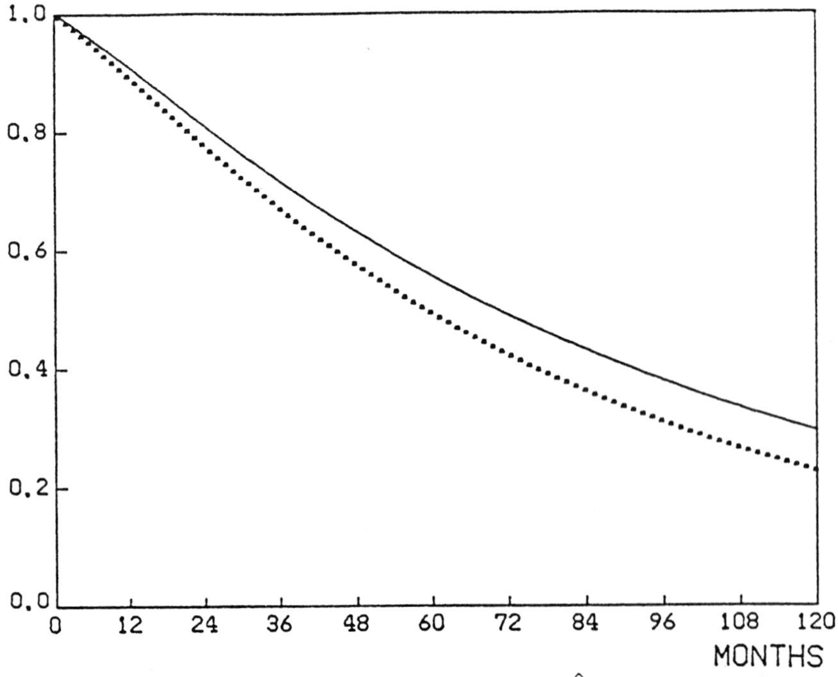


Figure 9. Estimated survival probabilities $\hat{S}_0(t)$ for patients with normal prothrombin at time 0 assuming constant transition intensities. (Prednisone treatment: ——— , placebo treatment: ···· .)

the results of Crowley et al [20] and Andersen [3]. We have

$$\hat{SE}\,(e^{\hat{\beta}_{pred}}) = 1.54$$

and

$$\hat{SE}\,(e^{\hat{\beta}_{plac}}) = 0.83\ .$$

In all the analyses reported so far the assumption has been made that the covariate value at any time t equals the value registered at the latest follow-up time $\tau$ for which $\tau < t$. Other definitions are possible. One could take the value at the follow-up time closest to t or one could make linear interpolation between the values at the follow-up times surrounding t, but it should be emphasized that the results of the analysis may depend on the choice that is made. We repeated the analysis of the effect of ascites on the death intensity redefining the ascites level at time t as the value recorded at the first follow-up time $\tau$ for which $\tau \geq t$. (If such a follow-up time did not exist the previous definition was used.) All estimates became smaller with the new definition, e.g., $\hat{\phi}_{pred} = 8.67$, and $\hat{\phi}_{plac} = 4.32$. This is probably due to the fact that more transitions (197) are observed from no ascites to ascites than from ascites to no ascites (137). So, at a given time t more patients will be alive with ascites with the new definition than with the old one and less patients will be alive without ascites, whereas the deaths will be observed from the same states with the two definitions.

## 5. MEASURING AND EVALUATING PROGNOSES BASED ON MULTISTATE MODELS

For the Cox regression model including only time-fixed covariates the survival function and the median survival time (and other quantiles of the survival time distribution) are functions of the hazard rate function only. Thus for the presentation of the results from such a model a graph can be drawn giving the median survival time or the $t_0$-year survival probability as a function of the prognostic index $PI = \hat{\beta}'z$. For the multistate models discussed in Section 3 the survival function depends on all transition intensities in the model. The transition probabilities can be estimated in simple multistate non-regression models as we saw it in Section 4. In the simple three state "disability" model (or cancer progression model) of Figure 3 the survival function can be estimated directly from estimates of the integrated intensities also when covariates are included. For patients in state 0 at time 0 we have for the simple disability model

$$S_0(t) = e^{-A_{01}(t)-A_{02}(t)} + \int_0^t e^{-A_{01}(u)-A_{02}(u)}\, e^{-(A_{12}(t)-A_{12}(u))}\, dA_{01}(u),$$

(see also Voelkel and Crowley, [28] ). Survival curves of this form were presented by Borch-Johnsen et al [ 8 ] in a study of the impact of diabetic nephropathy on the survival with insulin dependent diabetes and by Jansen and Jørgensen [ 23 ] in their study of infantile hydrocephalus. Andersen and Green [ 6 ] made similar calculations in an illness-death-emigration model with piecewise constant intensities.

For the general Cox regression model (1) with possibly several time-dependent covariates included, a model for the development of all covariates is, in principle, needed for the estimation of the survival function. From a practical point of view this is not feasible and some simpler approximations to the survival function are needed. One possibility is to restrict attention to short-term prognoses, that is to the estimation of conditional survival probabilities of the form

$$P(t,\Delta t) = \Pr(\text{alive at time } t+\Delta t \mid \text{alive at time } t,\ Z(u), 0 \le u \le t)$$

for $\Delta t$ relatively small. The conditional probability $P(t,\Delta t)$ can be estimated by assuming that $Z(u) = Z(t)$ for $t \le u \le t+\Delta t$ in which case

$$P(t,\Delta t) = \exp\{-\exp(\beta' Z(t))\ [A_0(t+\Delta t)-A_0(t)]\} \quad .$$

When the underlying intensity is constant $\alpha_0(u)\equiv\alpha_0$, $P(t,\Delta t)$ can be estimated by

$$\hat{P}(t,\Delta t) = \exp\{-\exp(\hat{\beta}' Z(t))\hat{\alpha}_0 \Delta t\} \tag{6}$$

which depends on t only via the prognostic index $PI(t) = \hat{\beta}' Z(t)$ at time t. Figure 1 shows that the assumption of a constant $\alpha_0$ was reasonable in the CSL1 study and the estimate (6) was applied to the estimation of P(t, 6 months). We did not, however, calculate the maximum likelihood estimate $\hat{\alpha}_0$ for $\alpha_0$ based on (5) (as only one type of transition is possible we drop the subscript h). Instead we used the estimate

$$\tilde{\alpha}_0 = \frac{N\ (1)}{\sum_{i=1}^{n} \int_0^1 Y_i(u)\exp(\hat{\beta}' Z_i(u)/du}$$

with $\hat{\beta}$ obtained from the Cox regression model (1). The estimate $\tilde{\alpha}_0$ is the maximum likelihood estimate if $\beta$ were known and equal to $\hat{\beta}$.

Figure 10 shows that P(t, 6 months) as a function of PI(t), based on the model in Table 1 and the estimate $\tilde{\alpha}_0 = 0.95$ years$^{-1}$. To evaluate the quality of the survival prediction based on this graph an evaluation procedure inspired by the one-sample logrank test of Breslow [ 11 ] also applied by Schlichting et al [ 27 ] was developed.

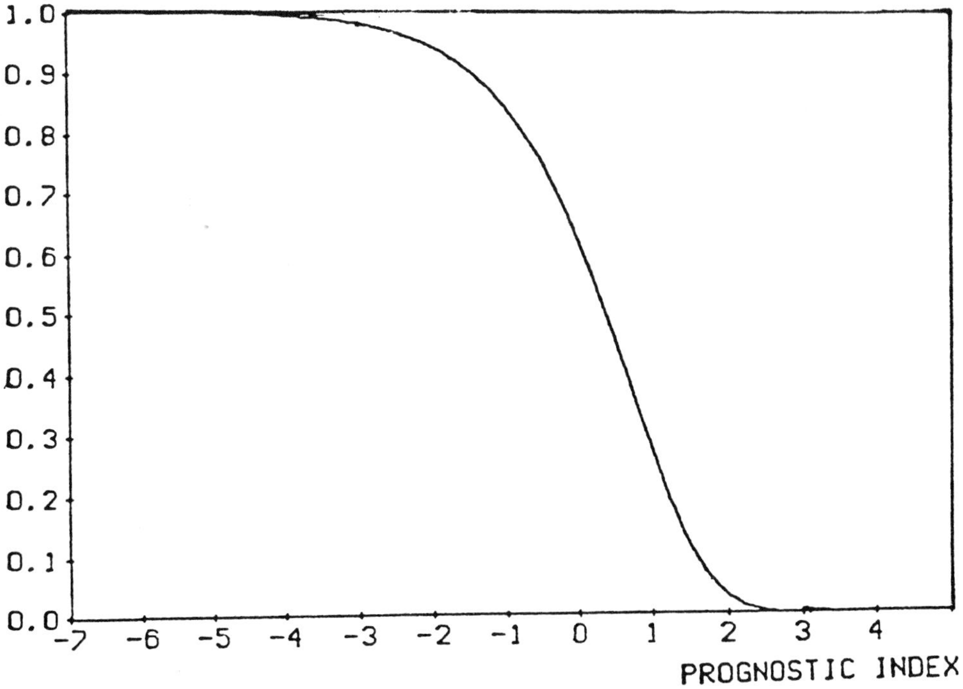


Figure 10. Estimated 6 months survival probability (7) as a function of the prognostic index PI(t), CSL1 study.

A random sample of approximately 75% of the patients was drawn and the regression coefficients corresponding to the covariates in the final model (Table 1) were estimated on the basis of the sample only. Also the underlying death intensity $\alpha_0$ (assumed constant) was estimated. The interval 0-10 years was divided into half year sub-intervals $[0,\frac{1}{2}),[\frac{1}{2},1),\cdots,[9\frac{1}{2},10)$ and for each sub-interval and for each of the remaining 25% of the patients alive and uncensored at the beginning of the sub-interval (at time t, say) the conditional probability of dying within the next six months was estimated as $1-\hat{P}_i(t, 6\text{ months})$ inserting that particular patient's covariates $z_i(t)$ and estimates $\hat{\beta}$ and $\tilde{\alpha}_0$ based on the random 75% sample. The 25% of the patients was (dynamically) divided into three groups according to their PI(t) value and within each of the three prognostic groups, j, observed ($O_j$) and "expected" ($E_j$) numbers of deaths were calculated, the contribution to $E_j$ from the sub-interval $[t,t+\frac{1}{2})$ being the sum over patients in prognostic group j at time t of the individual conditional probabilities $1-\hat{P}_i(t,\frac{1}{2})$ of dying in $[t,t+\frac{1}{2})$. A chi-squared goodness-of-fit statistic was then obtained as

$$\sum_{j=1}^{3}(O_j-E_j)^2/E_j \quad . \tag{7}$$

Table 3 shows the observed and expected numbers of deaths in the intervals [0,1 year), [1,5 years) and [5,10 years) and in the three prognostic groups $PI(t) \leq -3.7$, $-3.7 < PI(t) \leq -2.5$ and $-2.5 < PI(t)$. The statistic (7) takes the value 7.91 corresponding to $P = 0.05$, so there is some indication that it is insufficient to apply the estimate (6) to predict the number of deaths in a 6 month period. Particularly noticing the systematic differences between the observed and expected numbers of deaths: for the group with the best prognosis ($PI(t) \leq -3.7$) we have $O_1 > E_1$ and for the group with the worst prognosis ($PI(t) > -2.5$) we have $O_3 < E_3$. These tendencies are most marked during the first year where changes in the covariate values take place most rapidly (cf. Figures 6-7 and Christensen et al, [ 15 ]). Thus, for patients with a relatively good prognosis the fact that these patients may get worse is neglected in the calculation of E and vice versa: for patients with a relatively bad prognosis the fact that these patients may get better is neglected.

The simplest way of attempting to overcome these shortcomings of the prediction is to allow one time-dependent covariate to change during a sub-interval and we studied a model where also the prothrombin level was allowed to change. Thus for the 75% sample a Cox regression model with the prothrombin index dichotomized was considered and the estimates $\hat{\beta}$ and $\tilde{\alpha}_0$ were obtained. Also the transition intensities (assumed constant) between low and normal prothrombin were estimated from the 75% sample for both prednisone and placebo treatment, and P(t, 6 months) was estimated under the assumption of constant transition intensities as described in Section 4. Finally the expected numbers of deaths were calculated as before but with the new estimates $P^*_i$(t, 6 months) inserted. These expected numbers ($E^*$) are also shown in Table 3 and in this case the statistic (7) takes the value 7.13 corresponding to $P = 0.07$. Thus only a slight improvement is obtained by taking into account that the prothrombin index may change in a sub-interval. It is seen that the systematic differences are still present. A larger improvement would probably have been obtained if different transition intensities between low and normal prothrombin were used for $t < 1$ year and $t \geq 1$ year, respectively. In fact, for both transitions and for both treatments the intensity is significantly larger before than after the first year of observation.

TABLE 3

Observed numbers of deaths (O), expected numbers of deaths from Cox model alone (E) and expected numbers of deaths also taking into account the development of prothrombin ($E^*$).

| | $PI(t) \leq -3.7$ | | | $-3.7<PI(t)\leq-2.5$ | | | $-2.5 < PI(t)$ | | |
|---|---|---|---|---|---|---|---|---|---|
| Interval | O | E | E* | O | E | E* | O | E | E* |
| [0,1 year) | 4 | 3.64 | 3.70 | 5 | 5.25 | 5.05 | 14 | 20.66 | 20.02 |
| [1,5 years) | 10 | 9.38 | 9.59 | 8 | 9.09 | 8.84 | 8 | 16.23 | 15.96 |
| [5,10 years) | 7 | 4.33 | 4.57 | 4 | 2.30 | 2.22 | 2 | 4.26 | 4.18 |
| Total | 21 | 17.35 | 17.86 | 17 | 16.64 | 16.11 | 24 | 41.15 | 40.16 |

## 6. CONCLUSIONS

The Cox regression model with time-dependent covariates provides a flexible tool for the analysis of clinical and epidemiological survival data with follow-up information on the individual level. It should, however, be realized that this model describes only a small part of a larger and possibly much more complicated structure in that the Cox model specifies the individual death intensities for given values of the covariates whereas nothing is said about the development of the covariates in time.

In this paper some of the shortcomings of the model which are consequences of the above mentioned fact have been discussed and we have seen how some of these problems may be approached by considering a multi-state model instead of the simple two state model for survival data, cf. Figure 1. In this way it was possible to discuss in more detail the situation where the development of covariates was dependent on treatment and also it was possible to estimate survival probabilities and to evaluate the fit of the model. An advantage of this approach was that the large sample properties of the estimators could be derived rigorously using counting process and martingale results both in the case of models for homogeneous groups and in the case of regression models and both for parametric and for semi-parametric models. Among the limitations of the proposed multi-state model is the fact that few time-dependent covariates can be analyzed simultaneously in this way unless very large samples are available. This means that if other covariates are included than those defining the various alive states then the assumptions still have to be made that these other covariates develop in a deterministic way (they can for example be constant) during an interval of prediction. Thus only a small step towards a solution of some of the problems mentioned has been taken.

## ACKNOWLEDGEMENTS

Discussions with Erik Christensen, Niels Keiding, Bo V. Pedersen and Geert Schou are greatly appreciated. I wish to thank the Copenhagen Study group for Liver diseases for permission to use the CSL1 data.

## REFERENCES

[1] O.O. AALEN. Nonparametric inference for a family of counting processes. Ann. Statist., 6, (1985), 701-726.

[2] O.O. AALEN and S. JOHANSEN. An empirical transition matrix for non-homogeneous Markov chains based on censored observations. Scand. J. Statist., 5, (1978), 141-150.

[3] P.K. ANDERSEN. Comparing survival distributions via hazard ratio estimates. Scand. J. Statist., 10, (1983), 77-85.

[4] P.K. ANDERSEN and Ø. BORGAN. Counting process models for life history data: a review (with discussion). Scand. J. Statist., 12, (1985), 97-158.

[5] P.K. ANDERSEN and R.D. GILL. Cox's regression model for counting processes: a large sample study. Ann. Statist., 10, (1982), 1100-1120.

[6] P.K. ANDERSEN and A. GREEN. Evaluation of estimation bias in an illness-death-emigration model. Scand. J. Statist., 12, (1985), 63-68.

[7] J. BEGUN and N. REID. Estimating the relative risk with censored data. J. Amer. Statisti. Assoc., 78, (1983), 337-341.

[8] K. BORCH-JOHNSEN, P.K. ANDERSEN, T. DECKERT. The impact of proteinuria on the relative mortality in patients with Type I (insulin-dependent) diabetes mellitus. In press, Diabetologia, (1985).

[9] Ø. BORGAN. Maximum likelihood estimation in parametric counting process models, with applications to censored failure time data. Scand. J. Statist., 11, (1984), 1-16.

[10] N.E. BRESLOW. Covariance analysis of censored survival data. Biometrics, 30, (1974), 89-99.

[11] N.E. BRESLOW. Analysis of survival data under the proportional hazards model. Int. Statist. Rev., 43, (1975), 45-58.

[12] C.O. CHIANG. Introduction to stochastic processes in biostatistics. Wiley, New York, (1968).

[13] E. CHRISTENSEN, P. SCHLICHTING, P.K. ANDERSEN, et al. Updating prognosis and therapeutic effect evaluation in cirrhosis using Cox's multiple regression model for time dependent variables. Submitted for publication, (1985a).

[14] E. CHRISTENSEN, P. SCHLICHTING, P.K. ANDERSEN, et al. A therapeutic index predicting individual effect of prednisone in patients with cirrhosis. Gastroenterology, 58, (1985b), 156-165.

[15] E. CHRISTENSEN, P. SCHLICHTING, L. FAUERHOLDT, et al. Changes of laboratory variables with time in cirrhosis: prognostic and therapeutic significance. In press, Hepatology, (1985c).

[16] THE COPENHAGEN STUDY GROUP FOR LIVER DISEASES. Sex, ascites and alcoholism in survival of patients with cirrhosis. New England J. of Medicine, 291, (1974), 271-273.

[17] D.R. COX. Regression models and life tables (with discussion). J. Roy. Statist., Soc. B., 34, (1972), 187-220.

[18] D.R. COX, Partial likelihood. Biometrika, 62, (1975), 269-276.

[19] J. CROWLEY and M. HU. Covariance analysis of heart transplant survival data. J. Amer. Statist. Assoc., 72, (1977), 27-36.

[20] J. CROWLEY, P.-Y. LIU, J.G. VOELKEL. Estimation of the ratio of hazard functions. IN Survival Analysis, IMS Lecture Notes, 2, (1982), Crowley, J and Johnson, R.A., Eds., 56-73.

[21] V.T. FAREWELL. An application of Cox's proportional hazard model to multiple infection data. Appl. Statist., 28, (1979), 136-143.

[22] P. HOUGAARD and E.B. MADSEN. Dynamic evaluation of short-term prognosis of myocardial infarction. Stat. in Medicine, 4, (1985), 29-38.

[23] J. JANSEN and M. JØRGENSEN. Prognostic significance of signs and symptoms in hydrocephalus. Analysis of survival. In press, Acta. Neurol. Scand, (1985).

[24] J.D. KALBFLEISCH and R.L. PRENTICE. The statistical analysis of failure time data. Wiley, New York, (1980).

[25] D. OAKES. Survival times: aspects of partial likelihood (with discussion). Int. Statist. Rev., 49, (1981), 235-264.

[26] R.L. PRENTICE and S.G. SELF. Asymptotic distribution theory for Cox-type regression models with general relative risk form. Ann. Statist., 11, (1983), 804-813.

[27] P. SCHLICHTING, E. CHRISTENSEN, P.K. ANDERSEN, et al. Identification of prognostic factors in cirrhosis using Cox's regression model. Hepatology, 3, (1983), 889-895.

[28] J.G. VOELKEL and J. CROWLEY. Nonparametric inference for a class of semi-Markov processes with censored observations. Ann. Statist., 12, (1984), 142-160.

# Confidence Regions for Case-Control and Survival Studies with General Relative Risk Functions

*Suresh H. Moolgavkar* and David J. Venzon**

Abstract. Problems with Wald confidence regions are discussed. Geometric methods are used to construct confidence regions in curved exponential families. These methods are applied to case-control and survival studies with general relative risk functions. Simulations indicate that the geometric procedures have good coverage and power properties.

## INTRODUCTION

Much of this conference is concerned with the use of relative risk regression methods for the analysis of epidemiologic and survival data. In the original regression models, the relative risk $\rho(\beta,z)$ is an exponential function of a vector of known covariates z with unknown coefficients $\beta$; i.e.,

$$\rho(\beta,z) = \exp(\beta^* z) \quad .$$

More recently, there has been interest in considering more general models of the relative risk function, especially in the additive model

$$\rho(\beta,z) = 1 + \beta^* z \quad ,$$

where $\beta^*$ is the transpose of $\beta$. Various mixture models have also been suggested [11,21], in which a parametrized family of relative risk functions is considered, with the additive and exponential models being members of the family. Asymptotic results for a broad class of models have been obtained by Prentice and Self [19].

The purpose of this paper is to explore some of the small sample properties of various tests of inference with general relative risk functions. We find that, when the relative risk function is not exponential, the Wald test and the Wald confidence intervals may be

*Fred Hutchinson Cancer Research Center, 1124 Columbia Street, Seattle, Washington, 98104. This work was supported by NIH grant CA-39949.

very poorly behaved.

We use simple geometric methods to obtain corrected Wald regions. The results of simulations indicate that these regions have good coverage and power properties.

With the exponential form of the relative risk function, the Wald regions seem, in general, to be well-behaved. However, Hauck and Donner [13] have shown the Wald test can, in some circumstances, behave poorly. We recommend that a correction term be computed even when using the exponential relative risk. In most instances, this term will be small and may be ignored.

## THE PROBLEM

The problem is best illustrated by means of an example. We analyzed data from a case-control study of endometrial cancer. These data are in Appendix III of Breslow and Day [7]. There are 63 cases, each matched with four controls. For analysis we chose two covariates, history of gallbladder disease and length of estrogen use. Due to missing data in duration of estrogen use, the analysis actually consisted of 57 risk sets, with 4 controls in 49 risk sets and 3 controls in the other 8.

We were interested in analyzing these data using the mixture model proposed by Duncan Thomas [21]. In this model

$$\rho(\beta,z) = \{1+\beta^* z\}^{1-\alpha}\{\exp(\beta^* z)\}^{\alpha} \quad ,$$

where $\alpha$ is a real number, the mixture parameter. When $\alpha = 1$ or 0, respectively, the exponential and additive relative risk functions are recovered. Figure 1, taken from Lustbader et al [15] shows the 95% likelihood based confidence regions for $\alpha = 1$, 0 and $\hat{\alpha}$, where $\hat{\alpha}$ is the m.$\ell$.$e$. of $\alpha$. It is clear that except when $\alpha = 1$ (exponential relative risk), the likelihood regions are far from elliptical indicating that the sample size is probably not large enough for the asymptotic properties of $\hat{\beta}$ to hold. Table 1 also clearly indicates that the Wald test for $\beta=0$ is always smaller than the likelihood ratio test. Further, except with the exponential form of the relative risk function, the Wald test fails to reject $\beta=0$ at the 0.05 level of significance. Note that the score test is invariant under $\alpha$ for this family of models [15] and has good power.

Figure 2 is a further illustration of the problems with the Wald test. In this figure, the Wald test given by $I^{\beta} \cdot \beta^2$ is plotted against values of $\beta$ for the binary covariate presence or absence of gallbladder disease. Here $I^{\beta}$ is the Fisher (expected) information matrix at $\beta$. Note that $\hat{\beta}$, the m.$\ell$.$e$., depends on the pattern of failures in the risk sets (i.e., on the covariate values of the individuals who are the cases), but $I^{\hat{\beta}}$ does not. Thus it is not clear whether a particular value of the Wald statistic is achieved in these data. Nevertheless, the figure illustrates that there are major problems with the Wald statistic. Particularly for the additive relative risk model, the Wald statistic barely achieves significance over a narrow range of $\beta$-values, indicating that in this data set it is unlikely, even with true $\beta$ large that any configuration of cases (failures) would lead to a significant test. Even for the exponential relative risk model, the Wald test approaches 0 as $\beta$ becomes large indicating that $(I^{\beta})^{-1}$, the asymptotic variance, grows faster than $\beta^2$.

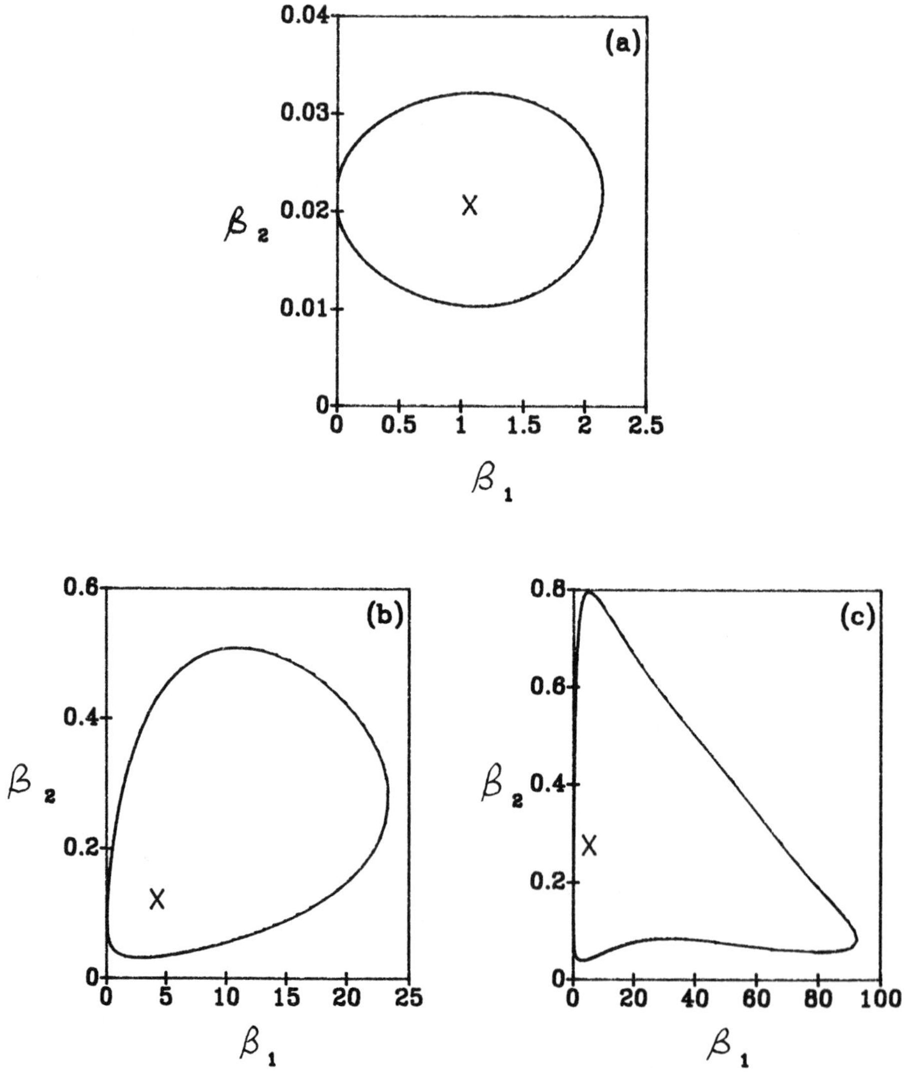


Figure 1. Likelihood contours defined by $\{\beta{:}2[\ell(\hat{\beta}) - \ell(\beta)] = 5.99\}$. The x indicates $\hat{\beta}$ for various values of $\alpha$ in the mixture model. Panels: (a) $\alpha$=1; (b) $\alpha$=0; (c) $\alpha = \hat{\alpha} = -0.034$.

TABLE 1

Test statistics using the mixture model

| $\alpha$ | L. Ratio Test | Wald Test |
|---|---|---|
| 1 (exponential model) | 33.7 | 27.9 |
| 0 (additive model) | 38.8 | 4.56 |
| $\hat{\alpha} = -0.034$ | 39.8 | 2.70 |

Score test = 36.4 for all $\alpha$.

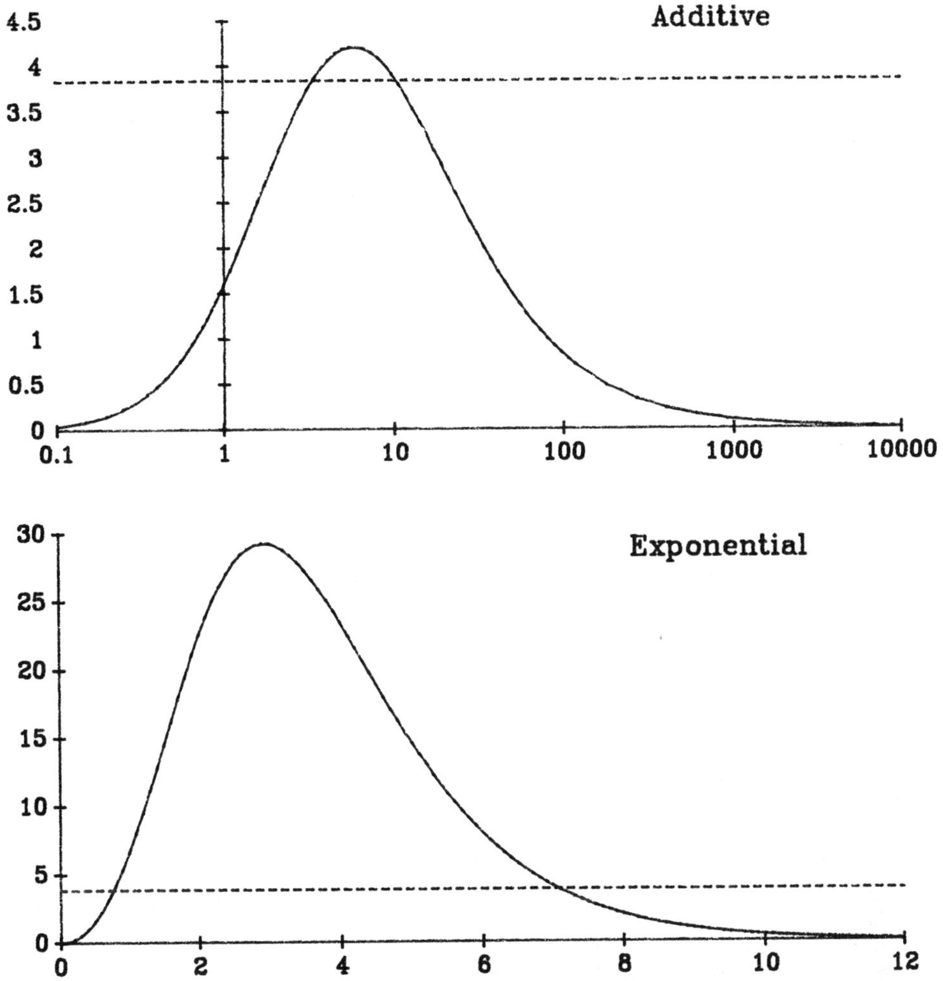


Figure 2. Plot of the Wald statistic for null hypothesis $\beta=0$ against $\beta$ for binary covariate (presence or absence of gallbladder disease) in data set from Appendix III of Breslow and Day [7]. The hatched horizontal line indicates a value of 3.84 for the Wald statistic. Upper panel: $\rho(\beta,z) = 1+\beta z$; lower panel: $\rho(\beta,z) = \exp(\beta z)$.

Note that the Wald statistic can be thought of as the square of the distance between two distributions. The "Wald distance" is equivalent to euclidean distance. In the next sections we introduce another distance function on finite dimensional spaces of distributions, and use this distance function to construct corrected Wald regions.

## SOME GEOMETRIC CONCEPTS

We need to introduce some concepts from differential geometry. Let $\gamma : [a,b] \to R^n$ be a $c^\infty$ curve, $[\gamma(s)]^* = (\gamma_1(s),\cdots,\gamma_n(s))$. Then, the tangent vector to $\gamma$ is given by $[\dot{\gamma}(s)]^* = (\dot{\gamma}_1(s),\cdots,\dot{\gamma}_n(s))$, and the arc length of the curve is $\mathrm{dis}_\gamma(a,b) = \int_a^b ([\dot{\gamma}(s)]^*[\dot{\gamma}(s)])^{\frac{1}{2}}\, ds$. Also, let us recall that it is always possible to reparametrize the curve so that $\mathrm{dis}_\gamma(a,b) = b-a$. Such a parametrization is called a parametrization by arc length and is characterized by

$$[\dot{\gamma}(s)]^*[\dot{\gamma}(s)] = |\dot{\gamma}(s)|^2 = 1 \quad .$$

Now, suppose that to each $\chi \in R^n$, there is attached in a $c^\infty$-manner, a symmetric positive-definite $n\times n$ matrix $\sum^\chi$. Suppose further that $\sum^\chi$ satisfies the following transformation law. Let $y(\chi)$ be a change of coordinates on $R^n$ (not necessarily linear), then $\sum^\chi = J_\chi^* \sum^{y(\chi)} J_\chi$, where $J_\chi$ is the Jacobian $(\partial y/\partial \chi)$. Then $\sum^\chi$ is called a tensor of type (0,2) and can be used to define a new metric on $R^n$ as follows.

First, the arc length of $\gamma$ is defined by

$$\mathrm{dis}_\gamma(a,b) = \int_a^b (\dot{\gamma}(s)^* \textstyle\sum^{\chi(s)} \dot{\gamma}(s))^{\frac{1}{2}}\, ds \quad .$$

Note that the arc length defined above is just a special case of this with $\sum^\chi$ the identity matrix. It is again possible to parametrize by arc length. In any case, let p,q be two points in $R^n$. Define the distance between p and q by

$$d(p,q) = \inf\{\text{lengths of differentiable curves from p to q}\} \quad .$$

If $\sum^\chi$ is the identity, we recover the usual metric; i.e., d(p,q) is just the length of the line segment joining p and q. More generally, under some regularity conditions, d(p,q) is realized as the arc length of a curve called a geodesic. We shall come back to this later after discussing exponential families.

## EXPONENTIAL FAMILIES

Consider an m-parameter exponential family of distributions with density functions

$$g(y,\theta) = \exp\{\theta^* y - a(\theta) + b(y)\}$$

where $\theta^* = (\theta_1, \theta_2, \cdots, \theta_m)$ is the vector of natural parameters. We note that $\dot{a}(\theta)$ is the expectation of Y and $\ddot{a}(\theta)$ is the covariance matrix of Y. We also note $\ddot{a}(\theta)$ is the Fisher information matrix which we denote by $\sum^{\theta}$. Note that $\sum^{\theta}$ is symmetric positive definite and that, under a change of parameters, it transforms like a tensor of type (0,2). Thus, $\sum^{\theta}$ can be used as in the last section to define a metric on $\theta$-space: given random variables $Y_1$ and $Y_2$ with parameters $\theta_1$ and $\theta_2$, the distance between $Y_1$ and $Y_2$ or $\theta_1$ and $\theta_2$, $d(\theta_1, \theta_2)$, is given by the infimum of the arc lengths of all curves in $\theta$-space joining $\theta_1$ and $\theta_2$.

Henceforth, $\Theta$ will denote the space of parameters $\theta$ equipped with the metric tensor $\sum^{\theta}$. Suppose that the model of interest is represented by a subfamily $\Omega$ of dimension d smoothly embedded in $\Theta$, $f: \Omega \to \Theta$, where f is 1-1. The triple $(\Theta, \Omega, f)$ is called a (m,d) exponential family. If $\Omega$ is an open subset of $R^d$ and f is affine, it is easy to see that $\Omega$ is the parameter space of a d-parameter exponential family. The likelihood function on $\Theta$ pulls back to $\Omega$ in the obvious way. Let $\ell$ be the log of the likelihood on $\Omega$. Then the Fisher information matrix at $\beta \varepsilon \Omega$, $I^{\beta}$, is given by

$$I^{\beta} = -E(\ddot{\ell}_{\beta}) = J_{\beta}^* \sum^{\theta(\beta)} J_{\beta} \quad ,$$

where $J_{\beta}$ is the Jacobian matrix $(\partial\theta/\partial\beta)$. Thus, the subfamily $\Omega$ inherits the geometry of $\Theta$ via $I^{\beta}$. The distance between two points (distributions) in $\Omega$ is defined in terms of $I^{\beta}$ as above.

Now, the Wald test of the hypothesis $\beta = \beta_0$ measures the distance (actually the square of the distance) between $\hat{\beta}$ and $\beta_0$ in an Euclidean metric: i.e., the one defined by the (constant) matrix $I^{\hat{\beta}}$. We would like to measure the distance in terms of the metric defined by $I^{\beta}$. One way of doing this is to find a variance stabilizing parametrization; i.e., a 1-1 transformation $\delta \mapsto \beta$ such that $I^{\delta} = J_{\delta}^* I^{\beta} J_{\delta} = \text{constant}$. In this new parametrization, the model $\Omega$ looks just like Euclidean space since the inner product matrix $I^{\delta}$ is constant, and the Wald test with $I^{\delta}$ measures the distance in terms of the desired metric. If $\Omega$ is one-dimensional, then such a variance-stabilizing transformation can always be found. However, if $\dim(\Omega) > 1$, then a very stringent condition must be satisfied for the existence of a variance-stabilizing transformation, and, in general, such a transformation cannot be found. In geometric terms, a variance-stabilizing transformation can be found if and only if a tensor constructed from $I^{\beta}$, the Riemannian curvature tensor, is identically zero.

Examples. (1) A multivariate normal family with unknown mean vector but known and constant covariance matrix has, by definition, a variance-stabilizing parametrization. This family is isometric to Euclidean space.

(2) Consider a univariate normal family with unknown mean and unknown variance. Then, it can be shown that this family has constant negative curvature [1]. A consequence is that the Riemannian curvature tensor is not zero and hence there does not exist any variance-stabilizing parametrization of this family. It is of interest to note that this family is isometric to the hyperbolic or the Lobachevski plane. In this geometry, Euclid's fifth postulate is violated: given a "straight line" and a point not on the "straight line", there exists an infinite number of "straight lines" passing through the point and not intersecting the given line.

(3) Consider a multinomial family $M(n,p_1,p_2,\cdots,p_k)$. Then this family has constant positive curvature, and, in fact, is isometric to an open subset of a sphere of radius $2n^{\frac{1}{2}}$ in $R^k$. This implies that there does not exist a variance-stabilizing parametrization for any model of dimension larger than one [17].

Although a variance-stabilizing parametrization cannot, in general, be found, another parametrization which is "almost variance-stabilizing" can be found. The first step to do this is to find the "straight-lines" or geodesics of the geometry defined by $I^\beta$. First, the Riemann-Christoffel symbols are defined by

$$\Gamma^i_{jk} = \sum_{s=1}^{d} \frac{1}{2}(\partial_j g_{ks} + \partial_k g_{js} - \partial_s g_{jk})\, g^{is} \quad ,$$

where $g_{ab}$ are the entries of $I^\beta$, $\partial_p$ denotes $\partial/\partial\beta_p$, and $g^{ab}$ are the entries of $(I^\beta)^{-1}$. A geodesic in the geometry defined by $I^\beta$ is then a curve $\beta(t) = (\beta_1(t),\cdots,\beta_d(t))$ which satisfies the system of quasi-linear differential equations (see [6] page 328)

$$\frac{d^2\beta_i}{dt^2} + \sum_{j,k} \Gamma^i_{jk}\frac{d\beta_j}{dt}\cdot\frac{d\beta_k}{dt} = 0;\ i=1,\cdots,d \quad .$$

For any point $\beta_0 \varepsilon \Omega$ and tangent vector v at $\beta_0$, the above system of differential equations has, for t small enough, a unique solution $\beta(t)$ such that $\beta(0) = \beta_0$ and $\dot\beta(0) = v$. That is, for any $\beta_0$ and any direction and velocity, there is a unique geodesic starting at $\beta_0$ in that direction and with the prescribed velocity. Under some regularity conditions, the geodesic can be defined for all t.

We now introduce a geodesic coordinate system based at $\beta_0$ as follows. The tangent space of $\Omega$ at $\beta_0$ can be identified with $R^d$. For any $v \varepsilon R^d$, let $\gamma_v(t)$ be the geodesic starting at $\beta_0$ and satisfying the condition

$\dot{\gamma}_v(0) = v$. Then, there exists an open neighborhood V of 0 in $\mathcal{R}^d$ and an open neighborhood W of $\beta_0$ in $\Omega$ such that the map Exp:$V \to W$ defined by $\text{Exp}(v) = \gamma_v(1)$ is a diffeomorphism. For historical reasons, the map Exp is called the exponential map, and defines the geodesic coordinate system at $\beta_0$. We then have the following proposition.

Proposition. Let $(u_1, \cdots, u_d)$ define a geodesic coordinate neighborhood centered at $\beta_0$: i.e., with $\beta_0 = (0, \cdots, 0)$. Let $h_{ij}$ be the entries of the Fisher information matrix in this coordinate system. Then $h_{ii} = c_i$, where $c_i$ is constant along $u_i$, and further $(\partial h_{ij}/\partial u_k)_{(0,\cdots,0)} = 0, \forall\, i,j,k$.

For a proof see reference [17]. The above proposition makes it clear in what sense the geodesic coordinate system is "almost variance-stabilizing". The diagonal entries of the Fisher information matrix are constant along coordinate curves, and the off diagonal entries are constant to first order at $\beta_0$. Further, in this parametrization, the "Wald distance" between $\beta_0$ and any other parameter $\beta$ is precisely the length of the geodesic joining $\beta_0$ and $\beta$, and hence corresponds to the definition of distance in Section 3.

Now if $\beta_0$ is the maximum likelihood estimate, an approximate confidence region for $\beta_0$ may be constructed as follows: First construct a Wald confidence region C in the tangent space to $\Omega$ at $\beta_0$, $C = \{v \in \mathcal{R}^d \mid v^* I^{\beta_0} v \leq c\}$, where c is some positive constant. Then confidence region R for $\beta_0$ is given by $R = \text{Exp}(C)$. This confidence region has the following interpretation. First, $\Omega$ is reparametrized in terms of a geodesic coordinate system centered at $\beta_0$, the Wald confidence region is computed in this parametrization, and then this region is re-expressed in terms of the original coordinates.

Of course, the above construction requires the solution of a system of quasi-linear differential equations. A Taylor series approximation to the mapping Exp is instructive. We obtain

$$[\text{Exp}(v)]_i \approx \beta_{0,i} + v_i - \frac{1}{2} \sum_{j,k} \Gamma^i_{jk}(\beta_0)\, v_j v_k \quad ,$$

where $\beta_{0,i}$ is the $i^{th}$ coordinate of $\beta_0$. Note that the first two terms in the Taylor series approximation yield the Wald confidence region in $\Omega$ in the original parametrization.

If $\Omega$ is one-dimensional, then there is a single Riemann-Christoffel symbol, which is given by

$$\Gamma = \frac{1}{2}(\partial g/\partial \beta) g^{-1} = \partial(\ln g^{\frac{1}{2}})/\partial \beta \quad ,$$

where the $1 \times 1$ Fisher information matrix is labelled g.

In order to construct confidence intervals for single parameters when $\Omega$ is multidimensional, we use the notion of profile likelihood ([8], page 88). Suppose, without loss of generality, that a confidence interval is to be constructed for $\beta_1$. Consider the profile likelihood for $\beta_1$; i.e., the function $\tilde{\ell}(\beta_1) = \ell(\beta_1, \hat{\beta}_{-1}(\beta_1))$, where $\hat{\beta}_{-1}(\beta_1) = (\hat{\beta}_2(\beta_1), \cdots, \hat{\beta}_d(\beta_1))$ is that value of $(\beta_2, \cdots, \beta_d)$ which maximizes the likelihood for a given value of $\beta_1$. The mapping $\beta_1 \mapsto (\beta_1, \hat{\beta}_{-1}(\beta_1))$ now becomes the (one-dimensional) model of interest, and a confidence interval can be constructed as above once g is computed. Note that, because of the tensorial property of the Fisher information, g is computed as follows,

$$g = J^*_{\beta_1} I^{\beta} J_{\beta_1} \quad ,$$

where $J_{\beta_1} = (1, \partial[\hat{\beta}_{-1}(\beta_1)]/_{\partial\beta_1})^*$ is the Jacobian of the mapping $\beta_1 \mapsto (\beta_1, \hat{\beta}_{-1}(\beta_1))$. An easy calculation shows that the vector $\partial(\hat{\beta}_{-1}(\beta_1))/_{\partial\beta_1}$ is given by $-A^{-1}w$, where A is the $(d-1) \times (d-1)$ matrix $(\partial^2\ell/\partial\beta_i\partial\beta_j)_{i,j>1}$, and w is the vector with entries $\partial^2\ell/\partial\beta_1\partial\beta_j$, with $j = 2, 3, \cdots, d$.

For more details of the geometry in this section see e.g., Boothby [6].

## MATCHED CASE-CONTROL AND SURVIVAL STUDIES AS CURVED EXPONENTIAL FAMILIES

The conditional likelihood of the logistic regression model for matched case-control studies is formally identical to the partial likelihood of the proportional hazards model for survival data. In either case, the appropriate likelihood function [21] is

$$L = \prod_{i=1}^{n} \frac{\rho(\beta, z_{i0})}{\sum_{j=0}^{m_i} \rho(\beta, z_{ij})}$$

where n is the number of risk sets, $\rho(\beta, z)$ is a generalized relative risk function, and $z_{ij}$ is a vector of covariates for the $j^{th}$ individual in risk set i, with j=0 corresponding to the case or the individual who failed. In this expression, $m_i$ is the number of controls for the $i^{th}$ case or the number of individuals whose survival time exceeds the $i^{th}$ failure time. For the usual logistic regression model and the original proportional hazards model proposed by Cox [9],

$$\rho(\beta, z) = \exp(\beta^* z) \quad .$$

The likelihood L can be viewed as arising from a multinominal sampling scheme as follows. Let $R_i; i=1,\cdots,n$ be multinominal random variables with sample size 1 and cell probabilities

$$p_{ij} = \frac{\rho(\beta, z_{ij})}{\sum_{\ell=0}^{m_i} \rho(\beta, z_{i\ell})} \quad ; \; j=1,\cdots,m_i; \; i=1,\cdots,n \quad .$$

Then L arises as the likelihood of this multinominal sampling scheme if the success for each $R_i$ is associated with $p_{i0}$. Now for each $R_i$, the natural parameter

$$\begin{aligned}\theta_i^*(\beta) &= \left(\ell n\left(\frac{p_{i1}}{p_{i0}}\right),\cdots,\ell n\left(\frac{p_{im_i}}{p_{i0}}\right)\right) \\ &= \left(\ell n\left(\frac{\rho(\beta,z_{i1})}{\rho(\beta,z_{i0})}\right),\cdots,\ell n\left(\frac{\rho(\beta,z_{im_i})}{\rho(\beta,z_{i0})}\right)\right) \quad .\end{aligned}$$

Let $\theta^* = (\theta_1^*,\cdots,\theta_n^*)$. Then the locus $\theta(\beta)$ defines, in general, a curved subfamily of the exponential family with natural parameter $\theta$ and covariance (Fisher information) matrix $\sum^{\theta}$, where $\sum^{\theta}$ is block diagonal with the $i^{th}$ block corresponding to the covariance matrix of $R_i$. In other words, $\Theta$-space is the Cartesian product of multinominal distributions with sample size 1. In matched case-control studies, the matrix $(\partial\theta/\partial\beta)^* \sum^{\theta(\beta)} (\partial\theta/\partial\beta)$ is the Fisher information matrix. This is not true for survival studies. However, this matrix has the appropriate asymptotic properties for inference and may be used to construct Wald-type confidence regions [19].

The Example Continued. Recall that in the endometrial cancer example with $\rho(\beta,z) = 1+\beta_1 z_1 + \beta_2 z_2$ discussed in the beginning of this paper, the null hypothesis $\beta=0$ is resoundingly rejected by the likelihood ratio test (Table 1), whereas it is not rejected by the Wald test at the 0.05 level of significance. Further, we saw that the likelihood based joint confidence region is far from elliptical. We applied the methods described in this paper to construct corrected confidence regions. The results are shown in Figure 3. The Adams-Gear algorithm was used to solve the system of quasi-linear equations. Further details can be found in [17,18]. Figure 3 shows that the corrected Wald region is in very good agreement with the likelihood based region. The first approximation to the corrected region, based on the Taylor expansion, is inadequate. Table 2 indicates that confidence intervals based on variance stabilization of the profile likelihood are in good agreement with likelihood based intervals. A $1-\varepsilon$ likelihood based interval for $\beta_1$ is defined by $\{\beta_1 | \tilde{\ell}(\hat{\beta}_1) - \tilde{\ell}(\beta_1) \leq \frac{1}{2}c\}$, where c denotes the upper ε point of the chi-square distribution on 1 degree of freedom.

With the exponential form of the relative risk function all methods yielded virtually identical results. See Table 2.

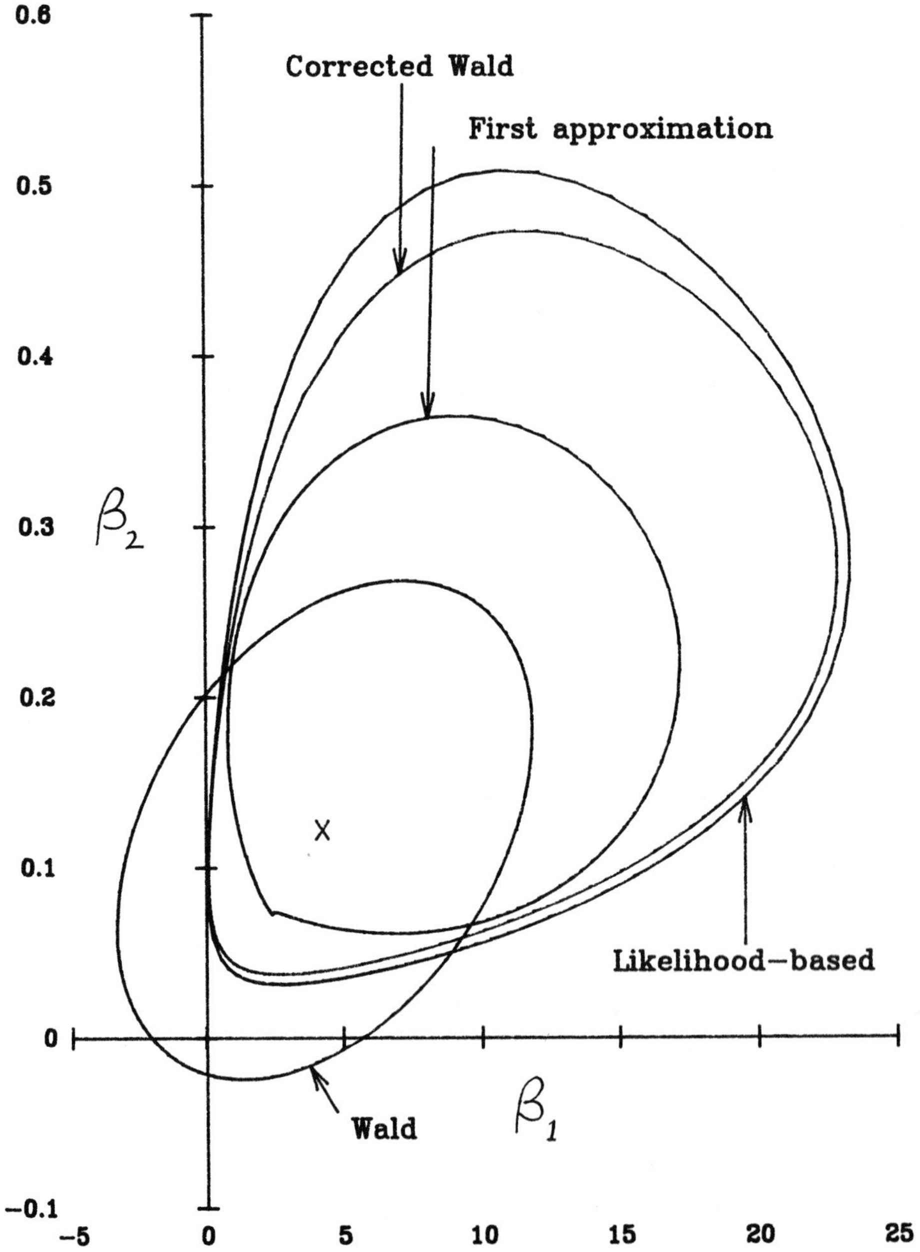


Figure 3. Ninety-five percent confidence regions with $\rho(\beta,z) = 1+\beta_1 z_1+\beta_2 z_2$. The 'x' denotes the maximum likelihood estimate.

TABLE 2

Results of analyses with $\rho(\beta,z) = 1 + \beta_1 z_1 + \beta_2 z_2$

m.ℓ.e. = $\hat{\beta} = (4.263,\ 0.122)$

Expected covariance matrix = $(I^{\hat{\beta}})^{-1} = \begin{matrix} 9.580 & 0.072 \\ 0.072 & 0.004 \end{matrix}$

95% confidence intervals for:

| | $\beta_1$ | | $\beta_2$ |
|---|---|---|---|
| Wald based | (-1.803, 10.329) | ; | (0.005, 0.239) |
| Likelihood based | ( 0.502, 16.67 ) | ; | (0.042, 0.374) |
| Variance stabilizing | ( 0.545, 16.11 ) | ; | (0.047, 0.347) |

Results of analyses with $\rho(\beta,z) = \exp(\beta_1 z_1 + \beta_2 z_2)$

m.ℓ.e. = $\hat{\beta} = (1.06302;\ 0.02070)$

Expected covariance matrix = $I(\hat{\beta})^{-1} = \begin{matrix} 0.18696 & 0.000016 \\ 0.000016 & 0.000019 \end{matrix}$

95% confidence intervals for:

| | $\beta_1$ | | $\beta_2$ |
|---|---|---|---|
| Wald based | (0.216, 1.911) | ; | (0.012, 0.029) |
| Likelihood based | (0.206, 1.918) | ; | (0.012, 0.030) |
| Variance stabilizing | (0.196, 1.928) | ; | (0.012, 0.030) |

## SOME SIMULATION RESULTS

We carried out simulations to investigate how well the various confidence regions did in the analysis of survival data. The details of the simulations can be found in Moolgavkar and Venzon [18]. First we briefly present the results with a single continuous covariate, and with $\rho(\beta,z) = 1 + \beta z$. Three different distributions were chosen for the covariate z: uniform, lognormal and normal. The total number of individuals in the simulation, here labelled n, was 50, 100, or 200. We also ran a simulation with n=200 and 50% censoring. We report here the two extreme cases, viz., the simulations with n=50 and n=200. The results with n=100 and n=200 with 50% censoring were quite similar.

The results of the simulations are presented in Tables 3-5, and are based on 1000 replicates for each value of n and each covariate distribution. For each of the three methods of constructing the 95% confidence interval, the coverage probability and the power, defined as the probability of excluding zero, were computed. As can be seen from the tables, the Wald region behaved poorly with respect to both coverage and power. This was especially noticeable with a normal covariate distribution. We note from the tables that the variance-stabilizing or corrected Wald region did about as well as the likelihood based region. The likelihood based intervals tended to be somewhat shorter than the corrected Wald intervals. However, none of the corrected Wald intervals were infinite, whereas a substantial number of likelihood based intervals were, especially with censoring.

TABLE 3

n=50

| | COVERAGE | | | POWER | | |
|---|---|---|---|---|---|---|
| $\underline{\beta}$ | Wald | ℓ-based | var. stab | Wald | ℓ-based | var. stab |
| | | | Covariate distribution: Uniform | | | |
| 0 | 0.914 | 0.956 | 0.960 | 0.086 | 0.044 | 0.040 |
| 2.5 | 0.896 | 0.958 | 0.950 | 0 | 0.658 | 0.640 |
| 5.0 | 0.892 | 0.961 | 0.957 | 0 | 0.900 | 0.906 |
| 10.0 | 0.874 | 0.977 | 0.966 | 0 | 0.985 | 0.987 |
| | | | Covariate distribution: Lognormal | | | |
| 0 | 0.919 | 0.954 | 0.946 | 0.081 | 0.046 | 0.054 |
| 2.5 | 0.928 | 0.932 | 0.936 | 0 | 0.498 | 0.438 |
| 5.0 | 0.916 | 0.944 | 0.954 | 0 | 0.828 | 0.802 |
| 10.0 | 0.904 | 0.960 | 0.956 | 0 | 0.972 | 0.968 |
| | | | Covariate distribution: Normal | | | |
| 0 | 0.898 | 0.958 | 0.966 | 0.102 | 0.042 | 0.034 |
| 2.5 | 0.880 | 0.962 | 0.949 | 0.002 | 0.418 | 0.404 |
| 5.0 | 0.850 | 0.968 | 0.960 | 0.002 | 0.655 | 0.651 |
| 10.0 | 0.780 | 0.966 | 0.978 | 0 | 0.821 | 0.830 |

We also did simulations with two covariates, one of them discrete and the other continuous. The results are presented in Table 5, and indicate once again that the Wald interval does poorly, but the other two methods yield similar and good results.

## DISCUSSION

For a large class of models of interest, the Wald test could be poorly behaved and yield misleading conclusions. While we did not encounter any problems with the Wald test when using the exponential form of the relative risk, the potential for problems does exist as pointed out in the beginning of this paper. We suggest that, when non-exponential forms of the relative risk function are used, either likelihood-based or corrected Wald confidence intervals be constructed as described in this paper. When the relative risk is exponential, we suggest the following procedure. First, the 95% Wald confidence inter-

TABLE 4

n=200

| | COVERAGE | | | POWER | | |
|---|---|---|---|---|---|---|
| $\underline{\beta}$ | Wald | $\ell$-based | var. stab | Wald | $\ell$-based | var. stab |
| | | | Covariate distribution: | Uniform | | |
| 0 | 0.949 | 0.958 | 0.970 | 0.051 | 0.042 | 0.030 |
| 2.5 | 0.933 | 0.945 | 0.962 | 0.963 | 0.995 | 0.998 |
| 5.0 | 0.928 | 0.945 | 0.952 | 0.991 | 1 | 1 |
| 10.0 | 0.914 | 0.950 | 0.960 | 0.762 | 1 | 1 |
| | | | Covariate distribution: | Lognormal | | |
| 0 | 0.947 | 0.960 | 0.966 | 0.053 | 0.040 | 0.034 |
| 2.5 | 0.948 | 0.955 | 0.958 | 0.545 | 0.849 | 0.844 |
| 5.0 | 0.953 | 0.958 | 0.958 | 0.959 | 0.995 | 0.996 |
| 10.0 | 0.942 | 0.956 | 0.964 | 1 | 1 | 1 |
| | | | Covariate distribution: | Normal | | |
| 0 | 0.934 | 0.955 | 0.952 | 0.066 | 0.045 | 0.048 |
| 2.5 | 0.905 | 0.946 | 0.946 | 0 | 0.864 | 0.872 |
| 5.0 | 0.891 | 0.948 | 0.949 | 0 | 0.970 | 0.980 |
| 10.0 | 0.855 | 0.963 | 0.956 | 0 | 0.997 | 1 |

TABLE 5

n=100

$\beta_2$=5 (Binary covariate, p=0.5)

Covariate distribution of $z_1$: Lognormal

Confidence intervals for $\beta_1$

| | COVERAGE | | | POWER | | |
|---|---|---|---|---|---|---|
| $\beta_1$ | Wald | $\ell$-based | var. stab | Wald | $\ell$-based | var. stab |
| 5.0 | 0.924 | 0.962 | 0.968 | 0 | 0.794 | 0.740 |
| 10.0 | 0.948 | 0.944 | 0.952 | 0 | 0.978 | 0.976 |

Confidence intervals for $\beta_2$

| | COVERAGE | | | POWER | | |
|---|---|---|---|---|---|---|
| $\beta_1$ | Wald | $\ell$-based | var. stab | Wald | $\ell$-based | var. stab |
| 5.0 | 0.940 | 0.960 | 0.948 | 0.812 | 1 | 1 |
| 10.0 | 0.944 | 0.964 | 0.948 | 0.438 | 1 | 1 |

val say $(\hat{\beta}-a, \hat{\beta}+a)$ should be constructed. If $2\{\ell(\hat{\beta}) - \ell(\hat{\beta}-a)\}$ and $2\{\ell(\hat{\beta}) - \ell(\hat{\beta}+a)\}$ are not approximately equal and equal to 3.84 then the likelihood-based or corrected Wald interval should be used. Alternatively, the Taylor series approximation to the corrected Wald confidence interval given in an earlier section should be routinely computed. If the first order correction to the Wald interval is large, then a likelihood-based or corrected Wald interval should be computed.

The methods presented in this paper stand at the confluence of several ideas in statistics. Geometric techniques, while not new to statistics, are only now being systematically investigated following a seminal paper by Efron [10]. Efron considered one dimensional hypotheses in that paper, defined the "statistical curvature" of such hypotheses, and studied the efficiency properties of statistics in terms of the curvature. Linear models in exponential families have zero curvature in Efron's definition. Thus, models with exponential relative risk have zero curvature (are uncurved) in the definition of Efron. In 1982, Amari [1] defined an entire one parameter family of geometries on finite dimensional families of distributions via what he called $\alpha$-connections. The Efron or exponential connection was one member of this family, viz. the one corresponding to $\alpha=1$. In this paper, we have used what is called the Riemannian connection, which corresponds to $\alpha=0$ in Amari's construction. We note that neither the exponential nor the additive relative risk model is uncurved in this geometry. We also point out here that the "statistical curvature" of Efron corresponds loosely to the notion of geodesic curvature or second fundamental form in differential geometry.

In his 1982 paper, Amari [1] shows how to construct a one-parameter family of consistent and first-order efficient estimators, the $\alpha$-estimators, of which the maximum likelihood estimator corresponding to $\alpha = -1$, is an example. The properties of the other $\alpha$-estimators need to be investigated for case-control and survival studies.

The work in this paper is also related to the vast literature on parameter transformations, and we direct the reader to the papers by Hougaard [14] and Sprott [20] as examples.

A discussion of curvature in the case of non-linear least-squares and its effect on confidence regions can be found in papers by Beale [5], Bates and Watts [3,4], and Hamilton, Bates and Watts [12]. We caution the reader, however, that the word "curvature" is used loosely in the statistical literature and often does not correspond to what would be called curvature by geometers.

The $\alpha$-geometries defined by Amari are based on the expected information matrix. More recently Barndorff-Nielsen [2] has constructed a parallel family of geometries, which he calls observed conditional geometries, based on the observed information matrix. In particular, he uses this construction to obtain a formula for the conditional distribution of the maximum likelihood estimator (conditioned on an appropriate ancillary). This formula can be used to derive confidence intervals for the m.ℓ.e. . Finally, McCullagh [16] has suggested yet another method for the construction of confidence regions based on the notion of local sufficiency. Both these methods need to be investigated in the context of case-control and survival studies.

## REFERENCES

[1] S.I. AMARI. Differential geometry of curved exponential families - curvatures and information loss. Ann. Statist., 10, (1982), pp. 357-385.

[2] O.E. BARNDORFF-NIELSEN. Differential and integral geometry in statistical inference. Research Reports No. 106, Department of Theoretical Statistics, University of Aarhus, (1984).

[3] D.M. BATES and D.G. WATTS. Relative curvature measures of nonlinearity. J.R. Statist. Soc. B, 42, (1980), pp. 1-25.

[4] D.M. BATES and D.G. WATTS. Parameter transformations for improved approximate confidence regions in nonlinear least squares. Ann. Statist., 9, (1981), pp. 1152-1167.

[5] E.M.L. BEALE. Confidence regions in non-linear estimation. J.R. Statist. Soc. B, 22, (1960), pp. 41-76.

[6] W.M. BOOTHBY. An Introduction to Differentiable Manifolds and Riemannian Geometry. Academic Press, New York, (1975).

[7] N.E. BRESLOW and N.E. DAY. Statistical Methods in Cancer Research. Vol. 1 - The Analysis of Case-Control Studies, International Agency for Research on Cancer, Lyon, (1980).

[8] D.R. COX. Analysis of Binary Data. Methuen, London, (1970).

[9] D.R. COX. Regression models and life tables (with discussion). J.R. Statist. Soc. B, 34, (1972), pp. 187-220.

[10] B. EFRON. Defining the curvature of a statistical problem (with applications to second order efficiency). Ann. Statist., 3, (1975), pp. 1189-1242.

[11] V.M. GUERRERO and R.A. JOHNSON. Use of the Box-Cox transformation with binary response models. Biometrika, 69, (1982), pp. 309-314.

[12] D.C. HAMILTON, D.G. WATTS and D.M. BATES. Accounting for intrinsic nonlinearity in nonlinear regression parameter inference regions. Ann. Statist., 10, (1982), pp. 386-393.

[13] W.W. HAUCK and A. DONNER. Wald's test as applied to hypotheses in logit analysis. JASA, 72, (1977), pp. 851-853.

[14] P. HOUGAARD. Parametrizations of non-linear models. J.R. Statist. Soc. B, 44, (1982), pp. 244-252.

[15] E.D. LUSTBADER, S.H. MOOLGAVKAR and D.J. VENZON. Tests of the null hypothesis in case-control studies. Biometrics, 40, (1984), pp. 1017-1024.

[16] P. McCULLAGH. Local sufficiency. Biometrika, 71, (1984), pp. 233-244.

[17] S.H. MOOLGAVKAR and D.J. VENZON. Confidence regions in curved exponential families: application to matched case-control and survival studies with general relative risk function (submitted), (1985a).

[18] S.H. MOOLGAVKAR and D.J. VENZON. Confidence regions for case-control and survival studies: a simulation study (in preparation), (1985b).

[19] R.L. PRENTICE and S.G. SELF. Asymptotic distribution theory for Cox-type regression models with general relative risk form. Ann. Statist, 11, (1983), pp. 804-813.

[20] D.A. SPROTT. Normal likelihoods and their relation to large sample theory of estimation. Biometrika, 60, (1973), pp. 457-466.

[21] D.C. THOMAS. General relative risk models for survival time and matched case-control analysis. Biometrics, 37, (1981), pp. 673-686.

# Relative Risk Regression Diagnostics

*Edward D. Lustbader*

Abstract. This paper suggests a number of techniques for detecting unusual observations that arise in matched case-control studies analyzed under the conditional likelihood of the logistic model and in survival studies analyzed under the partial likelihood of the proportional hazards model. Most of the suggested techniques are extensions of linear regression diagnostics. Appropriate generalizations of residuals, leverage, and influence are provided. In addition, diagnostic statistics related to hypothesis testing are discussed. Matched case-control and survival data present unique problems in interpretation of diagnostics due to the grouping of individuals in risk sets. In survival studies, the appearance of one individual in many risk sets presents another grouping problem for diagnostics. Reasonable approximations to minimize the computational burden of grouping are proposed. The diagnostics are illustrated using the data collected on patients enrolled in the Stanford Heart Transplant Program.

## INTRODUCTION

Observations which appear to stand apart from the bulk of the data are a constant concern of data analysts. Detection of these points might lead to their outright rejection, but this need not be the case. Detection might reveal new information that had gone unnoticed or suggest a weakness in the model or in the data.

In this paper, the data of interest arise in matched case-control studies analyzed under the conditional likelihood of the logistic model and in survival studies analyzed under the partial likelihood of the proportional hazards model. These likelihoods are formally

---

Fox Chase Cancer Center, 7701 Burholme Avenue, Philadelphia, PA, 19111. This work was supported by USPHS grants CA-06551, RR-05539, CA-39949 and CA-06927 from the National Institutes of Health and by an appropriation from the Commonwealth of Pennsylvania.

identical in that both are products over the probabilities of an individual failing or being a case. In turn, the probabilities are related to exposures or other risk factors, through the function which expresses relative risk. While the theoretical and computational aspects related to estimation and hypothesis testing under these likelihoods have received considerable attention, checking model adequacy is still relatively rudimentary. This paper suggests a number of detection techniques for unusual observations that might be of assistance in improving the fitted models.

Most of the suggested techniques are extensions of well-developed methods in linear regression diagnostics. Only the fundamental ideas of linear regression diagnostics such as residuals, leverage and influence are considered here because the intent is to provide a framework in which diagnostics for relative risk models can be derived. Many of the other linear regression ideas can also be extended. In fact, most of the diagnostics discussed here can be applied to a broad range of problems in non-linear regression.

Section 2 sets the notation for the likelihood of a general statistical model. In particular, it is shown that the maximum likelihood estimate (MLE) can be viewed as the solution of a weighted least squares problem under very general conditions. This least squares view allows for reasonable definitions of a "design" matrix and a "residuals" vector in this general setting. The design matrix and residual vector then serve as the basis for extending linear regression diagnostics to non-linear regression models. These definitions are given in section 3 along with the ANOVA decomposition of the weighted least squares problem. The explained sum of squares in this ANOVA is particularly interesting because it is identical to the score test of a global null hypothesis. This provides the basis for diagnostics related to hypothesis testing. Section 4 reviews the basic formulae of linear regression diagnostics and sets the stage for the application of these methods to relative risk regression models. In section 5, it is shown that the relative risk regression likelihoods can be viewed as a member of the exponential family, thereby providing the link with the weighted least squares problem that serves as the basis for diagnostic statistics.

Relative risk regression models present unique features for interpretation of diagnostics due to the grouping of individuals in risk sets. A risk set is a case along with its matched controls or a failure and all those whose survival time is greater than the given failure time. In addition, in survival analysis, the appearance of one individual in many risk sets presents yet another grouping problem for diagnostics. The major problem associated with grouping is in computation because the formulae require matrix inversion. However, a reasonable approximation is provided.

## 2. GENERAL LIKELIHOOD CONSIDERATIONS

Consider a statistical model with log likelihood $L(\eta)$ where $\eta$ is an m-dimensional vector. Assume enough regularity so that

$$E\left(\frac{\partial L}{\partial \eta}\right) = 0 \tag{1}$$

and

$$-E\left(\frac{\partial^2 L}{\partial \eta^2}\right) = i(\eta) \tag{2}$$

where $i(\eta)$ is positive definite. The parameter of interest is the vector $\gamma$ which is related to $\eta$ by a function $\eta(\gamma)$ in such a way that the matrix

$$J(\gamma) = \partial\eta/\partial\gamma \tag{3}$$

has full rank. The score vector for $\gamma$ is

$$U(\gamma) = \partial L/\partial\gamma = J(\gamma)^t \, \partial L/\partial\eta \tag{4}$$

Define "pseudo-observations" y by

$$y = \eta(\gamma) + [i(\eta)]^{-1} \, \partial L/\partial\eta$$

thereby permitting (4) to be written as

$$U(\gamma) = J(\gamma)^t \, i(\eta) \, \{y - \eta(\gamma)\} \tag{5}$$

The reason for the pseudo-observations is that $U(\gamma) = 0$ has the algebraic form of the normal equations of a weighted least squares problem because from (1) and (2)

$$E(y) = \eta(\gamma)$$

and

$$\mathrm{COV}(y) = [i(\eta)]^{-1}$$

In the most general settings this least squares view is tainted because y depends on $\gamma$. However, for the exponential family, we can let y be the actual observations. In minimal form, the log likelihood with natural parameter $\theta$ is proportional to

$$L(\theta) = y^t\theta - a(\theta) \tag{6}$$

so that

$$\partial L/\partial\theta = y - \partial a/\partial\theta$$

where $a(\theta)$ is some function of $\theta$.

If we parameterize with $\eta = E(y) = \partial a/\partial\theta$, then

$$\partial L/\partial\eta = (\partial\theta/\partial\eta)\{y-\eta\} \tag{7}$$

and $$\partial^2 L/\partial\eta^2 = -(\partial\theta/\partial\eta) + (y-\eta)\, \partial^2\theta/\partial\eta^2$$

Thus $i(\eta) = \partial\theta/\partial\eta$ and (7) becomes

$$\partial L/\partial\eta = i(\eta)\{y-\eta\}$$

Since $COV(y) = -\partial^2 L/\partial\theta^2 = \partial\eta/\partial\theta = [i(\eta)]^{-1}$, we have adopted a parameterization that makes $U(\gamma) = 0$ a legitimate least squares problem.

## 3. ANOVA DECOMPOSITION

For some fixed vector $\gamma_o$, make the first order approximation

$$\eta(\gamma) \approx \eta(\gamma_o) + J(\gamma_o)(\gamma-\gamma_o) \tag{8}$$

Define

$$X(\gamma) = [i(\eta)]^{\frac{1}{2}} J(\gamma) \tag{9}$$

$$e(\gamma) = [i(\eta)]^{\frac{1}{2}}\{y-\eta(\gamma)\} \tag{10}$$

and denote quantities evaluated at the MLE by circumflexes. Since $U(\hat{\gamma}) = 0$, substitution of (8) into (5) yields

$$\hat{\gamma} - \gamma_o \approx (X_o^t X_o)^{-1} X_o^t e_o \tag{11}$$

where $X_o = X(\gamma_o)$ and $e_o = e(\gamma_o)$.

### 3.1 SCORE TEST

Expression (11) has two very intuitive interpretations. First, one recognizes immediately that (11) is the solution of a linear regression of $e_o$ on $X_o$ in which the estimated parameter is $\hat{\gamma}-\gamma_o$. In this regression, $e_o$ contains the "observations" y which have been centered and scaled (based on $\gamma_o$). Therefore, the ANOVA decomposition of this regression has a total sum of squares of

$$e_o^t e_o = [y - E_o(y)]^t [COV_o(y)]^{-1} [y - E_o(y)] \tag{12}$$

where $E_o(y) = \eta(\gamma_o) = \eta_o$ and $COV_o(y) = [i(\eta_o)]^{-1}$. In the exponential family, or any other model in which y contains actual observations, (12) is the usual notion of a goodness-of-fit test under the hypothesis $\gamma=\gamma_o$.

The explained sum of squares for the ANOVA decomposition is

$$e_o^t X_o (X_o^t X_o)^{-1} X_o^t e_o \tag{13}$$

However, using (5), (9) and (10),

$$e_o^t X_o = U_o = (\partial L/\partial \gamma)_{\gamma=\gamma_o} \tag{14}$$

and from (2), (3) and (9)

$$X_o^t X_o = V_o = -E(\partial^2 L/\partial \gamma^2)_{\gamma=\gamma_o} \tag{15}$$

Hence, the explained sum of squares (13) is the score test for the hypothesis $\gamma=\gamma_o$, and (11) permits the score test to be viewed as the approximate length of the vector $\hat{\gamma}-\gamma_o$ in the metric of $V_o$.

Comment. The score test for $\gamma=\gamma_o$ is always the explained sum of squares of the regression of $e_o$ on $X_o$ even if (8) is a poor approximation. However, the view of the score test as the approximate length of $\hat{\gamma}-\gamma_o$ does require that (8) be reasonably good.

## 3.2 ITERATIVE ALGORITHM

The second interpretation of (11) depends on a slightly different linear regression. If we define

$$w = X\gamma + e \tag{16}$$

then (11) becomes

$$\hat{\gamma} \approx (X_o^t X_o)^{-1} X_o^t w_o \tag{17}$$

If (17) were an equality, the left-hand side would be a one-step approximation to the MLE of $\gamma$ starting from an initial guess of $\gamma_o$. Thus, (17) provides an iterative algorithm by simply redefining $\gamma_o$ to be the estimate of the MLE at iteration j. At convergence

$$\hat{\gamma} = (\hat{X}^t \hat{X})^{-1} \hat{X}^t w \tag{18}$$

where $\hat{X} = X(\hat{\gamma})$.

It is suggested from (16) and (18) that $e(\hat{\gamma})$ is an appropriate definition of residuals at the MLE for general models. Further, $X(\hat{\gamma})$ can be viewed as a "design" matrix. This view permits many familiar ideas from linear regression diagnostics to be extended to estimation in general settings.

Comment. A second justification for defining $e(\gamma)$ as the residuals for general models follows from noting that (5) is identical to $\partial e(\gamma)^t e(\gamma)/\partial\gamma$. That is, $U(\gamma) = 0$ minimizes the residual sum of squares. Further, $e(\gamma)$ has zero mean and unit covariance matrix.

## 4. LINEAR REGRESSION DIAGNOSTICS

Since diagnostics for general models are extensions of the linear regression diagnostics, it is worthwhile briefly reviewing the measures of adequacy for the usual linear model $Y = D\beta + u$ with $COV(u) = \sigma^2 I$. Examining the estimated residuals, $\hat{u}_k = Y_k - d_k\hat{\beta}$ (with $\hat{\beta} = (D^tD)^{-1}D^tY$ and $d_k$ = row k of D) is standard practice. However, it is well known that small values of $u_k$ can be associated with extreme values of $d_k$, whereas large values of $u_k$ are typically associated with extreme values of $Y_k$. Hence, a display of residuals should be considered along with a display of the position of $d_k$ in the covariate space. This latter display is most often based on the leverage values obtained from the diagonal elements, $h_{kk}$, of

$$H(D) = D(D^tD)^{-1}D^t \tag{19}$$

Residuals and leverage are valuable tools for detecting extreme points but provide little information as to the influence that these points have on parameter estimates. Influence assessment is most frequently accomplished by determining the change in $\hat{\beta}$ upon deletion of observation k. Let this quantity be denoted by $\Delta_k$. It can be shown [1] that

$$\Delta_k = (D^tD)^{-1}\, d_k^t\, \hat{u}_k/(1 - h_{kk}) \tag{20}$$

One immediate difficulty with $\Delta_k$ is that the elements of the vector need to be judged with respect to some measure of scale. There is considerable flexibility in the choice of scale, but those choices that use $\hat{\sigma}^2$ may have to accommodate the change in scale on deletion of observation k as well.

When the hypothesis $\beta=0$ is of interest, the change in the explained sum of squares upon deletion of each observation provides a direct measure of the impact of the observation on the null hypothesis. On deletion of observation k the change in explained sum of squares is [1]

$$Y_k^2 - \hat{u}_k^2/(1 - h_{kk}) \tag{21}$$

Comment: As can be seen from (18), the concepts of residuals, leverage and influence are easily defined in general settings. However, from (9) it should be noted that the "design matrix" $X(\gamma)$ depends on both the measure of scale, $i(\eta)$, and the Jacobian $J(\gamma) = \partial\eta/\partial\gamma$. Hence, unless $\eta$ is linear in $\gamma$, deletion diagnostics such as $\Delta_k$ will have to take account of both the change in $i(\eta)$ and $J(\gamma)$. If $\gamma=\gamma_o$ in (11) is an interesting null value, expression (21) provides an exact method of computing the change in the score test for this hypothesis. When the score test is a reasonable approximation to the distance between $\hat{\gamma}$ and $\gamma_o$, one could also interpret the score test diagnostic as an influence measure.

## 5. RELATIVE RISK REGRESSION

Relative risk regression models, of which the logistic regression model and the proportional hazards model are examples, are being increasingly used in the analysis of cohort studies. In the original formulation of these models, the relative risk $\rho(\beta,z)$ was "multiplicative," i.e. $\rho(\beta,z) = \exp(\beta^t z)$ where z is a vector of covariates and $\beta$ is a vector of parameters to be estimated. More recently, there has been interest in models with an additive form for relative risk, $\rho(\beta,z) = 1 + \beta^t z$, and in mixtures of additive and multiplicative components.

### 5.1 LIKELIHOOD

The conditional likelihood of the logistic model for matched case-control studies is formally identical to the partial likelihood of the proportional hazards for survival data. In either case, the appropriate log-likelihood function is [2]

$$L(\beta) = \sum_{q=1}^{n} \log \frac{\rho(\beta,z_{qo})}{\sum_{j=0}^{m_q} \rho(\beta, z_{qj})} = \sum_{q=1}^{n} \log \frac{\rho(\beta, z_{qo})}{S_q} \tag{22}$$

where $z_{qj}$ are the covariates for the $j^{th}$ individual in risk set q with j=0 corresponding to the case or the individual who failed. In this expression, $m_q$ is the number of controls for the $q^{th}$ case or the number of individuals whose survival time exceeds the $q^{th}$ failure time. Together these $(m_q+1)$ individuals constitute risk set q and n is the total number of risk sets.

In order to develop diagnostic statistics, it is best to define a parameterization that would permit the general considerations of section 2 to be applied. In particular, viewing $L(\beta)$ as a member of the exponential family is desirable. In this regard, define for individual j in risk set q

$$P_{qj} = \frac{\rho(\beta,z_{qj})}{S_q} \qquad j = 0, 1, \ldots, m_q \tag{23}$$

Now, in risk set q, an "observation" is made in the sense that every individual is identified as a case (failure) or not. Let $y_{qo} = 1$ and $y_{qj} = 0$ for $j = 1, \ldots, m_q$. Suppose that these observations are the realizations of independent Poisson random variables whose expectation is $P_{qj}$. The likelihood of these $(m_q+1)$ observations is

$$P_{qo} \exp(-P_{qo}) \sum_{j=1}^{m_q} \exp(-P_{qj}) = P_{qo} \exp(-\sum_{j=0}^{m_q} P_{qj})$$

$$= P_{qo} \exp(-1)$$

Thus, the log-likelihood of these Poisson observations is (apart from a constant) identical to (22).

## 5.2 DIAGNOSTIC STATISTICS

The Poisson view of $L(\beta)$ permits the straightforward extension of linear regression diagnostics to relative risk regression models. For the exponential family, the parameterization which permits (5) to be a legitimate least squares problem is $\eta = E(y)$. Specifically, for relative risk regression models,

$$\eta_{qj} = E(y_{qj}) = P_{qj}$$

$$\text{and} \qquad i(\eta) = [\mathrm{COV}(y)]^{-1} = \mathrm{diag}(1/P_{qj}) \ . \qquad (24)$$

With this parameterization, (23) provides the transformation between $\eta$ and the parameters of interest, $\beta$, so that the rows of $J(\beta) = \partial\eta/\partial\beta$ are given by

$$\partial P_{qj}/\partial\beta = P_{qj}(\kappa_{qj} - \bar{\kappa}_q)$$

$$\text{with} \qquad \kappa_{qj} = \partial \log \rho(\beta, z_{qj})/\partial\beta$$

$$\text{and} \qquad \bar{\kappa}_q = \sum_{j=0}^{m_q} P_{qj}\,\kappa_{qj} \ .$$

When $\rho(\beta, z) = \exp(\beta^t z)$, the rows of $J(\beta)$ are simply the covariates centered on the (weighted) risk set mean. The "design" matrix $X(\beta)$ is, from (9), just the scaled values of $J(\beta)$ so that with $\rho(\beta, z) = \exp(\beta^t z)$ relative risk regression models have a design matrix which has much in common with linear regression. In particular, the rows of $X(\beta)$ are given by

$$X_{qj} = \sqrt{P_{qj}}\,(\kappa_{qj} - \bar{\kappa}_q) \qquad (25)$$

The elements of the residuals for relative risk regression models are, from (10),

$$e_{qj} = \frac{y_{qj} - P_{qj}}{\sqrt{P_{qj}}} = \begin{cases} (1 - P_{qj})/\sqrt{P_{qj}} & j=0 \\ -\sqrt{P_{qj}} & j=1, \ldots, m_q \end{cases} \tag{26}$$

All quantities necessary for assessing the residuals, leverage and influence for relative risk regression models are now defined. However, relative risk regression departs from linear regression in terms of interpretation of these quantities because of the grouping of individuals in risk sets. In addition, for survival analysis, a separate row in $X(\beta)$ and an element in the residual vector $e(\beta)$ is computed for each person in each risk set. But it is quite common for one particular individual to appear in many risk sets, implying a second need for diagnostics based on more than one observation.

Comment: It is possible to view $L(\beta)$ as the sum of the log-likelihoods of the realization of a multinomial random variable with sample size 1 and cell probabilities $(P_{qo}, \ldots, P_{qm_q})$. In this view, the success is associated with $P_{qo}$. There are computational problems imposed by this view due to $i(\eta)$ being a block diagonal matrix. Furthermore, the diagnostics related to risk sets are identical for both the Poisson and multinomial views [3].

For survival studies, $i(\eta)$ in (24) has to condition on the risk sets to formally satisfy (2). Prentice and Self [4] have shown that (24) has the appropriate asymptotic properties and is satisfactory for use in computing diagnostics.

## 6. DIAGNOSTICS FOR RISK SET AND INDIVIDUALS

### 6.1 RESIDUALS

As is obvious from (25), cases always have positive residuals, whereas the controls have negative residuals. Hence, the sign is not informative, and it is sensible to define risk set 'residuals' as

$$r_q^2 = \sum_{j=0}^{m_q} e_{qj}^2 = (1 - P_{qo})/P_{qo}$$

As mentioned in the comment of section 3.2, maximizing $L(\beta)$ is identical to minimizing $\Sigma r_q^2$. It is also possible to view $r_q^2$ as the squared difference between the observed and expected values divided by the variance for a Bernoulli random variable with parameter $P_{qo}$ (and an observed value 1). However, when $m_q$ varies among risk sets (as in survival analysis), the interpretation of $r_q^2$ is difficult because, in general, the magnitude of $P_{qo}$ is highly dependent on $m_q$. For example, at $\beta = 0$, $P_{qo} = 1/m_q$ and $r_q^2 = m_q - 1$. Thus, risk set residuals are likely to be more valuable in case-control studies where the $m_q$ generally are about the same in each risk set.

Residuals for individuals in case-control studies are given by $e_{qj}^2$, but in survival analysis one needs to sum the appropriate $e_{qj}^2$ from each risk set in which the individual is at risk. For individuals who are ultimately censored, this sum will be identical to summing the probability of failure for that individual over all risk sets. For individuals with uncensored failure times, the residual will equal the sum of the probabilities of failure in the risk sets prior to the actual failure time plus $e_{ko}^2 - (1 - P_{ko})^2/P_{ko}$ for the contribution to the residual for failing in risk set k.

## 6.2 LEVERAGE

For an individual in a case-control study, the leverage is computed from the diagonal elements of $H(X) = X(\beta)\,[X(\beta)^t\, X(\beta)]^{-1}\, X(\beta)^t$. This is easily accomplished from (25). For risk sets, the equivalent concept is to isolate the elements of H(X) corresponding to all the individuals in the risk set. Then the leverage is $1 - \det\,(I - H_k)$ where $H_k$ is the appropriate submatrix corresponding to risk set k and I is the identity matrix. In survival analysis, the same calculation would yield the leverage for an individual with $H_k$ corresponding to the elements of H(X) contributed by that individual to all the risk sets in which he appears.

## 6.3 INFLUENCE

The calculation of $\Delta_k$ in (20) follows directly from (25) and (26) for any individual in a case-control study. For risk sets, a computational problem arises by the need to replace $1/(1-h_{kk})$ by $(I-H_k)^{-1}$. However, because H(X) is a projection matrix

$$(I-H_k)^{-1} = I + \sum_{j=1}^{\infty} (H_k)^j$$

and the first few terms of the series can be used as approximation to the inverse. For case-control and survival studies, experience has shown that $I + H_k$ is a suitable approximation.

As mentioned above, $\Delta_k$ is difficult to interpret without a measure of scale, and in case-control and survival studies the appropriate choice is not obvious. Asymptotically, $COV(\hat{\beta}) = (\hat{X}^t\hat{X})^{-1}$, but distance measures in this metric could be seriously misleading with general relative risk functions. Also $COV(\hat{\beta})$ changes on eliminating an observation.

## 6.4 HYPOTHESIS TESTING

As mentioned in the comment of section 4, (21) is an exact expression for the change in score test; and for relative risk functions of the form $\rho(\beta, z) = \rho(\beta^t z)$, the change in score will not depend on $\rho$. For risk sets or individuals in survival analysis, it will again be necessary to replace $1/(1-h_{kk})$ in (21) with $(I-H_k)^{-1}$ for which $I+H_k$ is recommended for computational simplicity [5].

For influence assessment, it is typical to focus attention on one parameter (or, in general, a subset of parameters) from the $\beta$ vector and treat the remainder as nuisance parameters. When $\Delta_k$ is used as an influence statistic, it is customary to ignore the covariance among parameters and simply scale the element of interest using the diagonal element of $(\hat{X}^t\hat{X})^{-1}$ [18]. With the change in score, associated with a subset of parameters, additional computations are needed. Let $\beta$ be partitioned into $\beta = [\beta_1^t, \beta_2^t]$ with $\beta_1$ the nuisance parameter. Compute $X_{qj}$ in (24) with $\beta_1 = \hat{\beta}_1$ and $\beta_2 = \beta_{20}$ where $\beta_{20}$ is a fixed vector and $\hat{\beta}_1$ is the MLE of $\beta_1$ when $\beta_2 = \beta_{20}$. When $\rho(\beta, z) = \rho(\beta^t z)$, usually $\beta_{20} = 0$ and $\hat{\beta}_1$ is the unrestricted MLE with fewer parameters in the model. Let $X_1$ be the matrix whose rows are given by the elements of $X_{qj}$ that involve derivatives with respect to $\beta_1$ and $X_2$ be the matrix whose rows are the remaining elements of $X_{qj}$. Then, the score statistic for $\beta_2 = \beta_{20}$ is given by

$$y_{2\cdot1}^t \, X_{2\cdot1} \, (X_{2\cdot1}^t X_{2\cdot1})^{-1} \, X_{2\cdot1}^t y_{2\cdot1} \qquad (27)$$

where $y_{2\cdot1}=Qy$, $X_{2\cdot1}= QX_2$ and $Q = I - X_1(X_1^t X_1)^{-1}X_1^t$.

In linear regression, this is the expression for the explained sum of squares from regressing y on $X_2$ after adjusting for $X_1$. An expression like (21) can yield the change in the score test on deletion of an individual or risk set where again an "(I+H)" approximation is recommended. The $e_{qj}$ needed for this calculation are given by (26) with $y_{2\cdot1}$ used in place of y and $P_{qj}$ is evaluated at $\beta_1 = \hat{\beta}_1$ and $\beta_2 = \beta_{20}$.

## 7. ADDITIONAL DIAGNOSTICS

For the proportional hazards model with background failure rate $\lambda(t)$, the quantities

$$\varepsilon_j = \Lambda(t_j)\ \rho(\tilde{\beta}, z_j)$$

are distributed as (possibly censored) exponential with parameter 1 where

$$\Lambda(t_j) = \int_0^{t_j} \lambda_0(u)du$$

with $t_j$ the survival time for the $j^{th}$ individual and $\tilde{\beta}$ the "true" parameter value. When $\beta$ is estimated from the partial likelihood and $\lambda_0(t)$ is unknown, the distribution of the $\varepsilon_j$ is less certain. Nonetheless, Crowley and Hu [6] suggested that the hazard rate estimate proposal of Breslow [7]

$$\hat{\Lambda}(t_j) = \sum_{q=1}^{n_j} 1/\hat{S}_q$$

be used so that

$$\hat{\varepsilon}_j = \hat{\Lambda}(t_j)\ \rho(\hat{\beta}, z_j) \tag{28}$$

In this expression, $n_j$ is the number of risk sets that individual j is at risk. It is clear that $\varepsilon_j$ is the sum of the appropriate $P_{qj}$ associated with one individual which in turn is the sum of the appropriate $e_{qj}^2$ for a censored individual. Hence, $\hat{\varepsilon}_j$ is identical to the definition of residuals proposed earlier for censored individuals. For uncensored individuals, $\hat{\varepsilon}_j$ will differ from the sum of the appropriate $e_{qj}^2$ as discussed in section 6.1.

Kay [8] used the exponentiality argument to recommend plotting the ordered values of $\hat{\varepsilon}_j$ against expected values of order statistics in a unit exponential sample. This is equivalent to constructing the plot recommended by Nelson [9]. Lagakos [10] considered the case of n=3 and one covariate and found that a complete enumeration of all possible orderings of the data did not yield $\hat{\varepsilon}_j$ that behaved like a sample from a unit exponential distribution. Arjas [11] showed that the unit exponential distribution for $\hat{\varepsilon}_j$ would hold for subset of individuals which was substantially smaller than the total number of individuals. Crowley and Storer [12] used displays of $\hat{\varepsilon}_j$ against potential covariates to assess whether a covariate has been omitted. Other techniques not based on $\hat{\varepsilon}_j$ for goodness-of-fit are given by Anderson [13], Schoenfeld [14], Wei [15] and their references.

Thomas [16] proposed a novel variation on residuals and goodness-of-fit when there is a specific quantitative exposure variable. The idea is to pick a threshold value of exposure, T, thereby defining a binary indicator $\delta_{qj} = 0$ or 1 depending on whether the exposure for individual j exceeds T or not for each member of risk set q. Then

$$\delta_{qo} - \sum_{j=0}^{m_q} \delta_{qj} \hat{P}_{qj} \tag{29}$$

is an equivalent of $y-\eta$ for individuals whose exposure is less than T. Thomas sums this "residual" over all the risk sets, scales the sum and plots the standardized value versus T. Thomas proposed this display for assessing whether the correct form for $\rho$ has been specified. However, it can be used more generally as a residual.

There have been alternative proposals to calculate deletion diagnostics for $\beta$, although none have resolved the aforementioned difficulties associated with a measure of scale. Storer and Crowley [17] propose augmenting the $\beta$ vector with additional parameters associated with indicator variables which delineate the included and excluded observations. Cain and Lange [18] introduce a matrix which includes a parameter that permits $\hat{\beta}$ to be expanded in such a way that the equivalent of $\Delta_k$ is obtained as a limit when the parameter approaches zero. In this regard, Cain and Lange extended the suggestion of Pregibon [19] for deriving diagnostics related to logistic regression.

8. An example. The Stanford Heart Transplant Program has received considerable attention from statisticians and serves as a good data set for illustration because of its familiarity. There are 103 patients of which 69 received a transplant. Upon entry, the age and calendar time for each patient was recorded as well as a binary indicator of previous heart surgery. For those transplanted, a measure of HLA matching (or, more accurately, mismatching) between donor and recipient is available. Only the 65 transplanted patients with full covariate information will be considered. Of these, 41 had died at the time of analysis [8].

Our analysis will be based on the likelihood (22) with $p(\rho, z) = \exp(\beta^t z)$. Four covariates--age, mismatch score, prior surgery, and waiting time--will be considered. Table 1 contains the parameter estimates, the standard errors from $(\hat{X}^t\hat{X})^{-1}$, and the t-ratios. Assessment of efficacy of transplantation is ultimately the goal of the analysis of these data, and, for this purpose, waiting time is a crucial covariate. One would hope that waiting time would not be predictive of post-transplant survival time. The t-test for waiting time, however, is equivocal. A likelihood ratio test and the score test (27) of the significance of waiting time treating the other three parameters as nuisance parameters were 2.6 and 2.8 respectively. Thus, the waiting time covariate merits further attention.

TABLE 1

Parameter estimates from fitting the proportional hazards models with exponential risk function to post transplant survival of patients in the Stanford Heart Transplant Program.

| | Age | Mismatch score | Prior surgery | Log waiting time |
|---|---|---|---|---|
| $\hat{\beta}$ | .049 | .491 | -.807 | -.213 |
| s.e. $(\hat{\beta})$ | .022 | .297 | .485 | .128 |
| ratio | 2.30 | 1.65 | 1.66 | -1.66 |

Figure 1 displays ranked survival time versus log waiting time and does not reveal any obvious association. In Figure 2, the residuals computed from (28) from the model which includes the three nuisance parameters (age, mismatch, prior surgery) are compared to theoretical distribution of exponential with parameter 1. This display indicates some departure from expectation, but the display of residuals versus

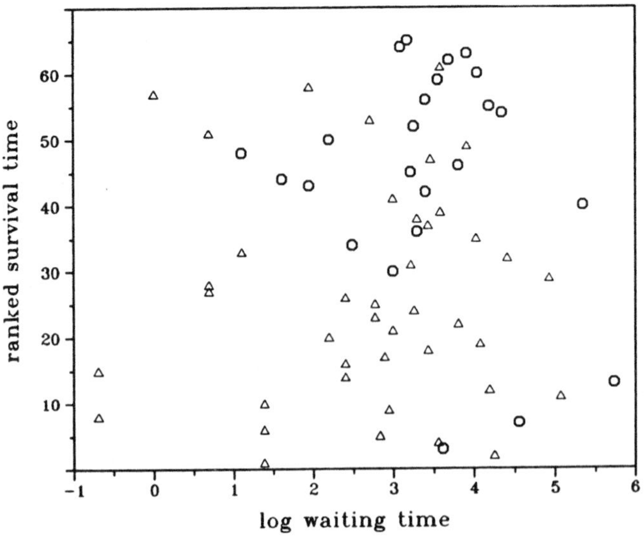


Figure 1. Rank of post-transplant survival versus the log of the waiting time for a transplant. A "delta" indicates an uncensored time whereas an "oval" indicates a censored time.

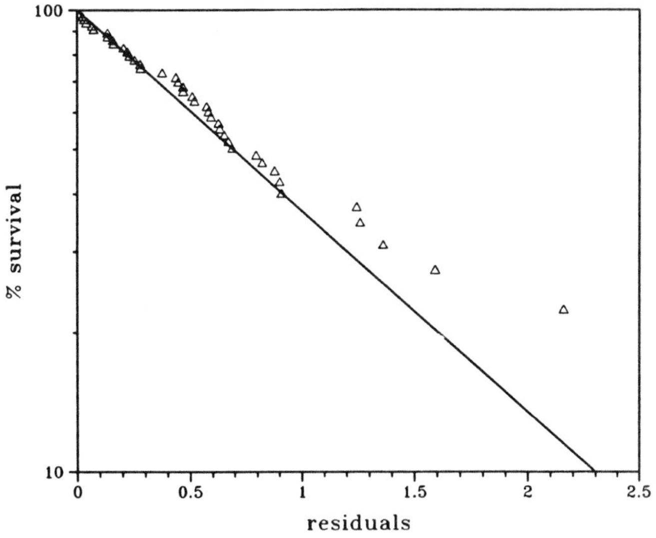


Figure 2. Residuals defined by (28) from a model which includes age, mismatch score, and prior surgery as covariates. The solid line is the theoretical curve with slope -1.

log waiting time in Figure 3 fails to suggest that waiting time covariate would be a useful addition. The Thomas residuals (29), on the other hand, seem to favor the addition of log waiting time by indicating a trend in Figure 4.

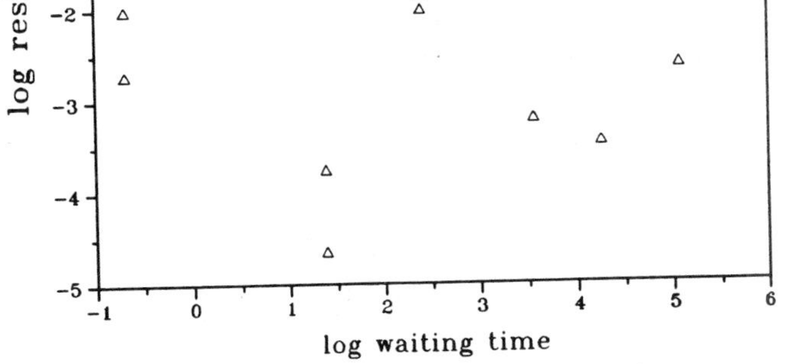

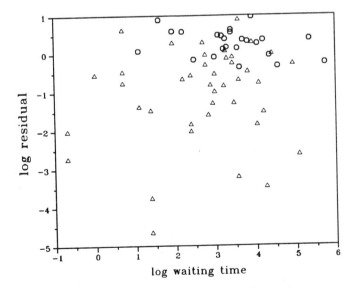

Figure 3. The log of the residuals defined by (26) accumulated for each individual versus the log of the waiting time for a transplant.

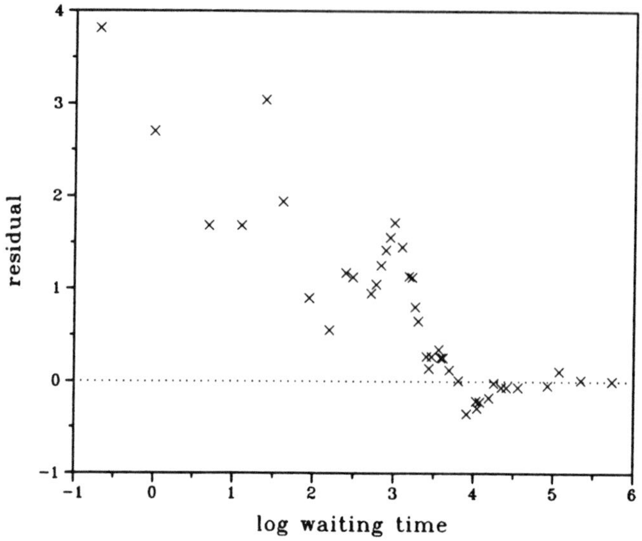


Figure 4. The residuals defined by (29) versus log waiting time.

The change in the $\hat{\beta}$ associated with waiting time upon deletion of each individual is given in Figure 5. Note from Table 1 that all the changes are apparently less than one standard error when the measure of scale is not adjusted by the deleted individual. The most revealing

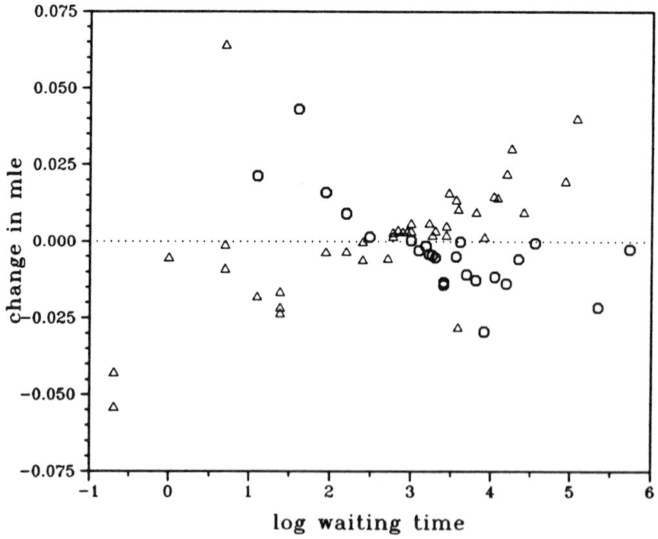


Figure 5. The approximate change in the mle of log waiting time upon deletion of each individual.

display is the score test upon deletion of each individual given in Figure 6. The pattern of change is identical to Figure 5, but the ordinate in Figure 6 has a clear interpretation. Deletion of either of two individuals is sufficient to make waiting time a significant covariate.

Terminating an analysis at this point is an unsatisfactory ending. However, the role of regression diagnostics is about complete. The tools provide insights that suggest further thought. For example, one might want to consider whether we have specified the correct form of the relative risk function, the proper functional form of the variables, the correct scale of measurements, or entertain the possibility of heterogeneity in the data. The list of consequences can be arbitrarily long.

Concluding that waiting time is not significant would be justified, but the conclusion is very unstable in the sense that minor alterations in the data would lead one to include waiting time in the model. This represents the most that one can reasonably expect from diagnostics. The methods are primarily descriptive, computationally convenient, lend themselves to graphical displays, and reveal "unusual" observations in a manner that can't be seen any other way.

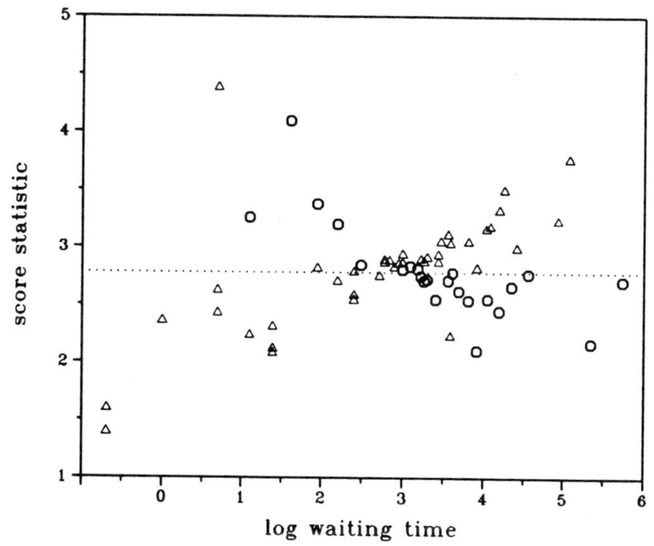


Figure 6. The approximate value of the score test for the significance of waiting time upon the deletion of each individual. The dotted line indicates the score test with no deletions.

## REFERENCES

[1] R.D. Cook and S. Weisberg, Residuals and influence in regression. Chapman, New York, 1982.

[2] D.C. Thomas, General relative risk models for survival time and matched case-control analysis. Biometrics 37 (1981), pp. 673-686.

[3] S.H. Moolgavkar, E.D. Lustbader, and D. Venzon, A geometric approach to non-linear regression diagnostics with application to matched case-control studies. Ann. Stat. 12 (1984), pp. 816-826.

[4] R.L. Prentice and S.G. Self, Asymptotic distribution theory for Cox-type regression models with general relative risk form. Ann. Stat. 11 (1983), pp. 804-813.

[5] E.D. Lustbader and S.H. Moolgavkar, A diagnostic statistic for the score test. J. Am. Stat. Assoc. 80 (1985), pp. 375-379.

[6] J. Crowley and M. Hu, Covariance analysis of heart transplant survival data. J. Am. Stat. Assoc 72 (1977), pp. 27-36.

[7] N. E. Breslow, Covariance analysis of censored survival data. Biometrics 30 (1974), pp. 89-99.

[8] R. Kay, Proportional hazard regression models and the analysis of censored survival data. Appl. Stat. 26 (1977), pp. 227-237.

[9] W. Nelson, Hazard plotting for incomplete failure data. J. Qual. Tech. 1 (1969), pp. 27-52.

[10] S.W. Lagakos, The graphical evaluation of explanatory variables in proportional hazards regression models. Biometrika 68 (1981), pp. 93-98.

[11] E. Arjas, On graphical methods for assessing goodness-of-fit in Cox's proportional hazards model. Unpublished manuscript (1985).

[12] J. Crowley and B.E. Storer, Contribution to the discussion on the paper by Aitkin, Laird and Francis. J. Am. Stat. Assoc. 78 (1983), pp. 277-281.

[13] P.K. Anderson, Testing goodness-of-fit of Cox's regression and life model. Biometrics 38 (1982), pp. 67-77.

[14] D. Schoenfeld, Chi-squared goodness-of-fit tests for the proportional hazards regression model. Biometrika 67 (1980), pp. 145-153.

[15] L.J. Wei, Testing goodness-of-fit for proportional hazards model with censored observations. J. Am. Stat. Assoc. 79 (1984), pp. 649-652.

[16] D.C. Thomas, Nonparametric estimation and tests of fit for dose-response relations. Biometrics 39 (1983), pp. 257-267.

[17] B.E. Storer and J. Crowley, A diagnostic for Cox regression and general conditional likelihoods. J. Am. Stat. Assoc. 87 (1985), pp. 139-147.

[18] K.C. Cain and N.T. Lange, Approximate case influence for the proportional hazards regression model with censored data. Biometrics 40 (1984), pp. 493-499.

[19] D. Pregibon, Logistic regression diagnostics. Ann. Stat. 9 (1981), pp. 705-724.

# An Example of Dependencies Among Variables in a Conditional Logistic Regression

*C. E. Davis, J. E. Hyde, S. I. Bangdiwala, and J. J. Nelson*

Abstract. Conditional logistic regression analysis of a matched case-control study investigating the relation between apolipoprotein A-1 and coronary death, adjusting for known risk factors, identified collinearity among the variables. Application of the Belsley, Kuh and Welsch diagnostic method to the X matrix, the pooled covariance matrix and the information matrix at the solution, indicates that the dependency would have been detected only by considering the information matrix at the solution.

## INTRODUCTION

The detrimental effects of collinearity in multiple linear regression are well known. Since the problem is one of ill-conditioning or near singularity of a matrix which must be inverted, it is clear that similar problems are likely to occur in non-linear regression situations such as logistic regression. A set of widely used procedures for detecting collinearity in linear regression has been described by Belsley, Kuh and Welsch (1). (For simplicity, these methods will henceforth be referred to as BKW.) To our knowledge, no such similar guidelines have been developed for logistic regression problems although other types of regression diagnostics have been and are being developed. See for example Lustbader (3) and Pregibon (4). In this paper, we describe a conditional logistic regression in a matched case-control data analysis in which dependency was detected, and describe our ad hoc attempts to adapt BKW methods to detect the cause of the problem. We make no claim that our analysis will allow for generalization to other settings since this is a case example.

---

From the Department of Biostatistics, University of North Carolina.
This research was supported by contract N01-HV-1-2243-L from the National Heart, Lung and Blood Institute.

## DESCRIPTION OF STUDY AND PRELIMINARY RESULTS

It has been established for many years that elevated blood cholesterol is a risk factor for the development of coronary heart disease; i.e. persons with high blood cholesterol have a high probability of developing heart disease. Cholesterol molecules are transported in the blood stream while attached to protein molecules called lipoproteins. It has now been further established that the concentration of cholesterol attached to the low density lipoprotein (LDL-C) is associated with the development of atherosclerosis, while there is an inverse association with the development of atherosclerosis for the high density lipoprotein cholesterol (HDL-C). Of late, the protein components of the various lipoproteins, the apolipoproteins, have been increasingly under investigation. It is hypothesized that some of the apolipoproteins will be associated with the increased development of atherosclerosis, while others may be negatively associated. In particular, apolipoprotein A-1 is predicted to be associated with decreased development of heart disease, since it is known to be correlated with HDL-C.

In 1972, the National Heart, Lung and Blood Institute established the Lipid Research Clinics Program, a series of collaborative epidemiologic and clinical studies of lipids, lipoproteins and heart disease. As part of this program, over 60,000 persons were screened for cholesterol. A subset of 8825 adults have been followed for mortality. During the initial screening apolipoproteins were not measured, but samples of serum were frozen and stored for later use. In 1979, it was decided to study the relation between apolipoproteins and heart disease using these frozen samples. Since it would have been prohibitively expensive to thaw all 8825 samples and measure the apolipoproteins, a case-control study was designed. All persons who were free of coronary disease at the time of the initial screening were considered eligible for the study. Cases were the 40 persons who had died due to coronary heart disease between the initial screen and July 1, 1979. Controls were matched on age group (30-39, 40-59, 60+), sex, race, screening clinic and length of storage of frozen sample ( to within 30 days of the case's storage time). Since the matching on age is rather coarse, it might be useful to include age in the regression function of the analysis. In this report we chosen not to since the data set is quite small. The design called for two controls per case; however, only one case could be matched for 10 of the cases. In the analysis described here, only the data from the 25 males and their corresponding 45 controls will be used. All of the statistical tests employed in this type of analysis are based on large sample results. With this small set of data the interpretation of any probability statements based on asymptotic results should be made with caution.

Table 1 contains a comparison of the established risk factors and apolipoprotein A-1 for the cases and controls.

Table 1: Mean Risk Factor Levels for Cases and Controls

| Variable | Controls(n=45) | Cases(n=25) |
|---|---|---|
| LDL-C (mg./dl.) | 148.4 | 166.8 |
| HDL-C (mg./dl.) | 42.8 | 39.2 |
| Systolic BP (mm. Hg) | 130.2 | 142.2 |
| Cigarettes (# daily) | 7.6 | 8.8 |
| Apolipoprotein A-1 (mg./dl.) | 94.8 | 80.4 |

As expected, the cases had higher LDL-C, higher systolic blood pressure, lower HDL-C and smoked more cigarettes than the controls. Note that the cases also have lower A-1 levels than the controls. A matched logistic regression model (2) was fitted for A-1 giving a coefficient of b=-0.041 with a standard error of 0.017. It thus appears that apolipoprotein A-1 is negatively associated with coronary death.

A question of interest is whether A-1 is related to coronary death after adjustment for the standard known risk factors. To investigate this, two matched logistic models were fitted, as reported in Table 2.

Table 2: Conditional Logistic Regression Coefficients

| | Model 1 | | Model 2 | |
|---|---|---|---|---|
| Variable | b | se(b) | b | se(b) |
| LDL-cholesterol | 0.023 | 0.009 | 0.118 | 0.055 |
| HDL-cholesterol | -0.089 | 0.038 | -0.154 | 0.099 |
| Systolic BP | 0.055 | 0.023 | 0.216 | 0.102 |
| Cigarettes | -0.020 | 0.027 | -0.076 | 0.054 |
| Apolipoprotein A-1 | | | -0.232 | 0.108 |

In the first model, the variables were LDL-C, HDL-C, systolic blood pressure, and number of cigarettes smoked daily. With the exception of cigarette smoking, where no significant effect was found, the results were as expected. When apolipoprotein A-1 was added to the model, the coefficients for all variables and the corresponding standard errors changed dramatically. This seemed to be a clear case of excessive dependency among the variables. However, a simple inspection of the correlations of the variables did not reveal any obvious source of collinearity. We then set out to look at the performance of the BKW methods on various versions of the 'X' matrix.

## BELSLEY, KUH AND WELSCH PROCEDURE

Before reporting the results, a brief description of the BKW methods will be presented.

1. Scale the X matrix to have unit column length.

2. Obtain the singular value decomposition of X, and from this calculate:

a. the condition indices (the square root of the ratio of the largest eigenvalue to the other eigenvalues) and

b. the matrix of variance decomposition proportions.

3. Determine the number and relative strengths of the near dependencies by the condition indices exceeding some chosen threshold such as 10, 15 or 30.

4. Determine the involvement of the variates in the near dependencies. For this step, some threshold variance decomposition proportion must be chosen. (BKW suggest 0.5).

In investigating the possible dependencies in the apolipoprotein data set we have applied the BKW method to three different matrices: 1) the X matrix of variables as though a linear regression were being performed, 2) the covariance matrix formed by combining the within matched samples covariance matrices and, 3) the information matrix at the solution. Since the conditional logistic regression is a form of nonlinear regression, application of the diagnostic procedures to the matrices 1) and 2) as described above may not detect dependencies that could adversely effect the estimates. On the other hand, if diagnostics applied to these matrices do identify problems successfully, application would be easier. In the next section we describe the results of these applications of the BKW method.

## REGRESSION DIAGNOSTICS

A. Linear Diagnostics The easiest and most straightforward approach to investigating possible dependencies in logistic regression is to use the diagnostics for linear regression; i.e. to use the X matrix in exactly the manner proposed by BKW. This can be justified because the logistic function can sometimes be approximated by a linear function and because the computations for the BKW method are available in statistical packages such as SAS. Table 3 gives the condition indices and "pi" matrix for the variance decomposition for the model with four variables (LDL-C, HDL-C, SBP and smoking) and with five variables (add apo A-1). Note that in each of these models an intercept term has been included (i.e. adjusted out) and that the method does not distinguish between cases and controls. Neither model indicates a possible problem with dependency. For example, in the four variable model, the largest index is 1.6, while in the five variable model, the largest condition index is also 1.6.

B. Within Matches Covariance Matrix. The above analysis with linear diagnostics ignores the matching used in the study design and in the matched logistic regression. In the matched logistic regression, case-control comparisons are made within matches and then combined across the matches to obtain the overall estimates. It should be the case that diagnostics applied to the covariance matrix computed taking into account the matching would provide more information about possible dependency problems in the matched logistic regression than the same diagnostics ignoring the matching.

Table 3: BKW Analysis of Linear Regression

Model 1

| Eigen-value | Condi-tion index | Variance Proportion for LDL | SBP | HDL | Cig. |
|---|---|---|---|---|---|
| 1.46 | 1.00 | 0.15 | 0.20 | 0.07 | 0.19 |
| 1.13 | 1.14 | 0.27 | 0.03 | 0.47 | 0.01 |
| 0.85 | 1.31 | 0.03 | 0.44 | 0.03 | 0.55 |
| 0.56 | 1.61 | 0.55 | 0.33 | 0.44 | 0.25 |

Model 2

| Eigen-value | Condi-tion index | Variance Proportion for A-1 | LDL | SBP | HDL | Cig. |
|---|---|---|---|---|---|---|
| 1.51 | 1.00 | 0.07 | 0.10 | 0.14 | 0.09 | 0.19 |
| 1.18 | 1.13 | 0.17 | 0.30 | 0.02 | 0.26 | 0.00 |
| 1.03 | 1.21 | 0.30 | 0.02 | 0.32 | 0.13 | 0.10 |
| 0.72 | 1.45 | 0.46 | 0.05 | 0.17 | 0.06 | 0.51 |
| 0.56 | 1.64 | 0.01 | 0.53 | 0.35 | 0.46 | 0.19 |

To investigate this, estimates of the covariance matrix were computed within the matched triplets or pairs and then combined to obtain an overall estimate of the covariance matrix. This matrix was then converted to a correlation matrix and the condition indices and variance decomposition matrix computed. The computations were done in SAS using PROC MATRIX (see the listing in the Appendix). Table 4 gives the results for both the four and five variable models. There is no indication from these statistics that any excessive dependency exists.

Table 4: BKW Diagnostics on Pooled Correlation Matrix

Model 1

| Eigen-value | Condi-tion index | Variance Proportion for HDL | LDL | Cig. | SBP |
|---|---|---|---|---|---|
| 1.30 | 1.00 | 0.02 | 0.31 | 0.21 | 0.15 |
| 1.14 | 1.06 | 0.40 | 0.06 | 0.10 | 0.25 |
| 0.93 | 1.47 | 0.33 | 0.09 | 0.36 | 0.22 |
| 0.61 | 1.82 | 0.25 | 0.54 | 0.33 | 0.38 |

Model 2

| Eigen-value | Condi-tion index | Variance Proportion for A-1 | HDL | LDL | Cig. | SBP |
|---|---|---|---|---|---|---|
| 1.53 | 1.00 | 0.21 | 0.22 | 0.00 | 0.00 | 0.08 |
| 1.30 | 1.09 | 0.00 | 0.00 | 0.36 | 0.24 | 0.08 |
| 0.98 | 1.25 | 0.03 | 0.03 | 0.02 | 0.40 | 0.44 |
| 0.63 | 1.56 | 0.22 | 0.01 | 0.55 | 0.30 | 0.33 |
| 0.56 | 1.66 | 0.53 | 0.74 | 0.06 | 0.06 | 0.06 |

C. Diagnostics at the Solution. The fitting of a model such as the matched logistic model can be thought of as iteratively re-weighted least squares fitting. In particular, if $b_{mle}$ is the maximum likelihood estimate, and b is a provisional estimate in a neighborhood of $b_{mle}$, then the final iteration to the solution is given by

$$\Delta = b_{mle} - b = (X'WX)^{-1}X'Wr$$

where W is a matrix of weights which depend on $b_{mle}$, and r is a vector of "residuals" defined so that X'Wr is the gradient of the likelihood at $b_{mle}$.

For the conditional logistic model, the matrix W is not diagonal, so there is not an exact parallel with weighted least squares. However, one can consider a transformed problem where $X^* = \sqrt{W}X$ and $r^* = \sqrt{W}r$,
then

$$\Delta = (X^{*\prime}X^*)^{-1} \quad X^*r^*$$

The variance of $\Delta$ for this linear model is proportional to

$$(X^{*\prime}X^*)^{-1} = (X'WX)^{-1}$$

which is the inverse of the information matrix for the original maximum likelihood problem.

Although the transformed linear model involves not only weighting observations, but combining them; the variables retain their original identity. Thus, one can intuitively apply one's experience with linear models by considering the information matrix to represent a covariance matrix of variables suitably "weighted" to correspond to the maximum likelihood problem.

Diagnostics applied to the information matrix (or its inverse ) will provide information about the possible ill-conditioning of X'WX and hence information about the possible pathological dependencies at the solution. For this reason the BKW methods have been applied to the information matrix at the solution. These results are contained in Table 5. For the four variable model the largest condition index is only 2.1, indicating no ill conditioning problem. However, when A-1 is added to the model the largest condition index becomes 10.5, indicating a modest amount of dependency among the variables. Inspection of the covariance decomposition matrix suggests that the dependency is among all five variables with particularly strong dependency among the three variables A-1, LDL-C and SBP. Looking at the correlations computed from the information matrix, one sees moderate correlations of A-1 with LDL-C and with SBP, while LDL-C and SBP are negatively correlated. There is no known reason for this set of variables to be dependent and it is likely that the dependency is just an unusual characteristic of this data set. This excessive dependency may in fact be a result of the small sample size.

Table 5: KBW Diagnostics on Information Matrix

Model 1

| Eigen-value | Condi-tion index | Variance Proportion for LDL | SBP | Cig. | HDL |
|---|---|---|---|---|---|
| 1.42 | 1.00 | 0.03 | 0.25 | 0.00 | 0.18 |
| 1.29 | 1.05 | 0.29 | 0.00 | 0.23 | 0.06 |
| 0.97 | 1.21 | 0.08 | 0.05 | 0.43 | 0.21 |
| 0.32 | 2.12 | 0.59 | 0.69 | 0.34 | 0.56 |

Model 2

| Eigen-value | Condi-tion index | Variance Proportion for A-1 | LDL | SBP | HDL | Cig. |
|---|---|---|---|---|---|---|
| 2.01 | 1.00 | 0.01 | 0.00 | 0.01 | 0.00 | 0.03 |
| 1.72 | 1.08 | 0.01 | 0.02 | 0.00 | 0.02 | 0.01 |
| 0.95 | 2.45 | 0.00 | 0.00 | 0.00 | 0.29 | 0.00 |
| 0.30 | 2.61 | 0.03 | 0.03 | 0.04 | 0.00 | 0.36 |
| 0.02 | 10.54 | 0.96 | 0.96 | 0.93 | 0.69 | 0.59 |

## CONCLUSION

It is, of course, dangerous to generalize too much from a case study such as this, but several comments seem warranted.

1. Application of the BKW method directly to the X matrix or to the within matched samples covariance matrix will not always allow detection of possibly detrimental dependencies. It should be pointed out that the use of the within matched samples covariance matrix is equivalent to using the X'WX matrix with b=0; i.e. its use here is equivalent to applying the BKW methods to the information matrix under the null hypothesis of no effect of any of the variables in the model.

2. This example illustrates that application of the BKW methods to the information matrix may be useful. However, even then the BKW cutpoints for detecting dependencies may not be large enough. In his paper at this conference, Lustbader (3) points out that the rows of X'WX are the variates centered on the weighted risk set mean. BKW do not recommend centering the variables in linear regression and their criteria for determining when a condition index is large is based on uncentered data. In the linear model, centering the data leads to smaller condition indices and thus the BKW criteria may be too stringent for straightforward application to conditional logistic regression.Some additional research into the use of the BKW methods in this case seems warranted.

## REFERENCES

(1) Belsley, David A, Kuh, Edwin, and Welsch, Roy E. Regression Diagnostics. John Wiley & Sons, New York, 1980.

(2) Breslow, N.E. and Day, N.E. Statistical Methods in Cancer Research Volume 1. The Analysis of Case-Control Studies. International Agency for Research on Cancer, Geneva, 1980.

(3) Lustbader, Edward D. "Relative Risk Regression Diagnostics." Proceedings of the 1985 SIMS Conference, John Wiley & Sons, New York, 1985.

(4) Pregibon, D. "Logistic Regression Diagnostics" Annals of Statistics, 9, 1982, pp. 705-724.

## APPENDIX

SAS Routine for BKW Diagnostics
on Information Matrix

```
PROC MATRIX PRINT;
   FETCH VC DATA = A (FIRSTOBS=2);
   EIG = EIGVAL(VC);
   VEC = EIGVEC(VC);
COVBINV = INV (VC);
SCALE = INV(SQRT(DIAG(COVBINV)));
R=SCALE * COVBINV * SCALE;
EIGEN MUSQR V R;
SROOTMUS = SQRT(MUSQR);
PHI = (V##2)*DIAG (MUSQR##(-1));
SUMPHI = PHI*J(NROW (PHI), 1,1);
PI= (PHI@¦(SUMPHI##-1)))';
```

## SECTION 3
On the Analysis of Correlated Disease Occurrence Data

The two papers in this section deal with the analysis of correlated failure time data. Such data may arise, for example, in the analysis of twin studies, or in the analysis of disease occurrence among family members more generally, or in an intervention trial using group randomization. Statistical methods for the regression analysis of correlated failure time data have been slow to develop, apparently because there is little to guide the specification of failure rates for a member of a 'block' (giving rise to correlated responses) after other members of the block have been censored.

The paper by David Oakes provides a comprehensive review of a bivariate failure time model proposed by Clayton. This model has the feature that the failure rate at time t for a subject whose pair member has been censored at $s < t$ is a constant times that for a subject whose pair member failed at s. The multiplicative constant linking these two rates characterizes the strength of the correlation between failure times within a pair. Both parametric and semi-parametric methods are described for estimating the correlation parameter and other parameters, and some comments on goodness-of-fit testing are made.

The bivariate model discussed by Oakes has a motivation in terms of a random relative risk factor shared by pair members. The paper by Self and Prentice builds upon this idea by considering random effects in general relative risk models that include stochastic covariates and that allow the number of subjects in a block to be variable. Such models lead to semi-parametric methods of estimation that reduce to partial likelihood methods in the univariate special case. These approaches potentially extend and unify relative risk regression methods as applied to environmental risk factors and regression methods used in genetic epidemiology (Section Five) as applied to various types of family data. As such, multivariate failure time methods seem an important area for further emphasis in epidemiology.

# A Model for Bivariate Survival Data

*David Oakes**

Abstract. A model proposed by Clayton for bivariate survival data is discussed. The joint distribution of the two survival times is absolutely continuous, a single parameter governs the association between the two survival times and the marginal distributions may be specified arbitrarily. Motivation for, and properties of, the model are given. Published and unpublished results for parametric and semi-parametric inference about the association parameter are surveyed. The techniques are illustrated by simple example, which includes a brief consideration of goodness-of-fit.

## INTRODUCTION

In chronic disease epidemiology we may be concerned with survival times, possibly subject to censoring, of individuals who are naturally or artificially paired. For example, in familial studies of disease incidence we may have data on the ages and causes of death of fathers and their sons. In a study of the incidence of thyroid tumors among subjects treated by radiation a control group was chosen from among the siblings of those exposed. One motivation for such individual matching is that genetic and environmental influences shared by siblings will result in an association between their risks of disease. Confirmation of this hypothesis and quantification of the association are of complementary interest to the results of the main comparison of the disease incidences in the two groups. Accurate modelling of the joint distribution may also permit recovery of some "interblock" information lost by the usual methods for the analysis of matched samples [18].

Unlike many bivariate distributions arising in reliability theory, the relevant distributions here are jointly (absolutely) continuous, and the natural graphical representation is as points in the positive quadrant of the plane.

---

*Department of Statistics and Division of Biostatistics, University of Rochester, Rochester, NY 14627.

In this paper I shall outline some published and unpublished results concerning one such model, proposed by D. G. Clayton. This model has two distinct motivations. First, it arises from a certain proportionality relation between bivariate hazard functions. Secondly, it has a simple interpretation involving an unobserved random frailty shared between the two members of a pair. Motivation and construction of the model are discussed in Section 2.

Given a fully parametric specification of the marginal distributions of the two components, inference about the parameter governing the association between them is in principle straightforward. The log-likelihood from a bivariate random sample can be maximised jointly in the unknown parameters. The likelihood ratio, score or Wald procedures may be used to obtain large - sample tests of simple or composite hypotheses, or inverted to give confidence intervals or regions (Cox and Hinkley [5]). Section 3 outlines some results on parametric inference for the model.

When the marginal distributions are left unspecified, giving a so-called semi-parametric problem, matters are less simple. Invariance arguments suggest that inference should be based on the rank statistic, but its exact distribution appears intractable. There seems to be no partial likelihood factorisation (Cox [3, 4]) that would simplify matters. Section 4 describes a number of approximate procedures.

In Section 5 we consider some extensions of the model to include explanatory variables and to allow for tests of goodness-of-fit. In Section 6 the various methods are illustrated and compared using a small data set of Lawless [12].

Of course, the model studied here is only one possible approach to the analysis of bivariate survival data, but it does have appealing properties, and also leads to interesting issues in statistical inference that may have wider application.

Much of the material surveyed here is contained in the papers by Clayton [1], Clayton and Cuzick [2] and Oakes [14, 15]. See also Cox and Oakes ([6], Chapter 10).

## THE MODEL: DEFINITION AND MOTIVATION

To fix ideas, suppose that we are interested in the ages S and T at death of a sister and brother. In a typical follow-up study we might have bivariate observations of four types. We may have (i) $S = s$, $T = t$ if both sister and brother have died, (ii) $S = s$, $T > t$ if the sister has died but the brother is still alive, (iii) $S > s$, $T = t$ if the reverse occurs and (iv) $S > s$, $T > t$ if both are still alive. Thus, we may have right - censoring in either or both components. If deaths from a specific cause are of interest, deaths from other causes may also be treated as censorings, although special care is then needed in the interpretation ([6], Chapter 9).

In principle it will be possible to estimate the age - specific mortality (hazard) rates $h(t|S > s)$ of brothers at age t, among those brothers whose sisters survive to at least age s. We may similarly estimate the hazard rate $h(t|S = s)$ of brothers at age t, among those brothers whose sisters die at age s. Both these hazard functions and their ratio will in general depend on both s and t. We restrict attention to the special family of bivariate distributions obtained by setting the ratio to a constant, not depending on s or t. Thus

$$h(t|S = s) = (1 + \phi)h(t|S > s). \tag{1}$$

Let $F(s,t) = \Pr\{S > s, T > t\}$ denote the joint survivor function of S and T, with marginals $G(s) = F(s,0)$ and $H(t) = F(0,t)$. For $i = 0,1$ and $j = 0,1$ write $(-1)^{i+j} F_{ij}(s,t)$ for the $(i,j)$'th derivative of $F(s,t)$, so that $F_{00} = F$ and $F_{11} = f$, the joint density of S and T. Then (1) is equivalent to the requirement

$$f(s,t)F(s,t) = (1+\phi)F_{01}(s,t)F_{10}(s,t) \tag{2}$$

so that $(1+\phi)$ is the odds ratio of the four probabilities associated with the shaded regions of Figure 1. From (2) the model is non-sexist; the relation (1) still holds if the roles of S and T are exchanged.

Equation (2) viewed as a partial differential equation in F with boundary conditions $F(s,0) = G(s)$ and $F(0,t) = H(t)$, has the explicit solution

$$F(s,t) = [\ \{G(s)\}^{-\phi} + \{H(t)\}^{-\phi} - 1]^{-1/\phi}. \tag{3}$$

It is easily seen that provided $\phi \geq 0$, (3) does define a joint survivor function with G and H as marginals. The special cases $\phi = 0$ and $\phi \to \infty$ correspond respectively to independence between S and $T(F=GH)$ and the Frechet bound $(F=\min\{G,H\})$ giving maximal positive association between G and H. For derivation of (3) see Clayton [1], Cox and Oakes [6], Chapter 10, or Clayton and Cuzick [2].

A number of attractive features of the distribution defined by (3) follow quickly from these results. First, a widely used measure of association is Kendall's [10] coefficient of concordance $\tau$.

Given an (uncensored) sample $\{(S_i,T_i),\ i=1,2,\dots,n\}$ from the bivariate distribution $\tau$ is defined as the average, over all pairs $i < j$, of the random variables

$$\Delta_{ij} = \mathrm{sgn}\{(S_i - S_j)(T_i - T_j)\}.$$

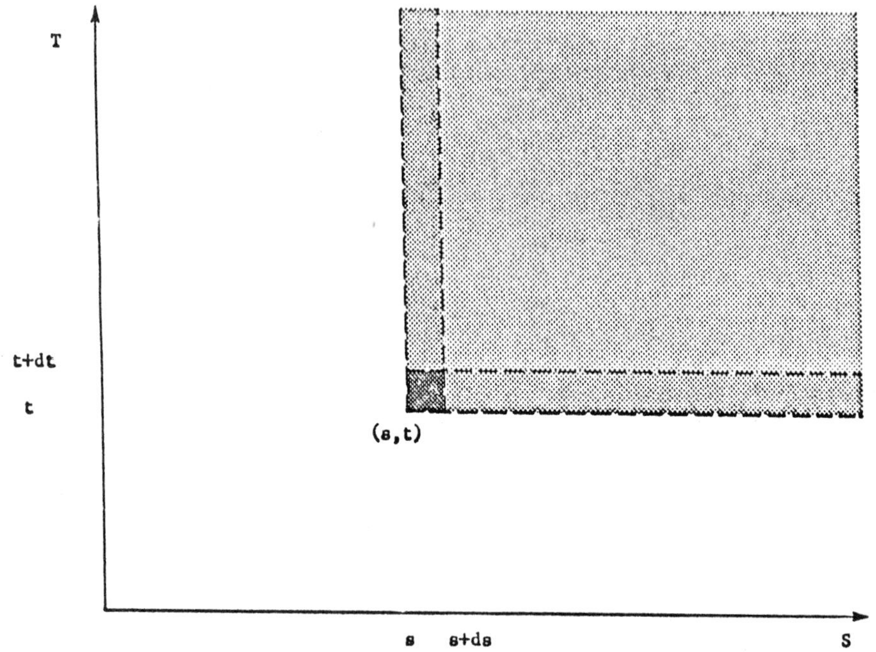


Figure 1: Illustration of the Model

Note that $\Delta_{ij} = +1$ if the two pairs are concordant, that is if they have the same ordering on both components, and $\Delta_{ij} = -1$ if the two pairs are discordant. For the distribution (3) it can be shown that $E(\tau) = E(\Delta_{ij}) = \phi/(\phi + 2)$, giving a simple interpretation of the association parameter.

Secondly, this interpretation extends to data subject to right - censoring in either or both components. With censored data, it may be impossible to determine the ordering of $S_i$ and $S_j$ or of $T_i$ and $T_j$. Thus, if $T_1 = 6^*$, $T_2 = 5$ ( $^*$ denotes censoring) then certainly $T_1 > T_2$. However, if $T_1 = 6$, $T_2 = 5^*$ then either $T_1 > T_2$ or $T_2 > T_1$ is possible. For a pair (i,j) to be classified as a definite concordance or a definite discordance, the smaller observation on both components must be uncensored. We may calculate a coefficient of concordance after discarding the indefinite pairs. For a general bivariate distribution the expectation of this quantity would depend in a complicated fashion on the censoring mechanism. If (3) is the joint survival distribution the expectation is still $\phi/(\phi + 2)$, whatever the censoring mechanism.

Thirdly, the model also behaves well under left-truncation. In many follow-up studies, observation on an individual does not start until certain criteria for entry to the study are satisfied. For example, in a study of occupational carcinogens observation might not begin until the worker had been employed in the industry in question for a defined period of time. In the present context, if observation on a sister - brother pair begins when their ages are $a_o$ and $b_o$ respectively, then the observed distribution of (S,T) is conditioned on $S > a_o$ and $T > b_o$. A simple calculation shows that the conditional survivor function $\tilde{F}(s,t) = \Pr\{S > s+a_o, T > t+b_o \mid S > a_o, T > b_o\}$ is related to the corresponding marginals $\tilde{G}(s) = \tilde{F}(s,0)$ and $\tilde{H}(t) = \tilde{F}(0,t)$ by

$$\tilde{F}(s,t) = [\ \{\tilde{G}(s)\}^{-\phi} + \{\tilde{H}(t)\}^{-\phi} - 1]^{-1/\phi},$$

an equation of the same form as (3), and with the same value of the parameter $\phi$. The notation here conceals a dependence of both $\tilde{G}$ and $\tilde{H}$ on both $a_o$ and $b_o$. In fact, the conditioning will in general change the form of the marginals. If for example, G and H are exponential, $\tilde{G}$ and $\tilde{H}$ will not be, unless $a_o = 0$ or $b_o = 0$ or S and T are independent ($\phi = 0$).

All the previous properties have flowed directly from the relation (1) between the bivariate hazard functions. The model (3) can be approached from a different direction. Suppose first that $G(s) = \Pr\{\ S > s\ \}$ and $H(t) = \Pr\{\ T > t\ \}$ are specified continuous univariate survivor functions and that $\phi > 0$ is also given. Then

$$G^*(s) = \exp[\ 1 - \{G(s)\}^{-\phi}], \qquad H^*(t) = \exp[1 - \{H(t)\}^{-\phi}]$$

will also be continuous univariate survivor functions. For example, if $G(s) = (1 + \alpha s)^{-1/\phi}$, a Pareto distribution, then $G^*(s) = \exp(-\alpha s)$, an exponential. If $G(s) = \exp(-\alpha s)$, then $G^*(s) = \exp[\ 1 - e^{\alpha\phi s}]$, the survivor function of an extreme value distribution. Now let **W** be a random variable having a gamma distribution with unit scale parameter and index $\eta = 1/\phi$, so that the density of **W** is $w^{\eta-1} \exp(-w)/\Gamma(\eta)$, and suppose that conditionally on the value w of **W**, S and T are independent with survivor functions

$$\Pr\{\ S > s \mid w\ \} = \{\ G^*(s)\ \}^w\ ; \quad \Pr\{\ T > t \mid w\} = \{H^*(t)\}^w.$$

Then it follows by simple integration that the unconditional joint survivor function $\Pr\{\ S > s,\ T > t\ \}$ is F(s,t), the same as (3).

The random variable W may be thought of as a multiplicative "frailty" [8, 17] that acts on the hazard functions of an (S, T) pair. In this representation W varies from pair to pair and is not itself observed. The coefficient of variation of W is $\phi^{1/2}$, so that, as we would expect, a large value of $\phi$ corresponds to a substantial within pairs component of variability in this random effects model.

## PARAMETRIC ESTIMATION

If the survivor function (3) is specified up to a low-dimensional vector $\underline{\theta}$ of unknown parameters, then standard procedures are available for inference about $\underline{\theta}$ from the likelihood function. Observations censored in neither, one or both components contribute terms $F(s,t;\underline{\theta})$, $F_{01}(s,t;\underline{\theta})$, $F_{10}(s,t;\underline{\theta})$ or $f(s,t;\underline{\theta})$ to the likelihood function. Subject to mild regularity conditions [5], Chapter 9, the usual large - sample properties of the estimators will obtain.

We take the view here that primary interest lies in the parameter $\phi$ governing the degree of association between S and T. If so, inferences about $\phi$ should not be contaminated by issues relating to the fit of the marginal distributions G(s) and H(t). We shall assume, therefore, that $\underline{\theta} = (\phi, \underline{\alpha}, \underline{\beta})$, where $\underline{\alpha}$ and $\underline{\beta}$ relate solely to G and H respectively, and that there is no functional relation between $\phi$, $\underline{\alpha}$, and $\underline{\beta}$. For example, the Pareto model, with $G(s) = (1 + \alpha s)^{-1/\phi}$ would not satisfy this requirement, since the sample $\{ S_i;\ i = 1,2,\ldots,n \} = \underset{\sim}{S}$ say of sisters ages would in itself provide information about $\phi$. The model $G(s) = (1 + \alpha s)^{-1}$ would be permissible, as would the more general model $G(s) = (1 + \alpha_0 s)^{\alpha_1}$.

Oakes [14] considered in detail the case where there is no censoring and both marginal survivor functions are assumed known up to Lehmann alternatives: $G(s) = \{G_0(s)\}^{\alpha}$; $H(t) = \{H_0(t)\}^{\beta}$, where G and H are specified continuous survivor functions. The substitutions $S' = -\log\{G_0(S)\}$, $T' = -\log\{H_0(T)\}$ transform the joint survivor function to

$$F(s,t) = \{ \exp(\alpha\phi s) + \exp(\beta\phi t) - 1 \}^{-1/\phi}, \qquad (4)$$

which has exponential marginals. Although there is no guarantee that the log-likelihood is concave for finite samples, large sample results can be derived in the usual way.

The expected information matrix for $(\phi,\alpha,\beta)$ can be found explicitly in terms of the Trigamma function $\Psi'(z) = \sum(n + z)^{-2}$. This allows a theoretical assessment of the loss of information about $\phi$

through lack of knowledge about $\alpha$ and $\beta$. At $\phi = 0$ the expected information matrix is diagonal, so that the parameter estimates are asymptotically independent and no information is lost. For large $\phi$, however, the situation is very different. In fact as $\phi \to \infty$, the asymptotic information about $\phi$ is more than doubled if $\alpha$ and $\beta$ are specified. A similar phenomenon was noted by Kendall and Stuart ([11], p. 75), for the correlation coefficient in the bivariate normal distribution with the two variances in the role of $\alpha$ and $\beta$. In specific applications it is possible, and for some purposes preferable to use the observed information, calculated directly from the second derivatives of the log-likelihood, rather than its theoretical expectation.

In view of the gross non-normality of the distribution (4) it is of some interest that the test statistic of the hypothesis $\phi = 0$ derived from the score statistic ([5], p. 323), turns out to be based on the usual product - moment $\sum S_i T_i$. Although $\phi = 0$ is a boundary of the parameter space, direct expansion of the log-likelihood function, its derivatives and their expectations, in powers of $\phi$ shows that the limiting operations are legitimate.

For $a > 0$ and $b > 0$, let $g_{ab}$ denote the transformation $g_{ab}(s,t) = (as,bt)$. The exponential model (4) is invariant under the group of all such transformations. One representation of the maximal invariant statistic is as $\{(U_j, V_j);\ j=2,3,\ldots,n\}$ where $U_j = S_j/S_1$ and $V_j = T_j/T_1$. The marginal likelihood of $(U_j, V_j)$ is a function of $\underline{\theta}$ only through $\phi$, and contains all the available information about $\phi$ in the absence of knowledge of $\alpha$ and $\beta$ [9]. To date this approach has not been explored. At first glance the calculations appear intractable. It should be noted also that the invariance arguments do not apply even in principle if there is censoring [9].

For more general parameterizations of the marginal distributions no detailed theoretical evaluations have been made. The orthogonality at $\phi = 0$ of the parameter estimates continues to hold, and a simple form is obtained for the test of independence [2].

The interpretation of the model (3) in terms of unobserved random frailties $W_i$ suggests a possible role for the EM algorithm [7] in parametric estimation. Suppose for the moment that the $\{W_i\}$ are observed and that the parameterizations of the marginal distributions are closed under Lehmann alternatives, in the sense that for each $\underline{\alpha}$, $\underline{\beta}$ and $\phi$ there are $\underline{\alpha}_\phi$ and $\underline{\beta}_\phi$ such that $\{G(s;\underline{\alpha})\}^\phi = G(s;\underline{\alpha}_\phi)$ and $\{H(t;\underline{\beta})\}^\phi = H(t;\underline{\beta}_\phi)$. Then in the absence of knowledge of $\underline{\alpha}$ and $\underline{\beta}$, the conditional distributions of S and T given W are uninformative about $\phi$; all the available information about $\phi$ is contained in the distribution of W. The full log-likelihood in $(\underset{\sim}{S}, \underset{\sim}{T}, \underset{\sim}{W})$ may be written

$$\ell_o(\underset{\sim}{W}; \phi) + \ell_o(\underset{\sim}{S}|\underset{\sim}{W};\underline{\alpha}_\phi) + \ell_o(\underset{\sim}{T}|\underset{\sim}{W};\underline{\beta}_\phi) \tag{5}$$

and each term may be maximized separately.

When $\underset{\sim}{W}$ is not observed, the E step of the EM algorithm involves calculation of the conditional expectation of (5) given the observed quantities $(\underset{\sim}{S}, \underset{\sim}{T})$, using current values of the parameter estimates. It can be shown that the calculation actually uses only the conditional expectations of $\underset{\sim}{W}$ and of the $\log(W_i)$, which both take simple forms, the latter involving the Digamma function. The M step of the algorithm, maximization of the conditional expectation of (5), gives new estimates exactly as if $\{W_i\}$ were observed.

Details of the application of the EM algorithm will be presented elsewhere. One further point is worth emphasizing here. In (5) the conditional likelihoods of $\underset{\sim}{S}$ and $\underset{\sim}{T}$ given $\underset{\sim}{W}$ use the distributions $G^*$ and $H^*$, not the marginal distributions G and H. Thus, if $G(s;\alpha) = e^{-\alpha s}$, at each iteration $\underline{\alpha}_\phi$ must be determined by solution of the likelihood equations from the extreme value distribution $G^*(s;\alpha)$.

## SEMI-PARAMETRIC INFERENCE

In this section we review various methods for inference about $\phi$, when no assumption is made concerning the form of the marginal distributions. The first suggestion, made by Clayton [1], is most easily described with the aid of a diagram (Figure 2). From now on we shall assume that there are no ties among the observed values of $S_i$ or among the observed values of $T_i$. Unless otherwise stated, we shall permit right-censoring in either or both components of the data.

As indicated in Section 2, each pair $\{(S_i,T_i),(S_j,T_j): \ (i<j)\}$ of bivariate observations may be classified as a definite concordance, a definite discordance, or (if there is censoring) as indefinite. We now construct a hypersample $\mathcal{H}$ of points $(X_h,Y_h)$, usually much larger than the original sample, in the following way. The point (X,Y) is a member of the hypersample if, for some i and j not necessarily distinct, $X = \min(S_i, S_j)$ and $Y = \min(T_i,T_j)$, and both $\min(S_i,S_j)$ and $\min(T_i,T_j)$ are uncensored. So $\mathcal{H}$ is a subset of the product set formed by arbitrarily pairing any sister's age at death with any brother's age at death.

The bivariate risk set at a point (s,t) consists of all sister-brother pairs who survive to ages s and t respectively. Formally, $R(s,t) = \{k : S_k \geq s, T_k \geq t\}$. For each hypersample point $(X_h,Y_h)$ let $R_h = R(X_h,Y_h)$ be the corresponding bivariate risk set and $r_h$ its size. Then it is easily shown that the conditional probability that $(X_h,Y_h)$ is an original point, given that it belongs to the hypersample and given $R_h$, is $\ell_h = (\phi + 1)/(\phi + r_h)$. Let $\Delta_h$ be an indicator variable, $\Delta_h = 1$ or $\Delta_h = 0$ for original or added points respectively. Clayton proposed that inference for $\phi$ should be based on the product

$$\text{lik} = \Pi_h\, \ell_h^{\Delta_h} (1-\ell_h)^{1-\Delta_h} = \Pi_h \frac{(\phi+1)^{\Delta_h}(r_h-1)^{1-\Delta_h}}{(\phi+r_h)} \tag{6}$$

viewed as a "conditional likelihood". Oakes [14] remarked that this likelihood does not correspond to a partial likelihood factorization of the full likelihood [3, 4] so that the usual information calculation will systematically underestimate the variance of the estimator. In recent work [15] I have derived a theoretical expression for the true asymptotic variance of Clayton's estimator. For uncensored data, an explicit expression can be obtained involving the Trigamma function (again!).

In fact, in the uncensored case the problem has an invariance structure reminiscent of that mentioned in Section 3 for exponential marginal distributions. Here, let a(s) and b(t) be any two monotonic increasing differentiable functions with a(0) = b(0) = 0, and write $g_{ab}(s,t) = (a(s),b(t))$. The rank statistic, defined as the permutation of the order statistic of $(T_1,T_2,\ldots,T_n)$ induced by the order statistic of $(S_1,S_2,\ldots,S_n)$ is invariant under the group of all such transformations $\{g_{ab}\}$, and its distribution depends only on $\phi$. If the invariance principle [13] is seen as compelling, then inferences about $\phi$ should depend on the data $(\underset{\sim}{S},\underset{\sim}{T})$ only through the marginal likelihood of the rank statistic. Oakes [14] calculated this marginal likelihood for the simplest non-trivial case, sample size n = 3, and showed that it did not equal the 'conditional' likelihood (6). The form of the calculations also suggested, unfortunately, that the exact marginal likelihood for larger samples would be intractable. It is important, however, that in principle the estimator obtained by maximizing this marginal likelihood would be asymptotically efficient among all rank invariant estimators of $\phi$.

An alternative non-parametric estimator based on the coefficient of concordance was proposed by Oakes [14]. The main merit of this estimator was the availability of a fairly simple valid estimator of its variance. Now that the true asymptotic variance of Clayton's estimator has been calculated, this advantage has been superceded and the concordance estimator should probably not be used, except for exploratory analyses as illustrated in Section 6. Theoretical calculations [15] and simulation results [2] show that the concordance estimator is much less efficient than Clayton's estimator. It is of some interest and importance in the theoretical calculations, however, that the latter estimator can be expressed as a weighted form of the former [2].

Recent work by Clayton and Cuzick [2] has concentrated on the search for an asymptotically efficient estimator. Their idea is to replace the actual sample values by expected values of order statistics calculated as if the data followed a specific parametric model. The likelihood is then maximized as if the data were sampled from that model. In the calculation of the expected order statistics, allowance must be made for the dependence between the samples (unless there is in fact no dependence, $\phi = 0$). Use of the order statistics from the marginal distributions alone leads to a consistent, but not efficient estimator. Judicious use of approximations allows efficient estimators and valid estimates of their variance to be derived in a tractable form. However, no explicit formula appears yet to be available for the expected information matrix.

In view of its simple structure and the availability now, of a valid variance estimator, the pseudo-likelihood function - as I prefer to call it - (6) is still a useful technique for the analysis of data from this model. Except at $\phi = 0$, however, and in certain limiting cases involving very heavy censorship, there is no reason to believe that it is asymptotically efficient.

## EXTENSIONS OF THE MODEL

We briefly mention two different generalizations of the model (1). First, the constant $\phi$ may be replaced by a function of s and t, possibly containing unknown parameters. In principle such an extension could be useful in devising formal procedures for assessment of fit. In practice it seems possible to devise explicit procedures only for the case that $\phi$ is constant over rectangles in the (s,t) plane. Here the partial differential equations for the joint survivor function F(s,t) in terms of the marginal survivor functions G(s) and H(t) and $\phi = \phi(s,t)$ are very easily solved. In fact each rectangle may be thought of as defining a separate distribution, subject to left truncation at the western and southern boundaries and right censoring at the northern and eastern boundaries. The availability of this simple reduction is a consequence of the insensitivity properties of the original model to right - censorship and left - truncation, discussed in Section 2.

The second generalization concerns the inclusion of covariates. These may play several roles:

(i) They may act on the marginal distribution of S and T or both

(ii) They may act on the association parameter

(iii) They may represent a specific assumed relation between the marginal distributions, for example $G(s) = \{H(s)\}^{\delta}$.

Clayton and Cuzick [2] discuss (i) and describe briefly how their semi-parametric procedure can be extended to this problem. Role (ii) is especially relevant in genetic applications, where, for example, the covariates might represent the familial relationship between the two members of a pair. In (iii) the entire character of the problem changes as the constraint imposes a relation between the two time scales. It would be of some interest to investigate the properties of the log-rank test of the hypothesis $\delta = 1$ for a non-zero $\phi$, and to derive alternative tests that explicitly allow for the dependence. The case that $\delta = 1$ corresponds to exchangeability between the two members of a pair [2].

## AN EXAMPLE

To illustrate the use of the model for a simple data set we consider the cable insulation failure times analyzed by Stone [16] and quoted in Lawless [12]. Here S denotes the time to inception of a fault and T the subsequent time to failure from inception. The data appear in Table 1. I have chosen to omit three data points for which no fault occurred. The remaining 17 points are uncensored in both components. Three ties among values of T were broken at random.

TABLE 1

Cable insulation failure times of Stone [16] quoted by Lawless [12], p. 477.

| S | rank(S) | T | rank(T) | S | rank(S) | T | rank(T) |
|---|---|---|---|---|---|---|---|
| 228 | 6 | 30 | 8 | 1227 | 16 | 39 | 10 |
| 106 | 1 | 8 | 3 | 254 | 8 | 46 | 11 |
| 246 | 7 | 66 | 12 | 435 | 11 | 85 | 14 |
| 700 | 13 | 72 | 13 | 1155 | 15 | 85 | 15 |
| 473 | 12 | 25 | 5 | 195 | 5 | 27 | 7 |
| 155 | 4 | 7 | 2 | 117 | 2 | 27 | 6 |
| 414 | 10 | 30 | 9 | 724 | 14 | 21 | 4 |
| 1374 | 17 | 90 | 16 | 300 | 9 | 96 | 17 |
| | | | | 128 | 3 | 4 | 1 |

Key: S = time to inception of fault
T = subsequent time to failure

Conventional tests for association all achieve statistical significance for these data. Pearson's correlation coefficient applied to the raw values is 0.505 (P = 0.02, one-sided), and more appropriately to the logarithms is 0.630 (P = 0.004). Spearman's rank correlation is 0.596 (P = 0.007). The means and standard deviations for the marginal distributions are respectively 484.2 and 411.7 for S and 44.6 and 31.2 for T. The approximate equality for both components suggests that an assumption of exponential marginal distributions may not be wildly unreasonable.

Figure 2 plots rank(T) against rank(S) and confirms the noticeable positive association between S and T. Of the 17 x 16/2 = 136 (i,j) pairs, 99 are concordant and 37 discordant. The concordance estimator of $\phi$ in (3) is $\hat{\phi}$ = 1.68, with standard error estimated from the calculations of Oakes [14] of 0.92. The theoretical results suggest that $\gamma = \log(1 + \phi)$ gives a more stable variance estimate, and on this scale the concordance estimate is $\hat{\gamma}$ = 0.99 (SE 0.34).

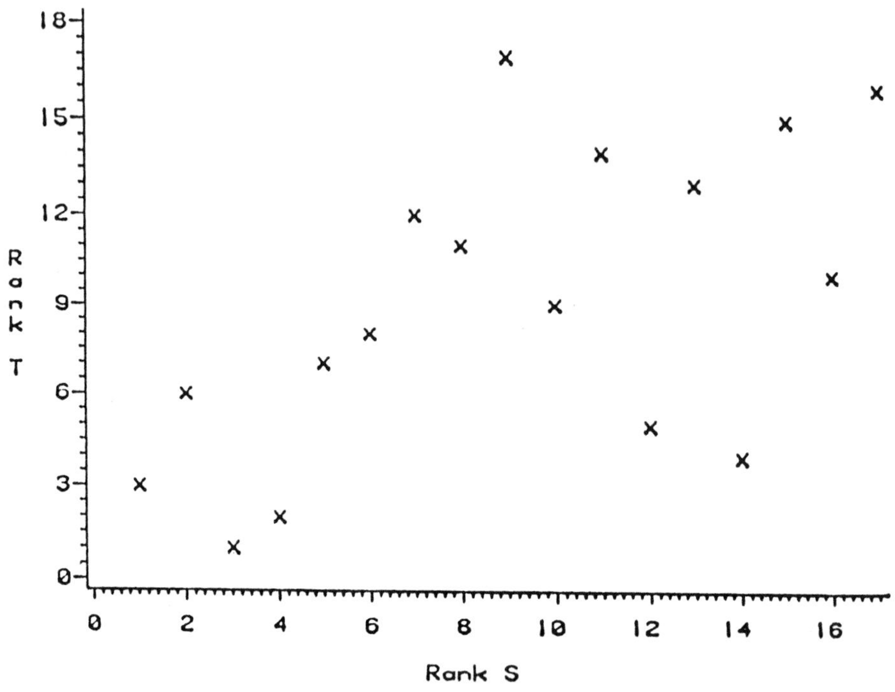


Figure 2: Rank(T) Against Rank(S)

Figure 3 shows the hypersample $H$ used to calculate Clayton's pseudo-likelihood estimator. Crosses mark the original sample points taken from Figure 2, and circles the added points for the 37 discordant pairs. The estimate is $\hat{\gamma}$ = 0.78. The calculations of Oakes [15] give an (asymptotic) standard error estimate of 0.31, which, perversely, agrees well with the invalid nominal estimate from the second derivative (0.32). The theoretical calculations show that in large samples the first standard error estimate should be on average 22% higher than the second, for this value of $\gamma$.

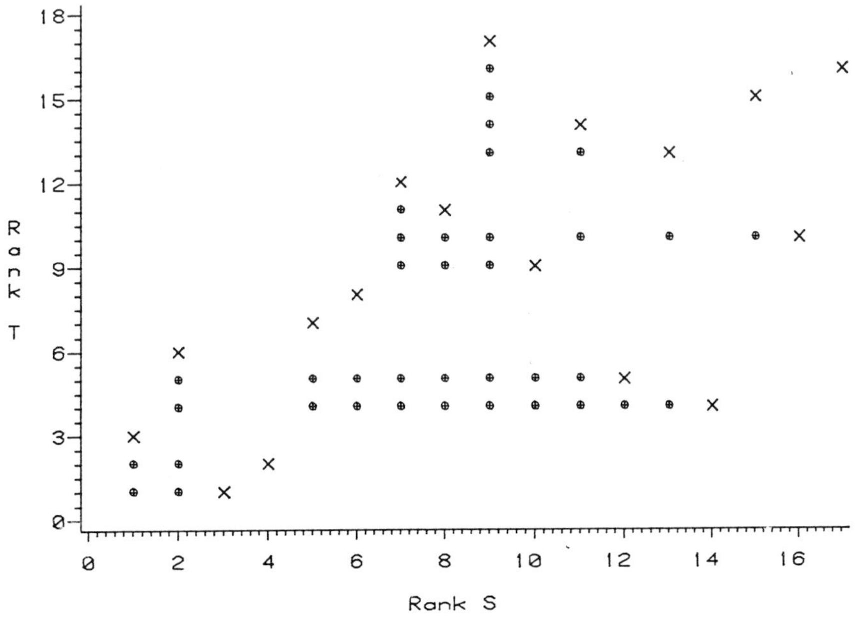


Figure 3: The Hypersample for the Pseudo-likelihood

Maximization of the parametric likelihood for exponential marginals gives estimates and standard errors of $\hat{\gamma} = 0.82$ (SE 0.28), $\hat{\alpha} = 0.00197$ (SE 0.00048) and $\beta = 0.0226$ (SE 0.0054). If $\alpha$ and $\beta$ were specified at these estimated values, the standard error for $\hat{\gamma}$ would decrease to 0.24. Here the observed and expected information matrices give the same estimated standard errors for $\hat{\gamma}$, to the accuracy reported. The change in log-likelihood from fitting $\gamma$ after $\alpha$ and $\beta$, is 2.95, giving $x_1^2 = 5.90$ for the likelihood ratio test of independence.

The parametric and pseudo-likelihood estimators agree well here. All analyses reveal an association between S and T that is significant at $P < 0.05$, but disagree somewhat on the precise magnitude and descriptive level of significance of the association.

Some insight into the reason for the slight disagreement between the concordance estimator ($\hat{\gamma} = 0.92$) and the pseudo-likelihood estimator ($\hat{\gamma} = 0.78$) can be gained from an informal test of fit (Figure 4). We divide the s and t axes at specified points $a_o$ and $b_o$ as shown (here $a_o = 8.5$, $b_o = 7.5$ for the ranks) and consider the separate concordance estimates of $\phi$ obtained from each of the four derived regions of the (s,t) quadrant. The south-west region corresponds to a sample subject to right censoring at $S = a_o$ and $T = b_o$. It yields 62 concordances and 14 discordances with $\hat{\phi} = 3.43$. Left truncation of S at $a_o$ combined with right censorship of T at $b_o$ gives the south-east region, with 7 concordances and 8 discordances ($\hat{\phi} = -0.125$). Similarly, the north-west region has 19 concordances and 5 discordances ($\hat{\phi} = 2.80$). Finally, the north-east region, corresponding to left truncation of S and T, has 11 concordances and 10 discordances ($\hat{\phi} = 0.10$). The discrepancy among the four estimates gives some evidence of lack of fit. Because of the dependence among the pairs, simple chi-square tests are not valid, and the variation shown is probably within the limits of sampling error. However, since the pseudo-likelihood estimator weights each (i,j) pair by (essentially) the reciprocal of the size of the corresponding risk set [2, 15], it gives more weight to the extremes of the distribution where the dependence is smaller, and therefore gives a lower overall estimate.

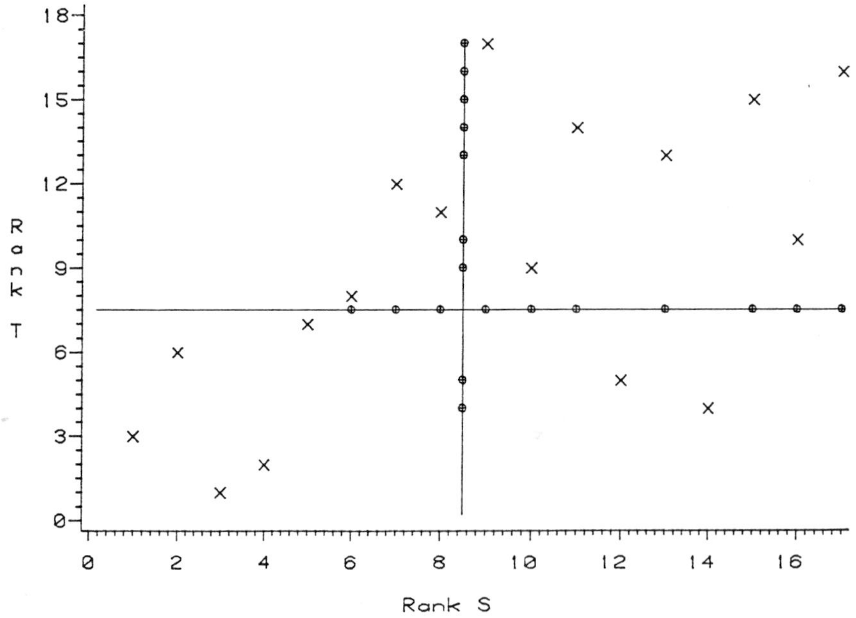


Figure 4: A Partitioning for a Test of Fit

## REFERENCES

[1] D. G. CLAYTON. A model for association in bivariate life-tables and its application in epidemiological studies of familial tendency in chronic disease incidence. Biometrika 65, (1978), pp. 141-151.

[2] D. G. CLAYTON and J. CUZICK. Multivariate generalizations of the proportional hazards model (with discussion). To appear in J. Roy. Statist. Soc. A.

[3] D. R. COX. Regression models and life tables (with discussion). J. Roy. Statist. Soc. B. 34, (1972), pp. 187-220.

[4] D. R. COX. Partial likelihood. Biometrika 62, (1975), pp. 269-276.

[5] D. R. COX and D. V. HINKLEY. Theoretical Statistics. Chapman and Hall, London, 1974.

[6] D. R. COX and D. OAKES. Analysis of Survival Data. Chapman and Hall, London, 1984.

[7] A. P. DEMPSTER, N. M. LAIRD and D. B. RUBIN. Maximum likelihood from incomplete data via the EM algorithm (with discussion). J. Roy. Statist. Soc. B. 39, (1977), pp. 1-38.

[8] P. HOUGAARD. Life table methods for heterogeneous populations: distributions describing the heterogeneity. Biometrika 71, (1984), pp. 75-83.

[9] J. D. KALBFLEISCH and R. L. PRENTICE. Marginal likelihoods based on Cox's regression and life model. Biometrika 60, (1973), pp. 267-278.

[10] M. G. KENDALL. A new measure of rank correlation. Biometrika 30, (1938) pp. 81-93.

[11] M. G. KENDALL and A. STUART. The Advanced Theory of Statistics, Vol. 2, 4th ed. Macmillan, New York, 1979.

[12] J. F. LAWLESS. Statistical Models and Methods for Lifetime Data. Wiley, New York, 1982.

[13] E. L. LEHMANN. Theory of Point Estimation. Wiley, New York, 1983.

[14] D. OAKES. A model for association in bivariate survival data. J. Roy. Statist. Soc. B. 44, (1982), pp. 414-422.

[15] D. OAKES. Semi-parametric inference in a model for association in bivariate survival data. Submitted.

[16] G. C. STONE. Statistical analysis of accelerated aging tests on solid electrical insulation. Unpublished M.A. Sc. Thesis, University of Waterloo, Waterloo, Ontario, Canada, (1978).

[17] J. W. VAUPEL, K. G. MANTON and E. STALLARD. The impact of heterogeneity in individual frailty on the dynamics of mortality. Demography 16, (1979), pp. 439-454.

[18] C. J. WILD. Failure time models with matched data. Biometrika 70, (1983), pp. 633-641.

# Incorporating Random Effects into Multivariate Relative Risk Regression Models

*Steven G. Self* and Ross L. Prentice**

Abstract. An approach for modelling multivariate failure time data is described in which random effects are incorporated into relative risk regression models. An 'ad hoc' method of estimation is proposed for these models which is very similar to the partial likelihood methods used in univariate problems. A large sample theory for the estimators is described. Possible extensions and potential applications of these models are discussed.

## INTRODUCTION

Many failure time regression problems involve the analysis of multiple failure times on individual study subjects. By viewing the data from such problems as a multivariate counting process, the relative risk regression models (e.g., Cox [4], Kalbfleisch and Prentice [7]) which have proved so useful in univariate problems generalize naturally to regression models for the intensity process. In these models, dependence of the intensity process on a subject's preceding failure and censoring history is accommodated into the relative risk model by additional terms in the regression function or by stratification of the baseline rate (Prentice, Williams and Peterson [12]). Partial likelihood estimation procedures and corresponding formal distribution theory also generalize readily to such multivariate models (Andersen and Gill [2], Prentice and Self [11]). With these methods, the dependence between failure times is usually modelled as though the actual occurrence of a failure has a direct effect on the intensity for the occurrence of subsequent failures.

Another important class of multivariate failure time problems arises because groups of study subjects have common characteristics that may relate to failure times and that are not captured by recorded covariates. Pairs of failure times arising from identical twins provide a classic example in which any attempt to describe the rele-

---

*Fred Hutchinson Cancer Research Center, 1124 Columbia Street, Seattle, Washington, 98104. This work was supported in part by NIH grants GM-24472 and GM-28314.

vant common genetic and environmental characteristics by means of covariates is likely to fall short. In these problems, a natural way of modelling the dependence among individuals is to incorporate random effects into the specification of the intensity process.

Incorporation of random effects into relative risk regression models has received relatively little attention in the literature. The main difficulty has been in devising a method for estimation that can accommodate the semiparametric nature of the models. In the special case of matched data, Holt and Prentice [6] proposed treating the matched sets as separate strata and using standard partial likelihood procedures for estimation. One disadvantage of this approach is that all regression information about covariates that are common to members of a matched set is unused. Also, some flexibility of modelling is lost in that all members of a matched set are required to have the same baseline intensity process. This may be unsuitable in modelling disease rates in families, for example, where it would be natural to permit both baseline rates and some regression coefficients to differ between fathers, mothers, sons and daughters. Also, characteristics common to family members (e.g., aspects of the household environment) could not be related to disease rates by this approach.

More recently, Clayton and Cuzick [3] have considered relative risk regression models with fixed covariates in which a single random effect enters the intensity process specification in a multiplicative way. They then suppose that the random effect arises from a (minus) log-gamma distribution and develop likelihood-based estimation procedures using the distribution of the generalized rank vector (e.g., Prentice [9]). A series of approximations are described in order to make this approach computationally feasible. In spite of these approximations, their procedures remain computationally complex and the relationship to established relative risk regression methods in the univariate failure time special case is obscure.

In this work, we consider relative risk regression models in which random effects terms enter the intensity process specification in a multiplicative way. The model described by Clayton and Cuzick [3] represents an important special case. Unlike Clayton and Cuzick, who focus on the shape of the multivariate distribution (e.g., multivariate Pareto), we focus on the form of the intensity process and propose estimation procedures that are very similar to the standard univariate procedures. A large sample distribution theory is outlined for the proposed estimators. Potential applications for these methods are discussed.

## INTENSITY PROCESSES WITH RANDOM EFFECTS

We will first consider data from a simple blocked experiment.

Using the counting process formulation and notation used by Andersen and Gill [2] the data for the $i^{th}$ subject $(1 \le i \le S)$ in the $k^{th}(1 \le k \le B)$ block may be written as $\{Y_{ik}(t), N_{ik}(t), Z_{ik}(t); t \in [0,1]\}$. The censoring process $Y_{ik}(t)$ takes value one if subject (i,k) is under observation at time t and takes value zero otherwise. The counting process $N_{ik}(t)$ counts failures observed in subject (i,k) prior to t and the covariate process $Z_{ik}(t)$ is a p-vector of data-analyst defined functions summarizing the concomitant information available about subject (i,k) prior to time t. Let $\{F_t; t \in [0,1]\}$ be the increasing right continuous family of sub $\sigma$-fields generated by the failure, censoring and covariate histories of all individuals under study prior to time t. Finally, let $\varepsilon_1, \cdots, \varepsilon_B$ be independent, identically distributed random variables that will represent the block effects. We will assume that the intensity process with respect to $F_t \vee \sigma(\varepsilon_1, \cdots, \varepsilon_B)$ for subject (i,k) is given by

$$Y_{ik}(t)\lambda_0(t)\exp\{Z_{ik}^T(t)\beta + \varepsilon_k\} \quad . \tag{2.1}$$

It follows from the innovation theorem (Aalen [1]) that the intensity process with respect to $F_t$ whose parameters are estimable from the data is given by

$$Y_{ik}(t)\lambda_0(t)\exp\{Z_{ik}^T(t)\beta\}\ E[\exp\{\varepsilon_k\}|F_t] \quad . \tag{2.2}$$

If it is assumed that innovations in the covariate and censoring processes are independent of the $\varepsilon_k$'s, then $E[\exp\{\varepsilon_k\}|F_t]$ may be written as

$$\frac{E_\varepsilon[\exp\{(\bar{N}_k(t)+1)\varepsilon - \bar{\Lambda}_k(t)\exp(\varepsilon)\}]}{E_\varepsilon[\exp\{\bar{N}_k(t)\varepsilon - \bar{\Lambda}_k(t)\exp(\varepsilon)\}]} \tag{2.3}$$

where $\bar{N}_k(t) = \sum_{j=1}^{S} N_{jk}(t^-)$ and $\bar{\Lambda}_k(t) = \sum_{j=1}^{S} \int_0^{t^-} Y_{jk}(s)\exp\{Z_{jk}^T(t)\beta\}d\Lambda_0(s)$.
Expression (2.3) depends on $\beta, \lambda_0$ and the distribution of $\varepsilon$. However, for well behaved censoring and covariate processes, the integrals in the expression for $\bar{\Lambda}_k(t)$ may be integrated by parts. Then (2.3) depends on $\lambda_0(t)$ only through the cumulative baseline intensity $\Lambda_0(t)$. Therefore in considering the family of random effects models for intensity processes given by (2.1) it is sufficient to study relative risk regression models in which the relative risk function is allowed to depend on the cumulative baseline hazard.

If it is assumed that the $\varepsilon_k$'s are drawn from a log-gamma distribution with variance $\theta$ then model (2.1) reduces, in the special case of fixed covariates, to the model considered by Clayton and Cuzick [3]. In this case, expression (2.3) has a particularly simple form given by

$$[1+\theta\bar{N}_k(t)]/[1+\theta\bar{\Lambda}_k(t)] \tag{2.4}$$

A more flexible approach to modelling (2.3) is to consider the $\varepsilon_k$'s to be drawn from a location/scale family of distributions. Then, by expanding the logarithm of (2.3) in a Taylor series and neglecting constants and higher order terms, an approximation to (2.3) is obtained as $\exp\{X_k^T(t)\theta\}$ where $X_k(t)$ represents a vector of collected terms in the Taylor expansion and $\theta$ is a vector of unknown parameters which are functions of the central moments of $\varepsilon$. The first two coordinates of $X_k(t)$ are given by $\bar{N}_k(t) - \bar{\Lambda}_k(t)$ and $(\bar{N}_k(t) - \bar{\Lambda}_k(t))^2 - \bar{\Lambda}_k(t)$, respectively.

A fairly straightforward interpretation of these terms follows upon noting that in the absence of the random effect they are almost martingales reflecting the failure history of the $k^{th}$ block. They fail to be martingales only by virtue of the left rather than right continuity of $\bar{N}_k(t)$. Thus, if $\bar{N}_k(t) - \bar{\Lambda}_k(t)$ is positive this indicates that members of block k are failing faster (prior to t) than expected. This is evidence the $\varepsilon_k$ is positive and the relative risks at t for individuals in block k are adjusted accordingly by the term $\exp\{X_k^T(t)\theta\}$.

In some situations the ability to model more complicated patterns of association is required. For example, in a study of disease rates in families, the different degrees of relationships among family members should be acknowledged when modelling familial aggregation due to putative genetic factors. Additional complexity is required if both common environmental and genetic effects are to be accommodated in the model. The natural generalization of model (2.1) to accommodate more complicated patterns of association would specify the $S \times 1$ vector of log relative risk processes for the $k^{th}$ family as $Z_k(t)\beta + \varepsilon$ where $Z_k(t)$ is the $S \times p$ matrix of covariate values for the $k^{th}$ family and $\varepsilon_k$ is an $S \times 1$ vector-valued random variable with a correlation structure that reflects the desired pattern of association. One approach to deriving the intensity process with respect to $\mathcal{F}_t$ from this model is to assume $\varepsilon_k$ to be drawn from a multivariate log-gamma distribution and try to obtain an exact evaluation of $E[\exp\{\varepsilon_k\}|\mathcal{F}_t]$ such as (2.4). One problem with this approach is that none of the multivariate gamma distributions available can accommodate complicated patterns of association. Also, there is no guarantee that a reasonably simple form for $E[\exp\{\varepsilon_k\}|\mathcal{F}_t]$ such as (2.4) will be obtained for any given multivariate gamma distribution.

Another approach for deriving the intensity process with respect to $\mathcal{F}_t$ is to specify $\varepsilon_k$ as arising from the variance components model

$$\varepsilon_k = V_{1k}\alpha_1 + V_{2k}\alpha_2 + \cdots + V_{qk}\alpha_q \tag{2.5}$$

where the $V_{ik}$'s are $S \times m_k$ matrices of known constants and the $\alpha_i$'s are independent $m_k \times 1$ vectors of independent random variables with mean zero and variance $\sigma_i^2$. An expansion of $\log E[\exp\{\varepsilon_k\}|\mathcal{F}_t]$ as above (retaining only the first significant terms) gives an approximation to the intensity process for the $i^{th}$ individual in the $k^{th}$ family as

$$Y_{ik}(t)\lambda_0(t)\exp\{Z_{ik}^T(t)\beta + X_{ik}^T(t)\theta\} \tag{2.6}$$

with $X_{ik}(t)$ a q-vector whose $j^{th}$ element is given by

$$\sum_{\ell=1}^{S} [N_{\ell k}(t^-) - \int_0^{t^-} Y_{\ell k}(s)\exp\{Z_{\ell k}(s)\beta\}d\Lambda_0(s)]V_{j\ell k}^T V_{jik}$$

where $V_{j\ell k}^T$ denotes the $\ell^{th}$ row of the matrix $V_{jk}$. The elements of $X_{ik}(t)$ may be interpreted as the weighted average over family members of observed deviations from the expected failure history where the weights are taken to be the contribution to the expected correlation between individual j and other family members by each of the random effects.

## PARAMETER ESTIMATION

In this section, we will propose a method for estimating parameters in the random effects models described above. A large sample distribution theory will be outlined for these estimators. A formal description of this theory will be presented elsewhere. We consider models for the intensity process of the $i^{th}$ individual in the $k^{th}$ block given by

$$Y_{ik}(t)\lambda_0(t)\exp\{Z_{ik}(t)\beta + X_{ik}(t;\theta,\beta,\Lambda_0)\} \tag{3.1}$$

where $X_{ik}$ is restricted to depend on $\Lambda_0$ through functions of the form

$$\int_0^t \sum_{j=1}^{S} w_{ijk}Y_{jk}(s)\exp\{Z_{jk}(s)\beta\}d\Lambda_0(s) \quad . \tag{3.2}$$

Note that in Clayton and Cuzicks' model, $X_{ik}(t;\theta,\beta,\Lambda_0)$ is given by $\log\{(1+\theta\bar{N}_k(t))/(1+\theta\bar{\Lambda}_k(t))\}$.

We will restrict the time-dependent covariates to be step-functions on a fixed, finite partition of the interval [0,1] and will consider only right censoring. With these restrictions, (3.2) may be rewritten as a linear function of $\Lambda_0$.

If $\Lambda_0$ were known, then $\beta$ and $\theta$ in model (3.1) could be estimated using standard partial likelihood techniques provided $X_{ik}$ is continuously differentiable with respect to $\beta$ and $\theta$. Specifically, these estimators could be defined as solutions to the score equations

$$0 = (SB)^{-1}\int_0^1 \sum_{i=1}^{S}\sum_{k=1}^{B}\left(U'_{ik}(t) - \frac{\sum_{j=1}^{S}\sum_{\ell=1}^{B} Y_{j\ell}(t)\exp\{Z_{j\ell}(t)\beta + X_{j\ell}(t;\theta,\beta,\Lambda_0)\}U'_{j\ell}(t)}{\sum_{j=1}^{S}\sum_{\ell=1}^{B} Y_{j\ell}(t)\exp\{Z_{j\ell}(t)\beta + X_{j\ell}(t;\theta,\beta,\Lambda_0)}\right)dN_{ik}(t) \tag{3.3}$$

where $U'_{ik}(t) = \frac{\partial}{\partial(\beta,\theta)}\,(Z_{ik}(t)\beta + X_{ik}(t;\theta,\beta,\Lambda_0))$. These equations are simply the partial likelihood score equations for general form relative models as described in Prentice and Self [11]. Since $\Lambda_0$ is not known, we propose augmenting the equations (3.3) by estimating equations for $\Lambda_0$ and thereby jointly estimating $\beta$, $\theta$ and $\Lambda_0$. Specifically, we propose using the estimating equations corresponding to the Nelson [8] estimator of $\Lambda_0$ given by

$$0 = \Lambda_0(t) - \int_0^t \frac{\sum_{i=1}^{S}\sum_{k=1}^{B} dN_{ik}(t)}{\sum_{j=1}^{S}\sum_{\ell=1}^{B} Y_{j\ell}(t)\exp\{Z_{j\ell}(t)\beta + X_{j\ell}(t;\theta,\beta,\Lambda_0)\}}, \quad t \in [0,1] \ . \tag{3.4}$$

Calculation of these estimators can be accomplished by iteration between equations (3.3) and (3.4). Given estimates of $\beta$ and $\theta$, equation (3.4) may be solved non-iteratively. After some simple modifications, computer programs that fit general relative risk regression models with time-dependent covariates can be used to perform these computations.

A large sample distribution theory for these estimators may be developed using techniques similar to those described in Tsai and Crowley [13]. First, the domain and range spaces of the score functions on the right-hand side of (3.3) and (3.4) are extended to be Banach spaces. Specifically, we take $(\beta,\theta,\Lambda_0)$ to be elements in the cartesian product of $\mathcal{R}^q$ equipped with the Euclidian norm (q is the sum of the dimensions of $\beta$ and $\theta$) and D[0,1] equipped with the supremum norm. The restrictions on the censoring and covariate processes described above are key in this extension.

Three conditions are then sufficient to demonstrate a Gaussian distribution of the estimators in large samples; i) the score functions on the right-hand side of (3.3) and (3.4), are continuously differentiable on a neighborhood of the true parameter values in

$\mathbb{R}^q \times D[0,1]$ and, at the true parameter values, this derivative is invertible, ii) the derivative of the score function converges uniformly on a neighborhood of the true parameter values to a function which is invertible at the true parameter values, and iii) the score functions evaluated at the true parameter values and scaled by $(SB)^{-\frac{1}{2}}$ converge to a Gaussian random variable in $\mathbb{R}^q \times D[0,1]$. Differentiability of the score functions follows from differentiability assumptions on $X_{ik}(t;\theta,\beta,\Lambda_0)$ with respect to $\theta$, $\beta$ and the function given in (3.2) together with the linearity of (3.2) and the chain rule for Fréchet derivatives. Conditions i) and ii) then follow from asymptotic stability and limiting regularity conditions for sample averages of a number of stochastic processes. Condition iii) follows under assumptions very similar to those described in Prentice and Self [11] which include finite interval, Lindeberg conditions and limiting stability and regularity of certain sample averages. The primary theoretical tools used in the proof of these results is the inverse function theorem and a martingale central limit theorem.

Under the conditions described above, the limiting values of estimators centered about the true parameter values and scaled by $(SB)^{-\frac{1}{2}}$ (denoted here simply as $\hat{\beta},\hat{\theta},\hat{\Lambda}_0$) are related to Gaussian random variables by equations of the form

$$\begin{bmatrix} Z_1 \\ \\ Z_2(t) \end{bmatrix} \doteq \begin{bmatrix} I\begin{pmatrix}\hat{\beta}\\ \hat{\theta}\end{pmatrix} + \int_0^1 \hat{\Lambda}(s)\,d\mu_1(s) \\ \\ A(t)\begin{pmatrix}\hat{\beta}\\ \hat{\theta}\end{pmatrix} + \hat{\Lambda}(t) + \int_0^t \hat{\Lambda}(s)\,d\mu_2(s,t) \end{bmatrix} \tag{3.5}$$

where $Z_1$ is a Gaussian random variable with mean zero and covariance matrix $I$ and $Z_2(t)$ is a Gaussian martingale with continuous sample paths which is independent of $Z_1$ and has variance function $V(t)$. The matrix $I$ is simply the covariance matrix of the scores for $\beta$ and $\theta$ which is given as the limiting value of

$$\int_0^1 \left[(SB)^{-1} \sum_{i=1}^{S} \sum_{k=1}^{B} Y_{ik}(t)\exp\{Z_{ik}(t)\beta + X_{ik}(t)\}\right]$$

$$\left[U'_{ik}(t) - \frac{\sum_{j=1}^{S}\sum_{\ell=1}^{B} Y_{j\ell}(t)\exp\{Z_{j\ell}(t)\beta + X_{j\ell}(t)\}U'_{j\ell}(t)}{\sum_{j=1}^{S}\sum_{\ell=1}^{B} Y_{j\ell}(t)\exp\{Z_{j\ell}(t)\beta + X_{j\ell}(t)\}}\right]^{\otimes 2} d\Lambda_0(t)$$

where for a vector $a = (a_1,\cdots,a_n)$, $a^{\otimes 2}$ denotes the matrix with

$(i,j)^{th}$ element $a_i a_j$. The vector $A(t)$ and variance function $V(t)$ are limiting values of the processes

$$\int_0^t \frac{\sum_{i=1}^{S} \sum_{k=1}^{B} Y_{ik}(w)\exp\{Z_{ik}(w)\beta + X_{ik}(w)\}U'_{ik}(w)}{\sum_{i=1}^{S} \sum_{k=1}^{B} Y_{ik}(w)\exp\{Z_{ik}(w)\beta + X_{ik}(w)\}} d\Lambda_0(w)$$

and

$$\int_0^t \frac{(SB)d\Lambda_0(w)}{\sum_{i=1}^{S} \sum_{k=1}^{B} Y_{ik}(w)\exp\{Z_{ik}(w)\beta + X_{ik}(w)\}} ,$$

respectively. The functions $\mu_1$ and $\mu_2$ are fairly complicated but estimable functions that are limiting values of sample averages of certain processes.

The invertibility of the limiting derivative of the score functions implies the existence of a matrix M and a measure $\phi$ such that $(\hat{\beta},\hat{\theta})$ may be written as

$$MZ_1 + \int_0^1 Z_2(t)d\phi(t) \quad . \tag{3.6}$$

Multivariate normality of $(\hat{\beta},\hat{\theta})$ follows immediately from this representation and calculation of the covariance matrix of $(\hat{\beta},\hat{\theta})$ from distributional properties of $Z_1$ and $Z_2(t)$ is straightforward. Derivation of explicit formulas for estimators of this covariance matrix is equivalent to obtaining explicit forms for the matrix M and measure $\phi$ in (3.6). This requires a representation for the solution of an integral equation and remains an open problem.

Finally, we note that there is no conceptual difficulty in extending this method of estimation to accommodate stratification of the baseline intensity. Additional score equations of the form (3.4) could be used to estimate the stratum specific baseline intensities and a representation for $(\hat{\beta},\hat{\theta})$ that is similar to (3.6) could be developed. Calculation of a covariance matrix for $(\hat{\beta},\hat{\theta})$ is slightly more complicated in this case because the score for $(\beta,\theta)$ and the scores for the stratum specific baseline intensities are no longer orthogonal. These covariances have a simple form, however, and are easily estimable.

## DISCUSSION

There is a wide variety of failure time regression problems which involve a dependence among failures that is most naturally described in terms of random effects. In some experiments, this type of dependence is induced by the design. For example, a randomized trial on smoking prevention in school children is currently being conducted at the Hutchinson Cancer Research Center in which school districts rather than individual children are randomized. This group randomization design will certainly induce dependence among group members that must be accommodated in the analysis of results from this Trial. Note that the methods described here permit the use of time to cigarette smoking or censorship data, and individual covariate data, in relative risk estimation. Random effects may also be used to model dependence among repeated events in a single study subject. For example, in the study of repeated infections in immunosuppressed patients, a model with a single random effect that represents an individual's underlying level of immunocompetence provides a reasonable alternative to the models described by Farewell [5]. In addition, random effects models can provide alternatives to the proportional hazards model in univariate problems.

The methods described have implications in the use of time-matched case-control studies to study familial aggregation of disease. The standard methodology for such studies as described in Prentice and Breslow [10] would prescribe a relative risk regression model which includes a 'family history' covariate. In most applications, this covariate is taken to be the number of relatives of the index case/control that are affected. If the familial aggregation is presumed to arise according to a random effects model, the "family history" covariate should be a contrast between the observed and expected disease history in the relatives possibly weighted by the degree of relation to the index case/control. Thus, the minimal information about family history obtained in such studies should include duration of disease free survival and disease incidence information on each family member. This information could then be combined with prior information about baseline incidence rates to construct a family history term in the relative risk function. Of course, in extremely rare diseases and in studies where the number of relatives is approximately the same for all index cases/controls, the expected disease history would make little contribution to the family history covariate and could be neglected.

In some case-control studies, more comprehensive information on relatives about disease history and risk factors is obtained. One use of this additional information is in calculating a more precise expected disease history for the "family history" covariate to be used in a traditional analysis of the data. Another more interesting possibility is in combining the information relating disease incidence to risk factors in the relatives with the information contained in the case/control contrasts in order to obtain more precise estimates of the effects of the putative risk factors. Finally, we note that it is possible to estimate the baseline disease rate from such a study. Given estimates of the other parameters in the relative risk process, the cumulative baseline hazard may be estimated by the Nelson estimator defined by equation (3.4) provided the index cases/controls are excluded from the summations. This may be a reasonable approach for estimating the age of onset curve even if the disease is rare, provided there is a strong familial aggregation.

There is still much work to do on the proposed method of estimation. There is a need to investigate their properties in finite samples. Presumably the approach to normality is slower than the usual partial likelihood estimators, however, the results from Clayton and Cuzick's [3] simulations comparing their method of estimation to parametric methods is encouraging. Sensitivity of the methods to the distribution of the random terms is another important question.

## REFERENCES

[1] O. AALEN. Nonparametric inference for a family of counting processes. Ann. Statist., 6, (1978), pp. 701-726.

[2] P.R. ANDERSEN and R.D. GILL. Cox's regression model for counting processes: a large sample study. Ann. Statist., 10, (1982), pp. 1100-1120.

[3] D. CLAYTON and J. CUZICK. Multivariate generalizations of the proportional hazards model. To appear, J.R. Statist. Soc. A, (1985).

[4] D.R. COX. Regression models and life tables (with discussion). J.R. Statist. Soc. B, (1972), pp. 187-220.

[5] V.T. FAREWELL. An application of Cox's proportional hazard model to multiple infection data. Applied Statist., 28, (1979), pp. 136-143.

[6] J.D. HOLT and R.L. PRENTICE. Survival analysis in twin studies and matched pair experiments. Biometrika, 61, (1974), pp. 17-30.

[7] J.D. KALBFLEISCH and R.L. PRENTICE. The Statistical Analysis of Failure Time Data. Wiley, New York, (1980).

[8] W. NELSON. Theory and applications of hazard plotting for censored failure data. Technometrics, 14, (1972), pp. 945-965.

[9] R.L. PRENTICE. Linear rank tests with right censored data. Biometrika, 65, (1978), pp. 167-179.

[10] R.L. PRENTICE and N.E. BRESLOW. Retrospective studies and failure time models. Biometrika, 65, (1978), pp. 153-158.

[11] R.L. PRENTICE and S.G. SELF. Asymptotic distribution theory for Cox-type regression models with general relative risk form. Ann. Statist., 11, (1983), pp. 804-813.

[12] R.L. PRENTICE, B. WILLIAMS and A.V. PETERSON. On the regression analysis of multivariate failure time data. Biometrika, 68, (1981), pp. 373-379.

[13] W. TSAI and J. CROWLEY. A large sample study of generalized maximum likelihood estimators from incomplete data via self-consistency. To appear, Ann. Statist., (1985).

# SECTION 4
## Relative and Absolute Risk Models

The two papers in this section pick up the topic of model form mentioned in Section Two, with an emphasis on additive and multiplicative models. Two distinct topics are discussed. Norman Breslow considers the use of mixture models in order to discriminate between, and more generally test the fit of, additive and multiplicative relative risk models. This work, including detailed worked examples, demonstrates that large numbers of subjects and disease events will typically be necessary to effect such discrimination. The importance of separating model departures due to relative risk form from departures due to the modelling of the 'marginal' relative risks for specific exposure variables is also brought out.

Duncan Thomas considers additive and multiplicative models not for the relative risk process, but for the disease rates themselves. Specifically, his multiplicative models are those in which the baseline rates, as a function of a suitable time variable, are acted upon multiplicatively by a function of covariates. In other words, his multiplicative models embody the class of relative risk models considered by other authors. In Thomas' additive models, on the other hand, the failure rate is the sum of the baseline rate (as a function of time) and a function of covariates. In view of the strong dependence of many chronic disease rates on age, which would often serve exactly or approximately as primary time variable, such additive models may not often be expected to yield descriptive models that are as simple as their relative risk counterparts. Nevertheless, the use of such models may provide additional insights into the data. Thomas describes some aspects of the fitting of such models. Such fitting requires the incorporation of external data if based on case-control data.

# Use of the Power Transform to Discriminate Between Additive and Multiplicative Models in Epidemiologic Research

*Norman Breslow*

Abstract. The Box-Cox power transform provides a convenient way to distinguish additive from multiplicative models for rates fitted to grouped cohort data, and additive from multiplicative relative risk functions fitted to grouped or continuous case-control data. The maximum likelihood calculations are programmed as a problem in iterated weighted least squares; by-products of those calculations are useful in assessing model stability and goodness-of-fit. The score test for the unknown exponent in the power transform coincides with Pregibon's goodness-of-link test for generalized linear models. An example shows that extensive data may be needed to reliably distinguish between such models.

## INTRODUCTION

Current approaches to the analysis of data from epidemiologic studies emphasize the fitting of explicit statistical models that express quantitatively the effects of risk factor exposure on disease incidence or mortality rates [6,13]. There has been a steady trend away from conventional linear or log-linear regression analyses towards the use of more flexible model structures [20,24], some of them suggested by mathematical theories of the disease process [15,26]. There has also been a growing realization that the new models may have certain undesirable statistical properties, and that model equations having substantially different mechanistic interpretations may give rather similar fits to the observed data.

This paper explores some possible uses of the power transformation as a means of adding flexibility to model equations now used to analyze data from both cohort and case-control studies. Originally proposed by Box and Cox [3], this transformation has a long history of

---

Department of Biostatistics, SC-32; University of Washington; Seattle, Washington, 98195. This work was supported in part by USPHS grants 5 K07-CA00723 and 1 R01-CA40644 from the National Cancer Institute.

use in applied statistics and remains a subject of keen theoretical interest [1,11]. It is employed here in conjunction with the maximum likelihood fitting of Poisson regression models to cohort data [10] and logistic regression models to case-control data [19]. Much of the material consists of an elaboration and extension of the work of McCullagh and Nelder [14] with generalized linear models; see especially Section 10.3 of their book dealing with parameters in the link function. The further development and application of these ideas presented here, largely by means of example, is intended mainly to stimulate discussion about the potential value of the approach.

## ABSOLUTE RISK ESTIMATION WITH COHORT DATA

Table 1 presents data reported by Rothman and Boice [21] from the Doll and Hill [9] study of mortality among British doctors. The data may be represented as a sequence of I=10 observations $(d_i, n_i, \underset{\sim}{x}_i)$ where $d_i$ are the number of coronary deaths in the $i^{th}$ category, $n_i$ the person-years denominators and $\underset{\sim}{x}_i$ a vector of explanatory variables, here age and smoking status. Note that the ratios of age-specific rates $d_i/n_i$ for smokers vs. nonsmokers generally decline with advancing age, whereas the rate differences increase. This suggests that neither the linear (constant rate differences) nor log-linear (constant rate ratio) models will provide an adequate summary of the effect of smoking on the age-specific rates, but that the smoking effect might be constant if expressed on some intermediate scale. The power transformation offers this flexibility.

As a model for the data we suppose that the $d_i$ have independent Poisson distributions with means $\mu_i = n_i h(\eta_i;\lambda)$ where $\eta_i = \underset{\sim}{x}_i \underset{\sim}{\beta}$ is the linear predictor and h is the inverse of a link function g that we assume depends upon a parameter $\lambda$. The power family of link functions will be written either in the simple form

$$g(\mu_i/n_i;\ \lambda) = (\mu_i/n_i)^{\lambda} = \eta_i \qquad (1)$$

or in a continuous version that contains both linear ($\lambda$=1) and log-linear ($\lambda$=0) models

$$g(\mu_i/n_i;\ \lambda) = \frac{(\mu_i/n_i)^{\lambda} - 1}{\lambda} = \eta_i. \qquad (2)$$

For some purposes we will want to think of the Poisson means $\mu_i$ as a function of $\underset{\sim}{\beta}$ alone for fixed $\lambda$ and for others as a function of both $\underset{\sim}{\beta}$ and $\lambda$, in which case $\lambda$ will simply be taken as the last component of an augmented parameter vector $\underset{\sim}{\beta}$.

TABLE 1.
Death Rates From Coronary Disease Among British Male Doctors[a]

| Age | Person-years Non Smokers | Person-years Smokers | Coronary Deaths Non Smokers | Coronary Deaths Smokers | Death Rates[b] Non Smokers | Death Rates[b] Smokers | Rate Difference[b] | Rate Ratio |
|---|---|---|---|---|---|---|---|---|
| 35-44 | 18,790 | 52,407 | 2 | 32 | 0.11 | 0.61 | 0.50 | 5.73 |
| 45-54 | 10,673 | 43,248 | 12 | 104 | 1.12 | 2.40 | 1.28 | 2.14 |
| 55-64 | 5,710 | 28,612 | 28 | 206 | 4.90 | 7.20 | 2.30 | 1.47 |
| 65-74 | 2,585 | 12,663 | 28 | 186 | 10.83 | 14.69 | 3.86 | 1.36 |
| 75-84 | 1,462 | 5,317 | 31 | 102 | 21.20 | 19.18 | -2.02 | 0.90 |
| Totals | 39,220 | 142,247 | 101 | 630 | 2.57 | 4.43 | 1.86 | 1.72 |

[a]Source: Doll and Hill [9] as quoted by Rothman and Boice [13].
[b]Per 1,000 person-years

Since the Poisson is a member of the exponential family of distributions, maximum likelihood estimation using Fisher's method of scoring may be considered as a problem in iterated weighted least squares (IWLS) regression [8,10,12]. Specifically, if $\mu=\mu(\beta)$ denotes the mean of the observation vector $d$, and $V = V(\beta)$ is the diagonal variance matrix with diagonal elements $V_{ii} = \mathrm{Var}(d_i)$, then the change in the $\beta$ coefficient is given in terms of the score vector $S$ and information matrix $I$ as

$$\Delta\beta = I^{-1}S = \left(\frac{\partial\mu'}{\partial\beta} V^{-1} \frac{\partial\mu}{\partial\beta}\right)^{-1} \frac{\partial\mu'}{\partial\beta} V^{-1} (d - \mu) \qquad (3)$$

where the primes denote transpose. At each cycle of iteration one evaluates the fitted values $\mu(\hat{\beta})$, their derivatives and the variances $V(\hat{\beta})$ that occur on the right hand side of (3) using the estimate $\hat{\beta}$ from the preceding cycle. An initial estimate of $\beta$ is needed to start the process. Writing $\theta$ for the vector of canonical parameters in the exponential family, we have further that $\partial\mu/\partial\beta = (\partial\mu/\partial\theta)\times(\partial\theta/\partial\beta) = V\partial\theta/\partial\beta$. Thus (3) may be expressed

$$\Delta\beta = (Z'VZ)^{-1}Z'Vy, \qquad (4)$$

where $y$ with components $y_i = (d_i - \mu_i)/v_i$ is a vector of "dependent" variables, $Z = \partial\theta/\partial\beta$ is a "design matrix" and $V$ is a diagonal weight matrix with variances on the diagonal.

For the special case of the Poisson distribution we have $v_i = \mu_i$ and $\theta_i = \log(\mu_i)$. Thus for model (1) the covariable value $z_{ij}$ corresponding to the $j^{th}$ component of $\underset{\sim}{x}_i$ is $\partial\theta_i/\partial\beta_j = x_{ij}/\{\lambda(\mu_i/n_i)^\lambda\}$ while that corresponding to the exponent of the power transform is $\partial\theta_i/\partial\lambda = -(\mu_i/n_i)^\lambda \log(\mu_i/n_i)/\{\lambda(\mu_i/n_i)^\lambda\}$. From this it follows that, providing one already has an algorithm available for fitting the model with fixed $\lambda$, that same algorithm may be used to fit the model with unknown $\lambda$ by including in the model an additional "constructed" covariable $-(\mu/n)^\lambda \log(\mu/n)$ whose value is updated at each cycle of iteration [3].

As demonstrated by Pregibon [16-18] for certain special cases, a number of important diagnostic procedures developed for least squares regression analyses extend approximately into the maximum likelihood domain via the IWLS relationship (4). For example, the diagonal elements $h_i$ of the projection matrix

$$\underset{\sim}{H}^{\frac{1}{2}} = \underset{\sim}{V}^{\frac{1}{2}}\underset{\sim}{Z}(\underset{\sim}{Z}'\underset{\sim}{V}\underset{\sim}{Z})^{-1}\underset{\sim}{Z}'\underset{\sim}{V}^{\frac{1}{2}} \tag{5}$$

identify observations that have a large potential influence on the fitted model. They are also useful intermediaries in the calculations of other diagnostic indices. The "one-step" approximation to the change in the ML estimate resulting from deletion of the $i^{th}$ observation is given by borrowing the usual formula from linear model theory,

$$(\Delta\hat{\underset{\sim}{\beta}})_{-i} \approx -(\underset{\sim}{Z}'\underset{\sim}{V}\underset{\sim}{Z})^{-1}\underset{\sim}{z}_i y_i v_i/(1 - h_i).$$

Furthermore, the score test for the significance of q regression variables added to a model that already contains p such variables is obtained by comparing the residual sum of squares $\underset{\sim}{y}'\underset{\sim}{V}^{\frac{1}{2}}(\underset{\sim}{I} - \underset{\sim}{H})\underset{\sim}{V}^{\frac{1}{2}}\underset{\sim}{y}$ obtained at convergence under the reduced model, i.e. after solving the least squares problem

$$\underset{\sim}{y} = \underset{\sim}{Z}'_p\underset{\sim}{\beta}_p + \underset{\sim}{\varepsilon}, \qquad \underset{\sim}{\varepsilon} \sim (0, \underset{\sim}{V}^{-1}),$$

with the residual sum of squares from the augmented model

$$\underset{\sim}{y} = \underset{\sim}{Z}'_p\underset{\sim}{\beta}_p + \underset{\sim}{Z}'_q\underset{\sim}{\beta}_q + \underset{\sim}{\varepsilon}, \qquad \underset{\sim}{\varepsilon} \sim (0, \underset{\sim}{V}^{-1})$$

where all quantities are evaluated at $\hat{\underset{\sim}{\beta}}_p$, the MLE under the reduced model. Thus if a ML fit has been obtained for a specific value $\lambda_0$ of the exponent in the power transform, the score test of $\lambda = \lambda_0$ is obtained after one iteration of the IWLS procedure using the augmented variable $z(\lambda_0) = -(\hat{\mu}/n)^{\lambda_0}\log(\hat{\mu}/n)$. Pregibon [16] calls it a "goodness-of-link" test. For testing the goodness of link of the log-linear model ($\lambda = 0$) we need the more general form of the link function given by equation (2), in which case $z(0) = -\frac{1}{2}\log^2(\hat{\mu}/n)$. An important consideration that has motivated much of the theoretical development is that all of the relevant calculations are easily performed in an interactive environment using the flexible program GLIM [2].

## APPLICATION TO THE BRITISH DOCTORS DATA

Table 2, reproduced from an earlier analysis [5] of the Doll and Hill data shown in Table 1, show the results of three fits of the power model corresponding to three distinct values of $\lambda$. It is evident that an intermediate model with $\lambda = 0.55$, a value originally determined by trial and error so as to minimize the deviance, fits substantially better than either of the more commonly used structures. Likelihood ratio (deviance) tests of the linear and log-linear hypotheses are $7.43 - 2.14 = 5.29$ and $12.13 - 2.14 = 9.99$, respectively, while the corresponding score (goodness of link) tests are 5.30 and 10.77. Thus we reject both conventional models in favor of one where the effects of smoking are expressed (approximately) on a square root scale. Since the regression coefficient for smoking is approximately equal to $\frac{1}{2}$ when $\lambda$ is equal to $\frac{1}{2}$, one may conclude that, roughly speaking, smoking increases by 1/2 the square root of the age-specific coronary death rates when these are expressed in units of deaths per 1000 person-years.

Part C of Table 2 displays the diagonal elements $h_i$ of the "hat" matrix defined in equation (3). These quantities sum to 6, the number of estimated parameters, for each of the three models. Large values of $h_i$ identify observations that exert a high degree of "leverage" on the overall fit of the model. These quantities are related to the degree of change in $\hat{\underset{\sim}{\beta}}$, relative to its confidence ellipsoid, that would be occasioned by deletion of each observation. Part D of Table 2 examines the specific effect of each observation on the smoking parameter of interest. Since an "observation" here means a cell defined by age and exposure, one would expect cells with large numbers of person-years and/or large numbers of deaths to have high leverage, and this is evident in Table 2C. However, there are also some interesting contrasts between models. The youngest age category with few deaths and many person-years appears to have the greatest influence on parameters that represent rate differences, whereas the older age groups with many deaths and fewer person-years are of greatest importance in estimating rate ratios. Note that there is little change in the smoking coefficient when individual observations are deleted from the power model ($\lambda = 0.55$), which confirms its goodness-of-fit from another viewpoint.

Table 3 presents additional results for the situation where $\lambda$ is explicitly estimated. As indicated earlier, this is accomplished via the introduction into the regression analysis of a "constructed"

TABLE 2.
Parameter Estimates, Fitted Values and Regression Diagnostics for Three Statistical Models for the Data in Table 1

| | | Statistical Model[a] | | | | |
|---|---|---|---|---|---|---|
| | Additive ($\lambda=1$) | | Power ($\lambda=0.55$) | | Multiplicative ($\lambda=0$) | |
| Age Group | Nonsmokers | Smokers | Nonsmokers | Smokers | Nonsmokers | Smokers |
| | | A. Parameter Estimates ± SE[b] | | | | |
| Parameter | | | | | | |
| 35-44 $\alpha_1$ | 0.084±0.066 | | 0.276±0.092 | | -1.012±0.192 | |
| 45-54 $\alpha_2$ | 1.556±0.214 | | 0.839±0.100 | | 0.472±0.130 | |
| 55-64 $\alpha_3$ | 6.219±0.454 | | 2.180±0.121 | | 1.616±0.115 | |
| 65-74 $\alpha_4$ | 13.440±0.963 | | 3.583±0.173 | | 2.338±0.116 | |
| 75-84 $\alpha_5$ | 19.085±1.704 | | 4.487±0.253 | | 2.688±0.125 | |
| Smoking $\beta$ | 0.591±0.125 | | 0.493±0.098 | | 0.355±0.107 | |
| | | B. Fitted Values[c] | | | | |
| 35-44 | 1.59 | 35.37 | 1.81 | 32.53 | 6.83 | 27.17 |
| 45-54 | 17.51 | 96.50 | 13.00 | 102.56 | 17.12 | 98.88 |
| 55-64 | 35.99 | 197.25 | 29.26 | 204.49 | 28.74 | 205.26 |
| 65-74 | 34.96 | 178.73 | 30.12 | 183.61 | 26.81 | 187.19 |
| 75-84 | 28.03 | 105.07 | 24.97 | 108.65 | 21.51 | 111.49 |
| Goodness-of-fit (Deviance) $\chi^2_4$ | 7.43 | | 2.14 | | 12.13 | |
| | | C. Leverage of $i^{th}$ Observation ($h_i$) | | | | |
| 35-44 | 0.98 | 0.93 | 0.67 | 0.86 | 0.25 | 0.81 |
| 45-54 | 0.31 | 0.77 | 0.42 | 0.85 | 0.29 | 0.88 |
| 55-64 | 0.19 | 0.82 | 0.28 | 0.85 | 0.38 | 0.91 |
| 65-74 | 0.18 | 0.83 | 0.22 | 0.84 | 0.36 | 0.91 |
| 75-84 | 0.22 | 0.78 | 0.24 | 0.79 | 0.34 | 0.87 |
| | | D. Approximate Change in $\beta$ Coefficient for Smoking on Omitting Corresponding Observation | | | | |
| 35-44 | 0.855 | 0.855 | 0.026 | 0.026 | -0.060 | -0.060 |
| 45-54 | -0.058 | -0.058 | -0.021 | -0.021 | -0.072 | -0.072 |
| 55-64 | -0.020 | -0.020 | -0.010 | -0.010 | -0.012 | -0.012 |
| 65-74 | -0.008 | -0.008 | -0.010 | -0.010 | 0.018 | 0.018 |
| 75-84 | 0.002 | 0.002 | 0.023 | 0.023 | 0.138 | 0.138 |

[a] Exponent ($\lambda$) of Power Function Relating Death Rates and Linear Predictor
[b] Person-years denominators expressed in units of 1,000.
[c] See Table 1 for observed values

variable $-(\mu/n)^{\lambda}\log(\mu/n)$ in addition to the five variables representing age effects and one variable representing smoking. The values of this constructed variable depend on the fitted values $\underset{\sim}{\mu}$ and the unknown parameter $\lambda$ and hence change at each cycle of iteration. At convergence, the regression coefficient corresponding to the constructed variable is the maximum likelihood estimate of $\lambda$.

The middle columns of Table 3 show the leverages $h_i$ for each observation for the model when $\lambda$ is estimated from the data. They thus sum to 7 rather than 6 as in Table 2. The last column shows the specific effects on the estimate of $\lambda$ from deletion of each observation. Note the decrease in $\hat{\lambda}$ towards additivity that accompanies deletion of data for the oldest age group, which had the most aberrant rate difference (Table 1), and the increase in $\hat{\lambda}$ when the youngest group is eliminated.

TABLE 3.
Parameter Estimates and Regression Diagnostics for Fitting the Power Model with Unknown Exponent to the Data in Table 1.

| PARAMETER | REGRESSION COEFFICIENTS ± STAND. ERROR | LEVERAGE ($h_i$) Non Smokers | Smokers | APPROXIMATE CHANGE IN $\hat{\lambda}$ Non Smokers or Smokers |
|---|---|---|---|---|
| Age 35-44 | 0.276 ± 0.178 | 0.94 | 0.97 | 0.183 |
| 45-54 | 1.115 ± 0.128 | 0.46 | 0.86 | 0.015 |
| 55-64 | 2.457 ± 0.702 | 0.47 | 0.89 | 0.028 |
| 65-74 | 3.861 ± 1.532 | 0.37 | 0.87 | 0.038 |
| 75+ | 4.766 ± 2.131 | 0.34 | 0.82 | -0.084 |
| Smoking | 0.493 ± 0.158 | | | |
| Exponent ($\lambda$) | 0.550 ± 0.144 | | | |

The 50% increase in the estimated standard error for the smoking coefficient when $\lambda$ is estimated from the data stems from the high correlation between $\hat{\lambda}$ and $\hat{\underset{\sim}{\beta}}$ and reflects the fact that the quantitative estimate of the smoking effect depends heavily on the scale of measurement. It does not imply that there is any greater uncertainty about the role of smoking *per se*. In conventional regression analyses, a high degree of correlation between estimated parameters would be indicative of model instability. It would suggest that one attempt to fix the values of one or more of the parameters on *a priori* grounds so as to reduce the uncertainty. Our suggestion here is to explore the goodness-of-fit for a variety of $\lambda$ and then, within the range of values that provide a reasonable fit, select one value for presentation of results on the basis of ease of interpretation (e.g. $\lambda=\frac{1}{2}$ in the example). Since the $\beta$ coefficients for different values of $\lambda$ are not comparable, it is appropriate to disregard the fact that $\lambda$ may have been estimated from the data when constructing confidence limits and tests for the $\beta$ parameters [4,11]. This contrasts with the situation when regression coefficients for two exposure variables are highly correlated due to a high degree of confounding. Then the uncertainty reflected in large standard errors is an appropriate warning that the data are insufficient to determine which of the two exposures are related to disease, or if they are both so related. Here the uncertainty has more to do with what is the best scale for achieving additivity of smoking and age effects, rather than with the magnitude of those effects per se.

## RELATIVE RISK ESTIMATION WITH CASE-CONTROL DATA

Case-control studies provide information about the ratio of incidence or mortality rates $R(\underset{\sim}{x})$ for persons who have a given set of exposures $\underset{\sim}{x}$ relative to those with a standard set of exposures ($\underset{\sim}{x}=0$). In a stratified analysis, the relative risk function $R(\underset{\sim}{x})$ is often assumed to be constant across strata, i.e. to act multiplicatively on background rates that are specific for age, calendar year or other factors used for matching or stratification of the case-control sample. However, this assumption may be relaxed by incorporation in $\underset{\sim}{x}$ of interaction terms involving both exposure and stratification variables. The data are represented as a series of I binomial observations $(r_i, n_i, s_i, \underset{\sim}{x}_i)$ where $r_i$ denotes the number of cases, $n_i$ the total of cases + controls, $s_i$ is a stratum indicator ($s_i = 1,\ldots,J$), and $\underset{\sim}{x}_i$ is a vector of covariables (including nuisance or stratum factors) that is constant for cases and controls in a given cell. If the covariables are continuous, then each cell as determined by a particular set of covariate values contains only one case or one control so that $n_i=1$ for all i.

The logistic disease incidence model for stratified data is written

$$\text{logit pr}(\text{"case"}|s_i, \underset{\sim}{x}_i) = \theta_i = n\alpha_{s_i} + \log R(\underset{\sim}{x}_i) \tag{6}$$

where the $\alpha_j$ are J unknown stratum parameters and the parametric form of the relative risk function has yet to be specified. It is well known that the fitting of this model to separate samples of cases and controls drawn at random from within each of the J strata yields asymptotically valid inferences about parameters in the relative risk function [19]. The model is widely employed with $R(\underset{\sim}{x}) = \exp(\underset{\sim}{x}'\beta)$, in which case the different risk factor effects combine multiplicatively not only with background but also with each other [6]. It has been demonstrated that the combined effects of alcohol and tobacco on oral and laryngeal cancer [22,27] and of asbestos and tobacco on lung cancer [23] are of this form. However, use of alternative model structures, in particular an additive relative risk of the form

$R(\underset{\sim}{x}) = 1 + \underset{\sim}{x}'\underset{\sim}{\beta}$, has been growing. Thomas [24] proposed discriminating between them by embedding them in the more general family of models $\log R(\underset{\sim}{x}) = \alpha\underset{\sim}{x}'\underset{\sim}{\beta} + (1-\alpha)\log(1+\underset{\sim}{x}'\underset{\sim}{\beta})$, where $\alpha$ is an unknown mixture parameter. Breslow and Storer [7] adapted the Box-Cox power transform for a similar purpose by defining

$$\log R(\underset{\sim}{x}) = \begin{cases} \dfrac{(1+\underset{\sim}{x}'\underset{\sim}{\beta}) - 1}{\lambda}, & \lambda \neq 0 \\ \log(1+\underset{\sim}{x}'\underset{\sim}{\beta}), & \lambda = 0 \end{cases} \tag{7}$$

so that the additive relative risk model occurs at $\lambda=0$ and the multiplicative one at $\lambda=1$.

Since the binomial distribution is a member of the exponential family with $\theta_i = \text{logit } p_i$ as the canonical parameter, the general theory set out in Section 3 also applies in this setting. Maximum likelihood estimation is accomplished via IWLS with "dependent" variables $y_i = (r_i - np_i)/v_i$, a diagonal "weight" matrix $\underset{\sim}{V}$ with variances $v_i = n_i p_i q_i$ on the diagonal, and a design matrix $\underset{\sim}{Z}$ whose entries are of the form $\partial\theta_i/\partial\alpha_j = 1$ or $0$ according as $s_i = j$ or not, $\partial\theta_i/\partial\beta_k = z_{ik}\{1+\underset{\sim}{x}_i\underset{\sim}{\beta}\}^{\lambda-1}$, and $\partial\theta_i/\partial\lambda = \lambda^{-2}\{\lambda(1+\underset{\sim}{x}_i\underset{\sim}{\beta})^{\lambda}\log(1+\underset{\sim}{x}_i\underset{\sim}{\beta}) - (1+\underset{\sim}{x}_i\underset{\sim}{\beta})^{\lambda} + 1\}$ ($\frac{1}{2}\log^2(1+\underset{\sim}{x}_i\underset{\sim}{\beta})$ when $\lambda=0$) if the exponent $\lambda$ is to be estimated from the data. All the preceding results concerning regression diagnostics and score tests for additional parameters, including goodness of link tests for $\lambda$, continue to apply.

## APPLICATION TO ILLE-ET-VILAINE DATA

Breslow and Storer [7] present three examples of the use of the transform (7) with case-control studies having both stratified and matched samples of cases and controls. Probably the most striking of these is their re-analysis of grouped data on esophageal cancer risk as related to alcohol-tobacco consumption in Ille-et-Vilaine [25]. Although these data had earlier been used to provide a textbook example of a multiplicative relationship [6], in fact the additive relative risk model fits equally well. Table 4 reproduces these findings with a grouping of age in six strata and alcohol/tobacco consumption in four levels each. The deviances are quite close over a range of $\lambda$ that encompasses both additive and multiplicative combination of relative risks. Nevertheless, the estimated risk ratio for heavy smokers and drinkers vs. light or non-smokers and light drinkers varies by a factor of two between the two models. Moreover, they have very different mechanistic interpretations. A particular drawback to the multiplicative model is the poor fit to the rather small number of cases in the critical baseline category. Application

TABLE 4
Comparison of Three Relative Risk Models Fitted to Stratified Data from the Ille-et-Vilaine Study of Alcohol, Tobacco and Esophageal Cancer*

| Alcohol (g/day) | Tobacco (g/day) | Total (cases + controls) | Cases Observed | Additive (λ=0) Cases Fitted† | Additive (λ=0) Relative Risk | Power (λ=0.33) Cases Fitted† | Power (λ=0.33) Relative Risk | Multiplicative (λ=1) Cases Fitted† | Multiplicative (λ=1) Relative Risk |
|---|---|---|---|---|---|---|---|---|---|
| 0-39 | 0-9 | 261 | 9 | 9.02 | 1.0 | 10.16 | 1.0 | 13.70 | 1.0 |
| " | 10-19 | 81 | 10 | 9.54 | 3.5 | 8.25 | 2.6 | 7.07 | 1.6 |
| " | 20-29 | 42 | 5 | 4.85 | 3.9 | 4.11 | 2.8 | 3.49 | 1.7 |
| " | 30+ | 28 | 5 | 7.40 | 15.1 | 6.41 | 11.1 | 4.78 | 5.2 |
| 40-79 | 0-9 | 179 | 34 | 33.31 | 7.2 | 31.45 | 5.9 | 30.96 | 4.2 |
| " | 10-19 | 85 | 17 | 18.33 | 9.7 | 19.32 | 9.3 | 18.86 | 6.6 |
| " | 20-29 | 62 | 15 | 15.29 | 10.1 | 16.20 | 9.9 | 16.02 | 7.0 |
| " | 30+ | 29 | 9 | 7.44 | 22.3 | 8.38 | 24.9 | 9.16 | 21.8 |
| 80-119 | 0-9 | 61 | 19 | 19.83 | 13.4 | 18.56 | 10.7 | 17.83 | 7.2 |
| " | 10-19 | 49 | 19 | 18.93 | 15.9 | 19.86 | 15.4 | 19.92 | 11.3 |
| " | 20-29 | 16 | 6 | 6.19 | 16.3 | 6.55 | 16.2 | 6.67 | 12.1 |
| " | 30+ | 12 | 7 | 5.03 | 28.5 | 5.82 | 36.1 | 6.59 | 37.3 |
| 120+ | 0-9 | 24 | 16 | 17.05 | 83.5 | 16.37 | 62.5 | 15.51 | 36.6 |
| " | 10-19 | 18 | 12 | 12.10 | 86.0 | 12.12 | 77.5 | 12.15 | 56.8 |
| " | 20-29 | 12 | 7 | 6.70 | 86.4 | 6.75 | 79.7 | 6.86 | 61.0 |
| " | 30+ | 13 | 10 | 9.00 | 98.6 | 9.69 | 134.6 | 10.47 | 188.7 |
| | | | | Goodness-of-fit statistics (DF=76) | | | | | |
| Deviance | | | | 82.32 | | 80.51 | | 82.77 | |
| | | | Chi-square | 79.49 | | 80.11 | | 88.18 | |

*Data from Tuyns et al. [25] as reported by Breslow and Day [6], Appendix I
†All estimates are adjusted for age in six strata

of the goodness of link tests by incorporation of the constructed covariables $\frac{1}{2}\log^2(1 + \underset{\sim}{x}'\hat{\underset{\sim}{\beta}})$ or $(1 + \underset{\sim}{x}'\hat{\underset{\sim}{\beta}})\{\log(1 + \underset{\sim}{x}'\hat{\underset{\sim}{\beta}})-1\}$ in the corresponding model equation yields $\chi_1^2 = 1.49$ and $\chi_1^2 = 1.60$, respectively. The regression coefficients of these variables are 0.24 and -0.70. Thus "first step" estimates of $\lambda$ are $\hat{\lambda} = 0.24$ starting from the additive model and $\hat{\lambda} = 0.30$ starting from the multiplicative model. These may be compared to the maximum likelihood estimate $\hat{\lambda} = 0.33$.

In their analysis of original data records from Ille-et-Vilaine, Breslow and Day (1) demonstrated that a satisfactory fit under the multiplicative model was achieved with two continuous exposure variables, $x_1$ = ALC and $x_2$ = log(TOB+1), where ALC denotes the reported daily consumption of alcohol (here expressed in units of 100 gm/day) and TOB is the amount of tobacco (gm/day). These analyses were repeated for this paper using a slightly different data set such that the one case and 117 controls under the age of 35 years were excluded and the remaining subjects were grouped into three age strata (35-54, 55-64 and 65+ years) instead of six. A series of models specified by equations (6) and (7) was fit with three stratum parameters ($\alpha$), two continuous regression variables $x_1$ and $x_2$, and various values for the exponent $\lambda$.

Figure 1 graphs the deviances obtained when $\lambda$ varies from 1.2 towards 0. In contrast to the situation with the grouped data, the minimum value of $\lambda$ was achieved at $\lambda$=0.67 with a deviance only 0.65 units away from that for the multiplicative model. The fit rapidly grew worse for smaller $\lambda$ and it proved impossible to achieve convergence with values of $\lambda$=0.1 or smaller. The estimated parameters and fitted values shown in Table 5 indicate clearly what was happening. The model was starting to estimate infinite relative risks for both alcohol and tobacco as $\lambda$ moved into the additive range. Stated another way, baseline risks for nondrinkers and nonsmokers (ALC=TOB=0), which are implicitly involved in the stratum parameters $\alpha$, were being estimated as 0. Investigation of the original data showed that there were in fact no cases among nonsmokers who consumed less than 25 grams of alcohol per day.

The standard errors of the parameter estimates shown in Table 5 consider $\lambda$ as a fixed variable. If instead it is explicitly estimated, we find $\hat{\lambda} = 0.670 \pm 0.291$, $\hat{\beta}_1 = 4.575 \pm 3.360$, and $\hat{\beta}_2 = 0.938 \pm 0.647$. Even though changes in $\lambda$ lead to markedly different estimates of $\underset{\sim}{\beta}$, a large range of ($\lambda$, $\underset{\sim}{\beta}$) give very nearly identical fits to these data. As already mentioned, however, we believe that it is not appropriate to attempt to account for the error of estimation in $\lambda$ when making inferences about $\underset{\sim}{\beta}$ since different values of $\lambda$ correspond to different scales of measurement and thus render the associated $\underset{\sim}{\beta}$ values incomparable.

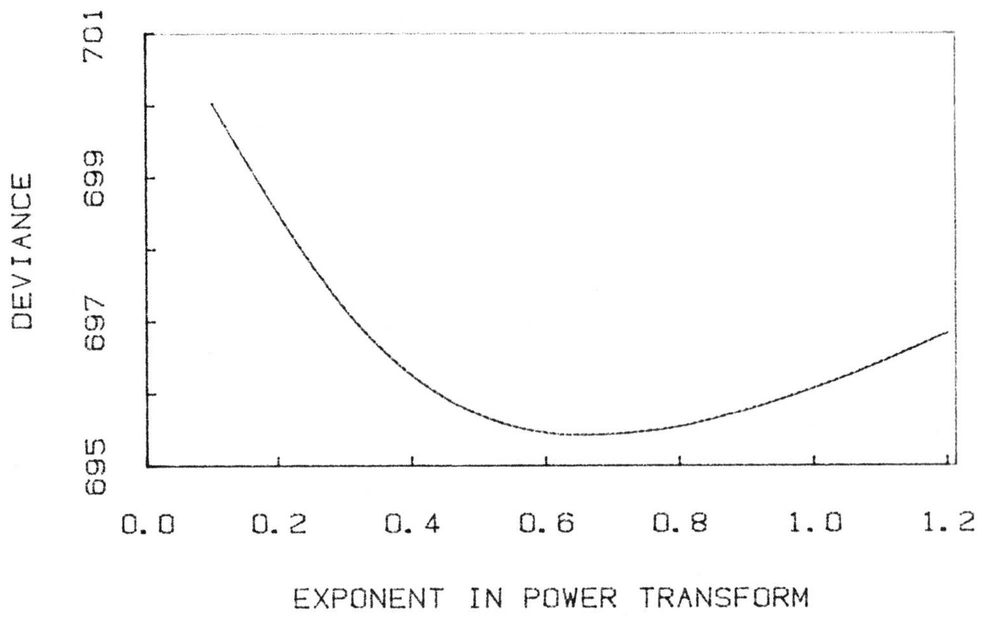


Figure 1. Deviances for fit of power model with continuous covariates to case-control data from Ille-et-Vilaine.

## CONCLUSIONS

Several conclusions may be drawn from our analysis of the Ille-et-Vilaine data. First, even with 200 cases and nearly 800 controls, the data are still not extensive enough to determine whether the effects of alcohol or tobacco on the relative risk of esophageal cancer combine in an additive or multiplicative fashion. Part of the problem may be the fact that very few members of the population (and no cases) abstain completely from the use of alcohol and tobacco. The relative risk for the "baseline" category, nominally set to one in the analysis, is thus quite ill-determined. We plan to analyze additional data from studies carried out in neighboring areas of France so as to attempt to settle the issue.

The lack of information for the baseline category also contributes to the problems in achieving convergence with the power model for continuous exposure variables when $\lambda$ starts to approach zero. Had the sample been sufficiently large so that a few cases (and presumably a much larger number of controls) had been found among abstainers, there would have been less of a tendency for the model to attempt to estimate a zero risk for this category.

Finally, this analysis points up an inherent limitation in the use of the power transform in order to attempt to distinguish between additive and multiplicative combinations of relative risks with

TABLE 5.
Results of Fitting Power Transform Models to Continuous Data From Ille-et-Vilaine

MODEL (FIXED λ)

| | | λ=1 (muliplicative) | λ=0.670 (minimum deviance) | λ=0.20 (∿ additive) |
|---|---|---|---|---|
| **A. Deviance** | | | | |
| | | 696.07 | 695.42 | 698.51 |
| **B. Estimated Stratum Parameters (α)** | | | | |
| Age group | | | | |
| 35-54 | | -4.719 | -5.354 | -10.047 |
| 55-64 | | -3.646 | -4.293 | -9.014 |
| 65+ | | -3.131 | -3.773 | -8.502 |
| **C. Regression Coefficients ± Standard Errors** | | | | |
| ALC/100 | | 2.507 ± 0.236 | 4.575 ± 0.588 | 120.23 ± 55.64 |
| LOG(TOB+1) | | 0.523 ± 0.092 | 0.938 ± 0.186 | 24.91 ± 12.88 |
| **D. Fitted Relative Risks** | | | | |
| ALC (gm/day) | TOB (gm/day) | | | |
| 0 | 0 | 1.0 | 1.0 | 1.0 |
| | 20 | 4.9 | 8.9 | 1007.1 |
| | 40 | 7.0 | 13.8 | 1623.7 |
| 40 | 0 | 2.7 | 4.5 | 362.7 |
| | 20 | 13.4 | 26.8 | 3398.9 |
| | 40 | 19.0 | 38.0 | 4742.0 |
| 80 | 0 | 7.4 | 14.8 | 1786.3 |
| | 20 | 36.5 | 71.7 | 8224.9 |
| | 40 | 51.8 | 98.6 | 10669. |
| 120 | 0 | 20.3 | 41.8 | 5087.0 |
| | 20 | 99.5 | 177.8 | 16639. |
| | 40 | 141.3 | 238.9 | 20640 |

continuous data. This is the fact that varying the exponent $\lambda$ changes the shapes of the individual relative risk functions as well as the manner in which those effects combine. This problem does not arise when the exposure variables are grouped into four or five categories each and separate parameters are estimated for each one relative to baseline, for then the effects of individual exposures are unconstrained whatever the value of $\lambda$. Thomas [24] presents a good discussion of this point. As a model for the relative risk of joint exposure to two quantitative variables $x_1$ and $x_2$, he suggests

$$R(x_1,x_2) = [1+x_1\beta_1 + x_2\beta_2]^{1-\lambda}[(1+x_1\beta_1)(1+x_2\beta_2)]^{\lambda}. \quad (8)$$

This has the desirable feature that $R(x_1,0) = (1+x_1\beta_1)$ and $R(0,x_2) = (1+x_2\beta_2)$, whatever the value of $\lambda$. Further work is needed on other models that separate the issue of the appropriate dose-response curves for exposure to individual agents from the issue of the appropriate scale on which to combine their effects.

## REFERENCES


[1] AC ATKINSON, Diagnostic tests for transformations, Technometrics (1985), (to appear).

[2] RJ BAKER and JA NELDER, The GLIM System: Release 3, Numerical Algorithms Group, Oxford, (1978).

[3] GEP BOX and DR COX, An analysis of transformations, J Roy Statist Soc, B 26 (1964), pp. 211-52.

[4] GEP BOX and DR COX, An analysis of transformations revisited, rebutted, J Amer Statist Assoc 77 (1982), pp. 209-10.

[5] NE BRESLOW, Cohort analysis in epidemiology, IN A Celebration of Statistics, (1985). Atkinson AC and Fienberg SE, Eds., Springer, New York, pp. 109-43.

[6] NE BRESLOW and NE DAY, Statistical Methods in Cancer Research I: The Analysis of Case-Control Studies, International Agency for Research on Cancer, Lyon, 1980.

[7] NE BRESLOW and BE STORER, General relative risk functions for case-control studies, American Journal of Epidemiology 122, (1985), pp. 149-62.

[8] C COX, Generalized linear models - the missing link, Appl Statist 33, (1984), pp. 18-24.

[9] R DOLL and AB HILL, Mortality of British doctors in relation to smoking: Observations on coronary thrombosis, National Cancer Institute Monograph 19 (1966), pp. 205-68.

[10] EL FROME, The analysis of rates using Poisson regression models, Biometrics 39 (1983), pp. 665-74.

[11] DV HINKLEY and G RUNGER, The analysis of transformed data (with discussion), J Amer Statist Assoc 79 (1984), pp. 302-20.

[12] JORGENSEN S, The delta algorithm and GLIM, Int Statist Rev 52 (1984), pp. 283-300.

[13] DG KLEINBAUM, LL KUPPER and H MORGENSTERN, Epidemiologic Research: Principles and Quantitative Methods, Lifetime Learning Publications, Belmont CA, 1982.

[14] P MCCULLAGH and JA NELDER, Generalized Linear Models, Chapman and Hall, London, 1983.

[15] SH MOOLGAVKAR and AG KNUDSON, Mutation and cancer. A model for human carcinogenesis, J Natl Cancer Instit 66 (1981), pp. 1037-52.

[16] D PREGIBON, Goodness of link tests for generalized linear models, Appl Statist 29 (1981), pp. 15-24.

[17] D PREGIBON, Logistic regression diagnostics, Annals of Statistics 9 (1981), pp. 705-24.

[18] D PREGIBON, Score tests in GLIM with applications, IN GLIM 82: Proceedings of the International Conference on Generalized Linear Models. Lecture Notes in Statistics 14, (1982). Gilchrist R, Ed., Springer-Verlag, New York, pp. 87-97.

[19] RL PRENTICE and R PYKE, Logistic disease incidence models and case-control studies, Biometrika 66 (1979), pp. 403-11.

[20] RL PRENTICE and S SELF, Asymptotic distribution theory for Cox-type regression models with general relative risk form, Annals of Statistics 11 (1983), pp. 804-13.

[21] KJ ROTHMAN and JD BOICE, Epidemiologic Analysis with a Programmable Calculator, NIH Publication 79-1649, Washington, US Government Printing Office, 1979.

[22] KJ ROTHMAN and AZ KELLER, The effect of joint exposure to alcohol and tobacco on risk of cancer of the mouth and pharynx, J Chronic Diseases 23 (1972), pp. 711-6.

[23] R SARACCI, Asbestos and lung cancer: An analysis of the epidemiological evidence on the asbestos-smoking interaction, Int J Cancer 20 (1977), pp. 323-31.

[24] DC THOMAS, General relative risk models for survival time and matched case-control analysis, Biometrics 37 (1981), pp. 673-86.

[25] AJ TUYNS, G PEQUIGNOT and OM JENSEN, LE CANCER DE L'OESOPHAGE EN ILLE-ET-VILAINE EN FONCTION DES NIVEAUX DE CONSOMMATION D'ALCOOL ET DE TABAC. DES RISQUES QUI SE MULTIPLIENT, Bull Cancer 64 (1977), pp. 45-60.

[26] AS WHITTEMORE and J KELLER, Quantitative theories of carcinogenesis, SIAM Review 20 (1978), pp. 1-30.

[27] EL WYNDER and IJ BROSS, A study of etiological factors in cancer of the esophagus, Cancer 14 (1961), pp. 389-413.

# Use of Auxiliary Information in Fitting Nonproportional Hazards Models

*Duncan C. Thomas**

Abstract. Alternatives to the proportional hazards model are considered, including models in which time and covariate effects combine additively, and models derived from the multistage theory of carcinogenesis. Such models can be fitted to cohort data without reference to external rates or parametric assumptions about the time dependence using the full likelihood by using the rates in the entire cohort. Some models may be fitted more easily by exploiting a factorization of the likelihood into the product of Cox's partial likelihood and a Poisson regression likelihood. In order to fit case-control data, external rates or control sampling fractions must be known. Applications to data on lung cancer in a cohort of Quebec asbestos workers are described.

## 1. INTRODUCTION

Cox's [1] proportional hazards model provides a means of drawing inferences about parameters describing covariate effects without requiring any assumptions about the effect of time (other than proportionality). Considering the generally strong and often complex dependence of the rates of most chronic diseases on age and to a lesser extent on calendar time, this is an important advantage. While there is considerable empirical support for the model, as reviewed by Breslow and Day [2, chapter 3], there are numerous examples where covariates and time do not act simply multiplicatively: an additive ("absolute risk") model is often advocated for radiation effects [3] and has been shown to fit lung cancer rates for nickel exposure better than a multiplicative model [4]; and indeed, the mere existence of "latent periods" guarantees that a simple multiplicative model will not apply unless a suitably lagged cumulative exposure variable is used as the covariate.

---

*Department of Preventive Medicine, University of Southern California, 2025 Zonal Avenue, Los Angeles, CA, 90033. This work was partially supported by NIH grants CA 17054 and CA 14089.

The term "proportional hazards models," includes any model that can be expressed in the form

$$h(t,\underset{\sim}{z}) = h_0(t)\, r[\underset{\sim}{z}(t),\underset{\sim}{\beta}] \tag{1}$$

where r depends on time t only through the action of time-dependent covariates, but is not an explicit function of t. A simple model which cannot be expressed in proportional hazards form is the additive model,

$$h(t,\underset{\sim}{z}) = h_0(t) + r[\underset{\sim}{z}(t),\underset{\sim}{\beta}],$$

where particular attention will be given to the linear-additive model,

$$h(t,\underset{\sim}{z}) = h_0(t) + \underset{\sim}{\beta}'\underset{\sim}{z}(t). \tag{2}$$

Another example is the multistage model

$$h(t,\underset{\sim}{z}) = t^{k-1} + \beta \int_0^t z(u)\, u^{i-1}\, (t-u)^{k-i-1}\, du \tag{3}$$

where z(u) is the intensity of exposure at time u, k is the number of stages, and i is the stage at which the carcinogen acts [5-7].

The line between proportional and nonproportional hazards models can be difficult to draw, however. For example, model (3) can be cast in proportional form if k is known:

$$h(t,z) = \alpha t^{k-1}\, [1 + \beta^* Z_{ik}(t)]$$

where $Z_{ik}(t) = \alpha t^{1-k} \int_0^t z(u)\, u^{i-1}\, (t-u)^{k-i-1}\, du,$

and $\beta^* = \beta/\alpha$, whereas if k is viewed as a nuisance parameter relating to the time dependence, then the requirement that r in equation (1) not be an explicit function of t no longer holds.

Aranda-Ordaz [8] has described a general family of models based on the Box-Cox transformation indexed by a single additional parameter $\lambda$ where $\lambda = 1$ reduces to the exponential multiplicative model and $\lambda = 0$ the linear-additive model. Methods of estimating $\lambda$ were described for grouped data. Unfortunately, for continuous covariates, this model confounds inferences about how time and covariate effects combine with inferences about the shape of dose-response relations and the interaction of covariates with each other. For this reason, mixture models along the lines described by Thomas [9] might be preferred.

In the next section, several ways the form of the time dependence might be specified are described. Section 3 compares the use of the full likelihood with a factorization into partial and Poisson likelihoods. Section 4 describes methods for fitting case-control data. Some applications to a nested case-control study in a cohort of Quebec asbestos workers are presented in the final section.

## 2. MODELS FOR TIME DEPENDENCE OF RISKS.

A general class of models for the joint effect of time and exposure can be constructed by considering functions of the form

$$h(t,\underset{\sim}{z}) = f\,[h_0(t,\underset{\sim}{\alpha}),\ r(z,\underset{\sim}{\beta})].$$

Thus, for example, a proportional hazards model is simply $f(x,y) = xy$ and an additive model is $f(x,y) = x + y$. The functions f, $h_0$ and r are assumed to be known and we wish to draw inferences about the parameters $\underset{\sim}{\alpha}$ and $\underset{\sim}{\beta}$. For proportional hazards models, use of Cox's partial likelihood obviates the need to specify $h_0$. For nonproportional models, the function $h_0$ must be specified, and in this section, three ways of doing so are considered.

2.1. Parametric models. The simplest method would be to specify $h_0$ as some parametric function involving one or more parameters to be estimated. For example, in fitting the multistage model, it would be natural to adopt the form

$$h_0(t,\underset{\sim}{\alpha}) = \alpha_0\, t^{\alpha_1 - 1}$$

where $\alpha_1 = k$, the number of stages in the process. Secular trends might be allowed for by estimating separate $\alpha_0$ coefficients in each birth cohort, though this might not be necessary if sufficient covariates were included. Whatever the choice, $h_0$ must be sufficiently general to allow a reasonable approximation to the true form without requiring an excessive number of nuisance parameters to be estimated.

2.2 External standards. If the form of the time dependence is thought to be complex, it may be preferable to use a set of external rates, say $h^*(t,u)$ where t now denotes age and u calendar year [10]. To control for possible selection bias or confounding factors that might make such external rates inapplicable to the population under study, one might consider multiplying these standard rates by a constant or function of time to be estimated, i.e.,

$$h_0(t,\underset{\sim}{\alpha}) = g(t,\underset{\sim}{\alpha})\, h^*(t,u)\ . \tag{4}$$

For example, to allow for the possible dilution of the "healthy worker effect" after selection into the cohort, one might select a model of the form

$$g(t,\underset{\sim}{\alpha}) = \exp\,[\alpha_0 + \alpha_1 (t-t_0)^{-\alpha_2}]$$

where $t_0$ is the age at first employment. Alternatively, Breslow and Langholz [11] have considered non-parametric methods of estimating g in the context of proportional hazards models.

Note that the function $g(t,\underset{\sim}{\alpha})$ must include adjustments for the average exposure of the reference population to any covariates included in the model. The form of the adjustment, however, depends on the form of the underlying model. For example, if cumulative smoking is included as a linear-multiplicative effect on $h_0$ and we wish to model the cohort rates as a constant multiple $\alpha$ of the reference population rates (adjusted for smoking), then it is natural to take $g(t,\alpha) = \alpha/[1 + \underset{\sim}{\beta}'\bar{\underset{\sim}{z}}(t,u)]$ where $\bar{\underset{\sim}{z}}(t,u)$ is the average value of the covariate in the reference population. This leads to the model

$$h(t,\underset{\sim}{z}) = \alpha h^*(t,u)\ [1 + \underset{\sim}{\beta}'\underset{\sim}{z}]\ /\ [1 + \underset{\sim}{\beta}'\bar{\underset{\sim}{z}}(t,u)].$$

On the other hand, if cumulative smoking is included as a linear-additive effect on $h_0$, then $g(t,u)$ becomes $\alpha - \underset{\sim}{\beta}'\bar{\underset{\sim}{z}}(t,w)/h_0(t,u)$ and the model is

$$h(t,z) = \alpha h^*(t,u) + \underset{\sim}{\beta}'[\underset{\sim}{z} - \bar{\underset{\sim}{z}}(t,u)]. \tag{5}$$

To the extent that g is in fact constant (or properly modelled if not), the use of external rates may improve the efficiency of the analysis. Breslow et al. [12] showed that for multiplicative models, the gain in efficiency is small unless the covariates are highly correlated with time; for additive models, Breslow [13] showed that the gain could be substantially larger.

2.3 Internal standards. Alternatively we could define a partition of the time scale into K intervals and assume that the rate was a constant within each interval, i.e.,

$$h_0(t,\underset{\sim}{\alpha}) = \alpha_k \quad . \qquad \tau_{k-1} < t \leq \tau_k$$

Thus, if $D_k$ denotes the number of failures in interval k and $T_k$ the total person-time in that interval, the rate in the total cohort would be $\bar{h}_k = D_k/T_k$. For example, in the linear-additive model (2), $h_0$ would then be given by

$$\hat{\alpha}_k = \bar{h}_k - \underset{\sim}{\beta}'\bar{\underset{\sim}{z}}_k \tag{6}$$

where $\bar{z}_k$ denotes the mean of $z_i(t)$ over the set $R(t)$ of subjects at risk at time t, averaged over the time interval. The additive model can therefore be expressed in the form

$$\hat{h}(t,\underset{\sim}{z}) = D_k/T_k + \underset{\sim}{\beta}'(\underset{\sim}{z} - \bar{\underset{\sim}{z}}_k) \ . \quad \tau_{k-1} < t \leq \tau_k \tag{7}$$

Equation (7) can be thought of as an intermediate step in an estimation process using the method of moments rather than maximum likelihood to estimate $\alpha_k$. An inherent difficulty with any additive model, however, is that it could lead to negative hazards for some subjects unless constraints were placed on $\underset{\sim}{\beta}$ or the model reformulated to set the hazard to zero in such cases; the latter would require redefinition of $\bar{z}_k$ so that the average hazard was still equal to $\bar{h}_k$.

This problem of negative hazards, when it arises, is simply a sign of model misspecification.

Another approach to incorporating internal standards, described by Holford [14], is to use maximum likelihood to estimate the $\alpha_k$ as functions of $\beta$ and then substitute these functions back into the likelihood to obtain a maximum relative likelihood [15] as a function only of $\beta$. When applied to multiplicative models, allowing the intervals to become infinitesimal, this approach leads directly to Cox's partial likelihood. For additive models, allowing the intervals to be defined by observed failure times, as done by Breslow [16] for proportional hazards models, leads to a likelihood that is linear with respect to $\beta$, so that $\hat{\beta}$ is infinite. The approach is applicable provided the number of intervals is kept small compared with the number of failures, but then requires iterative calculation to obtain $\alpha_k$ whereas equation (6) does not.

## 3. LIKELIHOOD CONSTRUCTION.

3.1 Full likelihood. The full likelihood is

$$L = \prod_{i=1}^{D} h[t_i, z_i(t_i)] \prod_{i=1}^{N} \exp\{-\int_0^{t_i} h[t, z_i(t)]\, dt\} \qquad (8)$$

where $i=1,\ldots,D$ are the failures and $i=D+1,\ldots,N$ the censored observations. Equation (8) can be used to estimate $\alpha$ and $\beta$ simultaneously. For example, under the linear-additive model with $h_0$ specified parametrically or using external standards (4), the likelihood becomes

$$L = \{\prod_{i=1}^{D} [h_0(t_i) + \beta' z_i]\}$$

$$\times \exp\{-\sum_{i=1}^{N} H_0(t_i) - \sum_{i=1}^{N} \beta' Z_i(t_i)\}$$

where $H_0(t) = \int_0^t h_0(u)\, du$ and $Z_i(t) = \int_0^t z_i(u)\, du$. For internal standards, substitution of (7) into (8) and rearranging terms produces

$$L = e^{-D} \prod_{k=1}^{K} \prod_{i=1}^{D_k} \{(D_k/T_k) + \beta'[z_i(t_i) - \bar{z}_k]\}. \qquad (9)$$

This likelihood is conditional on the $D_k$ and $T_k$ which were used in arriving at the internal standards, and as noted above is valid only for grouped data.

3.2. Conditional and Poisson likelihoods. Following an argument of Oakes [17], the full likelihood can be written as $L = L_1 L_2$, where

$$L_1 = \prod_{i=1}^{D} \frac{h[t_i, \underset{\sim}{z}_i(t_i)]}{\sum_{j \in R_i} h[t_i, \underset{\sim}{z}_j(t_i)]}$$

is Cox's partial likelihood and

$$L_2 = \prod_{i=1}^{D} \{ \sum_{j \in R_i} h(t_i, \underset{\sim}{z}_j(t_i)] \} \exp\{ -\sum_{i=1}^{N} H[t_i, \underset{\sim}{z}_i(t_i)] \} \tag{10}$$

is the probability of observing exactly one death at each of the observed times $t_i$. It may be more convenient to work with the grouped times, for which (10) is proportional to the Poisson probability of observing the $D_k$ deaths given the $T_k$ person-times at risk,

$$L = \prod_{k=1}^{K} e^{-E_k} E_k^{D_k} / D_k! \tag{11}$$

where $$E_k = \prod_{i=1}^{N} h[\tau_k, \underset{\sim}{z}_i(\tau_k)] \; T_{ik}.$$

and $T_{ik}$ is the contribution of subject i to the person-years in cell k.

This suggests that one should seek a separation of parameters into two sets which might be more efficiently estimated in one part or the other, even if the two sets are not independent. For example, in Cox's approach to the proportional hazards model, $\underset{\sim}{\beta}$ is estimated using $L_1$ and $h_0(t)$ is then estimated conditional on $\underset{\sim}{\beta}$ using $L_2$. A similar approach will sometimes be possible for nonproportional models.

Consider for example the linear-additive model using external standards (5). This model can be written in proportional form as

$$h(t, \underset{\sim}{z}) = [1 + \underset{\sim}{\beta}^{*\prime} \underset{\sim}{z}^*(t)] \, \alpha \, h^*(t) \tag{12}$$

where $\beta^* = \beta/\alpha$ and $z^*(t) = [z - \bar{z}(t)]/h^*(t)$. Since $h_0(t)$ is known with no unknown parameters (except the constant $\alpha$), $\underset{\sim}{\beta}^*$ can be estimated using $L_1$ and then $\alpha$ can be estimated using $L_2$. More complex functions $g(t,\alpha)$ could probably not be estimated efficiently without exploiting the information in the absolute rate, using the full likelihood.

Using internal standards, the partial likelihood $L_1$ is proportional to the expression derived in (9) by constraining the model to reproduce the average rate in the cohort as a whole.

Once $\underset{\sim}{\beta}^*$ has been estimated, $h_0$ can be computed directly from (6) without any need for further fitting.

## 4. CASE-CONTROL STUDIES.

For cohort data, there is probably little advantage to splitting the likelihood in the above way. However, considerable economy can be obtained by analyzing the data as a nested case-control study [12,13,18]. Thus $L_1$ would be applied to the case-control data to estimate covariate effects, and $L_2$ would then be used to estimate time effects, using the covariate information from the controls to estimate the cohort values and exploiting the known sampling fractions.

Consider for example the linear-additive model where a set of external rates is available. Again, provided we assume $g(t,\alpha)$ is a single constant $\alpha$, one could first estimate $\beta^*$ in (12) by applying the conditional likelihood $L_1$ to the case-control data, after having transformed the covariates from z to z*. The proportionality constant $\alpha$ can then be estimated from the Poisson likelihood (11) using the controls and person-years to estimate the cohort values. Thus, letting $C_k$ denote the total numbers of controls in interval K, $E_k$ becomes

$$E_k = (T_k/C_k) \sum_{i=1}^{C_k} h[t_i, \underset{\sim}{z}_i(t_i)].$$

The maximum likelihood estimate of $\alpha$ is therefore simply

$$\hat{\alpha} = D \Big/ \sum_{k=1}^{K} [h_k^* T_k + (\underset{\sim}{\beta}/C_k)' \sum_{i=1}^{C_k} \underset{\sim}{z}_i(\tau_k)] \qquad (13)$$

A slight refinement is possible by replacing the mean of $\underset{\sim}{z}$ over the controls by a weighted average of case and control means, exploiting the control sampling fractions; in practice, the difference is generally negligible.

To use internal standards with the linear-additive model (7), one would simply estimate $D_k/T_k$ from the full cohort and estimate $\underset{\sim}{z}_k$ from the weighted average of case and control values using the sampling fractions. As for cohort data, $h_0$ can then be estimated from (6).

This approach to fitting non-multiplicative models has obvious computational advantage over fitting the full cohort data on individuals. Breslow et al. [10,13] have advocated the use of Poisson regression techniques for grouped data as another means of reducing the computational burden; that approach, however, still requires that covariate information be assembled on the entire cohort, whereas the approach proposed here requires covariate information only on the cases and controls and only the distribution of person-years for the entire cohort. Another alternative would be to fit the model using a "case-cohort" analysis [19]; though the discussion of this design has so far been limited to proportional hazards models, this should be possible with more general models but would be somewhat more computationally intensive and complex than the approach proposed here.

The same approach could be applied to population-based case-control studies. Here the control sampling fractions are not known, but can be estimated from population rates. However, for this to be possible, it is necessary to assume that the population rates $h^*(t)$ apply exactly to a subject with covariate values equal to the mean of the controls, as the proportionality function g is no longer estimable. Fitting the model then proceeds directly from the conditional likelihood $L_1$.

## 5. APPLICATIONS.

In this section, the approaches described above are applied to a nested case-control study of lung cancer in Quebec asbestos workers [9,18,20-22]. The original cohort consisted of approximately 11,000 males born 1891-1920 who had worked for at least a month in the Quebec chrysotile mining and milling industry. Follow-up commenced one month after first employment and continued until death, loss to follow-up, or the end of 1975. The distribution of the 245 lung cancer deaths and person-years by age and calendar year is given in Table 1. For each lung cancer death, three controls were selected at random from those born in the same year who worked in the same mining area and outlived the case, thus effectively sampling from the person-years in Table 1. (To save space, the table is presented in ten-year intervals, but in the actual fitting, five year intervals were used.)

TABLE 1
Lung Cancer Deaths / Person Years in the Quebec Asbestos Mining Cohort

| Age | 1926-35 | 1936-45 | 1946-55 | 1956-65 | 1966-75 |
|---|---|---|---|---|---|
| 15-24 | 0/12,059 | 0/ 6,851 | --- | --- | --- |
| 25-34 | 0/26,783 | 0/23,750 | 0/14,850 | --- | --- |
| 35-44 | 0/11,016 | 2/28,509 | 2/30,618 | 1/17,296 | --- |
| 45-54 | --- | 0/10,979 | 2/28,576 | 16/30,606 | 11/16,751 |
| 55-64 | --- | --- | 10/10,019 | 32/24,432 | 47/26,570 |
| 65-74 | --- | --- | --- | 22/ 7,454 | 76/16,937 |
| 75-84 | --- | --- | --- | --- | 24/ 3,716 |

TABLE 2

DERIVATION OF SIMPLE MULTIPLICATIVE AND ADDITIVE RISK COEFFICIENTS

| Age | Years | Lung Cancer Deaths | | Person Years | Relative Risk | Excess Rate x $10^6$ | Average | | Excess Risk Coefficients | |
|---|---|---|---|---|---|---|---|---|---|---|
| | | Obs | Exp | | | | Dust | Smoking | Relative | Absolute |
| 20-54 | 1926-55 | 6 | 16.61 | 189,775 | 0.36 | -5.6 | 97 | 268 | -0.00656 | -0.06 |
| | 1956-65 | 17 | 17.09 | 47,902 | 0.99 | -0.2 | 168 | 520 | -0.00003 | 0.00 |
| | 1966-75 | 11 | 11.75 | 16,751 | 0.94 | -4.5 | 179 | 683 | -0.00036 | -0.02 |
| 55-64 | 1946-55 | 10 | 8.62 | 10,019 | 1.16 | 13.7 | 159 | 245 | 0.00100 | 0.09 |
| | 1956-65 | 32 | 33.87 | 24,432 | 0.94 | -7.7 | 243 | 581 | -0.00023 | -0.03 |
| | 1966-70 | 20 | 21.74 | 12,953 | 0.92 | -13.4 | 239 | 635 | -0.00033 | -0.06 |
| | 1971-75 | 27 | 25.99 | 13,617 | 1.04 | 7.5 | 246 | 711 | 0.00016 | 0.03 |
| 65-74 | 1956-65 | 22 | 16.20 | 7,454 | 1.36 | 77.9 | 204 | 584 | 0.00175 | 0.38 |
| | 1966-70 | 38 | 23.27 | 8,075 | 1.63 | 182.4 | 224 | 511 | 0.00281 | 0.81 |
| | 1971-75 | 38 | 30.91 | 8,862 | 1.23 | 80.0 | 235 | 634 | 0.00097 | 0.34 |
| 75-84 | 1966-75 | 24 | 13.63 | 3,716 | 1.76 | 279.1 | 184 | 464 | 0.00414 | 1.52 |
| Total | | 245 | 219.68 | 343,556 | 1.11 | 73.7 | 143 | 337 | 0.00081 | 0.52 |

We have previously described the fits of several general relative risk models to the case-control data [9,21,22]. These models investigate various hypotheses about the shape of the dose-response relationship, the form of the interaction between asbestos and smoking, and the effect of latency using time-weighted indices of "effective" exposure. Conditional on the choice of covariates, however, all these models assume that their effects are multiplicative on time. To test this hypothesis, interaction variables involving products of smoking and asbestos with various time-related variables were added to the multiplicative model, and a strong negative interaction of asbestos with age at risk was noted [22]. This suggested that asbestos might act more nearly additively on time, but such a model could not be fitted to the case-control data without knowledge of the underlying rates as described below. For this purpose, consideration is limited to the indices of cumulative asbestos and "cigarette-years" up to nine years before the death of the case described in earlier reports. Conclusions from this analysis might not apply to other forms of exposure indices.

Epidemiologists often explore the constancy of risks over time on additive and multiplicative scales by examining the excess relative and absolute risks per unit of exposure over various subgroups of the data, as illustrated in Table 2. The overall risk, relative to the U.S. rates used as the standard, is 1.11 leading to a relative risk slope coefficient for asbestos of 0.00081 (assuming smoking is similarly distributed in the cohort and the U.S. population). However, it is clear that the excess is confined to the older age groups, and the difference in excess risks cannot be explained simply by differences in cumulative exposure. Possibly a different choice of exposure index, or a joint examination of asbestos and smoking effects, might provide an explanation, but an obvious problem is the probable overestimation of expected deaths by the external rates, either because of lack of comparability of the U.S. and Quebec population rates or because of the "healthy worker" effect. To the extent that the expected deaths have been overestimated by a constant factor, all risk coefficients will be underestimated, but the degree of underestimation will be much greater in the low risk groups. There is no simple method to correct for this bias other than simultaneous estimation of $\alpha$ and $\beta$ coefficients, either by trial and error or by the regression techniques described here.

To illustrate how one might explore these effects systematically, the eight possible combinations of additive and multiplicative relations among the three factors asbestos (A), smoking (S), and time (T) were formalized for external standards as follows:

AST : $\alpha h_k^* (1 + \beta_1 A)(1 + \beta_2 S) / (1 + \beta_2 \bar{S}_k)$

(A+S)T : $\alpha h_k^* (1 + \beta_1 A + \beta_2 S) / (1 + \beta_2 \bar{S}_k)$

AT+S : $\alpha h_k^* (1 + \beta_1 A) + \beta_2 (S - \bar{S}_k)$

$$A{+}ST: \quad \alpha h_k^* (1 + \beta_2 S) / (1 + \beta_2 \bar{S}_k) + \beta_1 A$$

$$(A{+}T)S: \quad [\alpha h_k^* / (1 + \beta_2 \bar{S}_k) + \beta_1 A] (1 + \beta_2 S)$$

$$(S{+}T)A: \quad [\alpha h_k^* + \beta_2 (S - \bar{S}_k)] (1 + \beta_1 A)$$

$$AS{+}T: \quad \alpha h_k^* + [(1 + \beta_1 A)(1 + \beta_2 S) - 1 - \beta_2 \bar{S}_k]$$

$$A{+}S{+}T: \quad \alpha h_k^* + \beta_1 A + \beta_2 (S - \bar{S}_k)$$

Similar expressions were derived for use with internal standards. The $\tilde{\beta}$ coefficients were estimated (as $\beta$ *) from the case-control data using the conditional likelihood, recasting each in multiplicative form in the manner of equation (12). Using external standards, the $\alpha$ coefficients were then estimated from the deaths and person-years using the Poisson MLE in equation (13).

For all the models in which smoking acts additively on time, nonsmokers with low asbestos exposures and low baseline rates were estimated to have negative risks, thereby putting a constraint on the parameter space. In none of these models did iteratively reassigning such subjects to zero risk produce a likelihood that was remotely close to that obtained for multiplicative effects of smoking and time; the best fitting of these additive smoking models was A+S+T, which produced conditional and Poisson log likelihoods of -282.12 and -144.66 respectively with external standards. With internal standards, the estimates from the model AT+S were not constrained, but its likelihood was no better. Table 3 is therefore limited to those four models in which smoking and time combine multiplicatively. The fit of these four cannot be distinguished on the basis of the conditional likelihood. However, the two models in which asbestos acts additively on time produced far worse agreement between the numbers of observed and predicted deaths, as indicated by the Poisson likelihood. Basically, this model predicts far too many deaths at young ages and too few at older ages, as apparent from the descriptive statistics in Table 2. Though the differences between models AST and (A+S)T by each likelihood are small, both criteria slightly favor a multiplicative joint effect of asbestos and smoking over an additive one.

For multiplicative models, the standard rates do not enter into the fitting of the conditional likelihood, so no comparison of the two standards is possible. Using internal standards, constraints were needed for the model A+ST. The model (A+T)S produced an estimate of $\beta_1$ about one-third the value obtained using external standards and a substantially poorer likelihood.

TABLE 3
Comparison of Additive and Multiplicative Models for Asbestos (A), Smoking (S), and Time (T) Effects Using External Standards

| Model | Estimates (s.e.) | | | Log Likelihoods | |
|---|---|---|---|---|---|
| | Alpha | Asbestos | Smoking | Conditional* | Poisson+ |
| AST | .760 (.049) | .00185 (.00065) | .00251 (.00080) | -272.28 | -92.69 |
| (A+S)T | .853 (.055) | .00365 (.00177) | .00353 (.00145) | -273.74 | -93.27 |
| A+ST | .725 (.046) | 2.05# (0.74) | .00423 (.00172) | -271.92 | -130.69 |
| (A+T)S | .660 (.042) | 1.14# (0.45) | .00253 (.00080) | -272.77 | -133.62 |

* Null = -304.25
\+ Null = -56.31 (df=64)
\# Estimate is $\beta^*$ in units of rate per $10^6$ PY-A. To obtain $\hat{\beta}$, multiply $\hat{\beta}^*$ by $\hat{\alpha}$.

For all four models, the estimate of $\alpha$ is significantly less than unity, implying that risk coefficients derived by the simple method in Table 2 would be considerably underestimated. Rescaling the expected deaths by $\hat{\alpha}$ = 0.76 for the relative risk model and 0.66 for the absolute risk model increased these average risk coefficients by about three and four-fold respectively, but the tendency for both coefficients to increase strongly with age remained. Paradoxically, as noted above, there is a strong dose-response relationship with asbestos at ages less than 65, but few excess deaths, whereas at older ages, there is only a weak dose-response relation but many excess deaths. This anomaly remains unexplained, but suggests that cumulative asbestos exposure, even lagged nine years, is not the right covariate, or that some other factor needs to be considered.

In our search for more appropriate covariates, we have considered exposure indices based on the multistage model of carcinogenesis (amongst others). Because cases and controls had been age matched, it was not possible to estimate the number of stages k with any precision and this parameter was therefore fixed at 6, in accordance with the shape of the age incidence curve for the general population. We would therefore like to know if incorporation of either the person-years (internal standards) or the population rates (external standards), would improve the estimation of this parameter. Similar methods may prove useful and are currently being explored.

## REFERENCES

[1] D. R. COX, Regression models and life tables (with discussion), J. Roy. Statist. Soc., Ser. B, 34, (1972), pp. 187-220.

[2] N. E. BRESLOW and N. E. DAY, Statistical Methods in Cancer Research I: The Analyses of Case-Control Studies. International Agency for Research on Cancer, Publ. 32, Lyon, France, (1980).

[3] COMMITTEE ON THE BIOLOGICAL EFFECTS OF IONIZING RADIATION, The effects on populations of low levels of ionizing radiation. National Academy of Sciences, Washington DC, (1980).

[4] J. KALDOR, J. PETO, N. DAY, et al., Models for respiratory cancer in nickel workers. Submitted for publication.

[5] P. ARMITAGE and R. DOLL. Stochastic models for carcinogenesis, Proc. 4th Berkeley Symp. on Math. Statist. and Prob. 4, (1961), pp. 19-38.

[6] A. WHITTEMORE, The age distribution of human cancer for carcinogenic exposures of varying intensity, Am. J. Epidemiol. 106, (1977), pp. 418-432.

[7] D. C. THOMAS, Temporal effects and interactions in cancer: implications of carcinogenic models, in: Environmental Epidemiology: Risk Assessment (R. Prentice, A. Whittemore, eds. ), SIAM Institute for Mathematics and Society, Philadelphia, PA, (1981), pp. 107-121.

[8] F. J. ARANDA-ORDAZ, An Extension of the proportional-hazards model for grouped data, Biometrics, 39, (1983), pp. 100-107.

[9] D. C. THOMAS, General relative risk models for survival time and matched case-control analysis. Biometrics 37, (1981), pp. 673-686.

[10] G. BERRY, The analysis of mortality by the subject-years method. Biometrics 39, (1983), pp. 173-184.

[11] N. E. BRESLOW and B. LANGHOLZ. Estimation of relative mortality functions. J. Chron. Dis. (1986) in press.

[12] N. E. BRESLOW, J. H. LUBIN, P. MAREK, and B. LANGHOLZ. Multiplicative models and the analysis of cohort data, J. Am. Statist. Assoc. 78, (1983), pp. 1-12.

[13] N. E. BRESLOW, Cohort analysis in epidemiology, Univ. of

Washington, Dept. of Biostatistics, Tech. Rep. No. 65.

[14] T. R. HOLFORD, Life tables with concomitant information. Biometrics 32, (1976), pp. 587-597.

[15] J. D. KALBFLEISCH and D. A. SPROTT, Applications of likelihood methods to models involving large numbers of parameters, (with discussion). J. Roy. Statist. Soc., Ser. B, 32, (1970), pp. 175-208.

[16] N. E. BRESLOW, Contribution to the discussion of the paper by Cox [1] cited above.

[17] D. OAKES, Survival times: aspects of partial likelihood. Int. Statist. Rev. 49, (1981), pp. 235-264.

[18] F. D. K. LIDDELL, J. C. MCDONALD, and D. C. THOMAS, Methods of cohort analysis: appraisal by application to asbestos mining, (with discussion) J. Roy. Statist. Soc., Ser A, 140, (1977), pp. 469-491.

[19] R.L. PRENTICE, S. G. SELF, and M. W. MASON, Design options for sampling within a cohort, in: Modern Statistical Methods in Chronic Disease Epidemiology (S. Moolgavkar and R. Prentice, eds.), New York, Wiley, this volume, (1985).

[20] J. C. MCDONALD, F. D. K. LIDDELL,G. W. GIBBS, et al., Dust exposure and mortality in chrysotile mining, 1910-75. Br. J. Ind. Med. 37, (1980), pp. 11-24.

[21] D. C. THOMAS, Nonparametric estimationa and tests of fit for dose-response relations. Biometerics 20, (1983), pp. 263-268.

[22] D. C. THOMAS, Statistical methods for analyzing effects of temporal patterns of exposure on cancer risks. Scand. J. Work Environ. Health 9, (1983), pp. 173-184.

# SECTION 5
## Statistical Methods in Genetic Epidemiology

As mentioned above this conference sought to provide a forum for exchange of statistical methods between scientists concerned with genetic factors in relation to disease and scientists primarily concerned with environmental factors. The papers by Elston and Rice in this section provide a summary of certain key methods in genetic epidemiology, using terminology that is readily followed by the environmental epidemiologist.

Bob Elston describes methods used in segregation analysis using large pedigrees. Such analyses aim to identify and elucidate Mendelian inheritance in relation to disease occurrence. This presentation brings out the impact of ascertainment procedure on estimation and testing when studying sibships or other family data. It also points out the difficulty of distinguishing among competing genetic hypotheses while allowing for environmental factors, based on such data. For example, models that allow both monogenic and polygenic transmission as well as environmentally caused transmission from one generation to the next, may be fraught with serious identifiability problems. As Elston points out, segregation analysis provides only a first step to more detailed genetic analysis.

The paper by John Rice describes some basic approaches to partitioning the variation in a quantitative trial into genetic and environmental components based on family data. In the multifactoral model approach both genetic and environmental factors are assumed to act additively to determine a liability for a subject, which in turn relates directly to disease risk or other endpoint. Selected models for both the genetic and environmental components lead to correlation structures among family members which can be compared to available data. Some of the ideas of Section Three may provide valuable extensions of such methods by allowing the use of, possibly censored, time to disease endpoints, and by relaxing parametric assumptions.

# Modern Methods of Segregation Analysis

*Robert C. Elston*

Abstract. Classical segregation analysis was concerned with the detection of Mendelian inheritance by analyzing dichotomous variables observed on the members of sibships. Modern segregation analysis is similarly concerned with the detection of Mendelian inheritance, but the variables may be quantitative and they may be observed on members of larger family structures. Two general models that each subsume monogenic Mendelian inheritance as a special case have been proposed for hypothesis testing and parameter estimation, using likelihood methods. There are four components to each model: the joint genotypic distribution of mating individuals, the distribution of phenotype conditional on genotype, the distribution of offspring genotypes conditional on parental genotypes, and the mode of sampling from the population. These components are described for particular cases of each model, and a general formulation of the likelihood presented in terms of them. The advantages and disadvantages of the two models are discussed, and it is seen that they are largely complementary with respect to power and robustness. A more general model that combines features of both these models is thus more useful than either, but even such a model can falsely indicate the presence of a major gene.

## INTRODUCTION

Segregation analysis is concerned with the detection of Mendelian ratios due to the segregation of genes when they are transmitted from one generation to the next. Man has 22 pairs of homologous autosomal chromosomes and two sex chromosomes; genes on the sex chromosomes will not be considered in this paper. Genes occur in pairs in linear sequence along the homologous chromosomes, each pair occupying a locus. Different genes that occur at the same locus are termed alleles. Although each individual can have at most two different alleles at any one locus, more than two alleles can be present at a locus in the whole population. A parent transmits just one of the two alleles at any given

Department of Biometry and Genetics, Louisiana State University Medical Center, 1901 Perdido St., New Orleans, Louisiana 70112, U.S.A.
This work was supported in part by U.S. Public Health Service research grant GM 28356 from the National Institute of General Medical Sciences.

locus, chosen at random, independently to each offspring: this, essentially, is Mendel's "law of segregation."

The two alleles that an individual has at a given locus comprise the genotype at that locus, whereas an observed characteristic or trait is termed the phenotype. If variability of the phenotype in a family is caused by genotypic differences at a single locus, the phenotype is mongenic; if, on the other hand, it is caused by the segregation of genes at many loci, it is termed polygenic. Classical segregation analysis was largely concerned with the study of rare diseases, in which the phenotype is a dichotomous variable ("affected" versus "unaffected"), in an attempt to determine whether observed familial distributions are consistent with monogenic inheritance. Two special cases were commonly considered: dominant inheritance, in which the presence of a single abnormal allele in a individual is sufficient to produce the affected phenotype, and recessive inheritance, in which the presence of two abnormal alleles is necessary for an individual to be affected.

## CLASSICAL SEGREGATION ANALYSIS

Consider a rare autosomal dominant disease, due to the presence of the abnormal allele $\underline{A}$ that has a gene frequency q in the population; and let the normal allele be $\underline{a}$, with gene frequency 1-q. (The use of the word "frequency" where "proportion" or "probability" is meant is entrenched in the genetics literature). If there is random mating with respect to this locus, the three possible genotypes will be distributed in the population as follows:

$$\begin{array}{lccc} \text{genotype}: & \underline{AA} & \underline{Aa} & \underline{aa} \\ \text{frequency}: & q^2 & 2q(1-q) & (1-q)^2 \end{array} \quad . \tag{1}$$

Since q is small, virtually all affected individuals (who must have genotypes $\underline{AA}$ or $\underline{Aa}$) have genotype $\underline{Aa}$, and when these marry unaffected individuals ($\underline{aa}$), half their children will be affected and half unaffected. Thus, to test for autosomal dominant inheritance, we can observe the children of affected × unaffected matings and test whether the observations fit binomial distributions with p, the probability of a child being affected, equal to a half. The likelihood of observing r affected children in a family of s children is simply the binomial probability

$$\binom{s}{r} p^r (1-p)^{s-r} , \tag{2}$$

and if our sample is made up of independent families we can base inferences about p on the product of such quantities.

In the above example, the allele $\underline{A}$ is said to be dominant to the allele $\underline{a}$ (with respect to the phenotype being considered), reflecting the fact that $\underline{AA}$ and $\underline{Aa}$ individuals have the same phenotype. Let us now consider an autosomal recessive disease, but at the same time maintain the convention that a capital letter is used for a dominant allele. To do this we let a be the abnormal allele and A the normal one: thus aa individuals are affected, and AA and Aa individuals again have the same phenotype, but now they are unaffected. Thus for a rare recessive disease 1-q is small, and we see from (1) that virtually all the individuals who are capable of transmitting the abnormal allele have genotype Aa, and so are unaffected. It follows that for a rare recessive disease nearly all affected individuals arise as a result of Aa × Aa matings, which give rise to an affected child with probability $p=\frac{1}{4}$. We can therefore test for recessive inheritance by testing the null hypothesis $p=\frac{1}{4}$ in a sample of families in which the disease is segregating among the children, but neither parent is affected. It is, however, necessary to allow for the fact that a sample of such families does not consist of a random sample of all Aa × Aa matings: those Aa × Aa matings that by chance give rise to only unaffected children are certainly not part of the sample, and the probability that a family is sampled may depend upon the number of affected children it contains.

Let $\pi$ be the probability that an affected individual is ascertained and so brings the family into the sample. Such an individual is called a proband. Assuming independent ascertainments, the probability that a family with r affected children contains at least one proband, and so is sampled, is $1-(1-\pi)^r$. This multiplied by (2) is thus the joint probability that a sibship of size s from an Aa × Aa mating contains r affected children and is sampled, if p is the probability that an Aa × Aa mating gives rise to an affected child. Also, the probability that any sibship of size s from an Aa mating includes at least one proband, i.e., the probability that the sibship enters the sample, is $1-(1-\pi p)^s$. Thus the likelihood that the sibship contains r affected children and s - r unaffected children, conditional on it being sampled, is

$$\binom{s}{r} p^r (1-p)^{s-r} [1-(1-\pi)^r]/[1-(1-\pi p)^s] \ , \ r=1,\ 2,\ \ldots\ ,\ s\ , \qquad (3)$$

which can be thought of as the binomial probability (2) multiplied by a "correction for ascertainment." Again, for a sample of families independently ascertained in this way, the likelihood is a product of such terms, one for each family. In particular it should be noted that if $\pi=1$ the ascertainment is termed complete, and (3) becomes the truncate binomial

$$\binom{s}{r} p^r (1-p)^{s-r} \ /[1-(1-p)^s] \ , \ r=1,\ 2,\ \ldots\ ,\ s\ .$$

On the other hand, as $\pi \to 0$ we have what is called single ascertainment, and (3) becomes (noting $(1-\pi)^r \to 1 - r\pi$ and $(1-\pi p)^s \to 1 - s\pi p$)

$$\binom{s-1}{r-1} p^{r-1} (1-p)^{s-r} \ , \ r=1,\ 2,\ \ldots\ ,\ s\ .$$

The likelihood appropriate for complete ascertainment is also appropriate for any situation in which we have a random sample of all Aa x Aa matings with at least one affected offspring; and the likelihood appropriate for single ascertainment is also appropriate for any situation in which, for fixed s, the probability that a sibship enters the sample is proportional to the number of affected children it contains.

The above is a brief synopsis of classical segregation analysis. Further details and extensions of these approaches to the analysis of dichotomous traits in sibships can be found in various reviews (see, e.g., [6], [17], [18], [19], [21], [22] and [23]).

## GENERAL LIKELIHOOD FOR PEDIGREE DATA

Elston and Stewart [9] formulated the likelihood of data on a randomly chosen simple pedigree under various genetic models, allowing for a distribution of phenotypes that can be either discrete or continuous. (A simple pedigree was defined precisely using graph theoretic terms in [15]; basically, it is a pedigree that, for any two persons connected by marriage, contains a most one line of ascent to the previous generation). Later papers extended this approach to allow for complex pedigree structures and the ascertainment of pedigrees through probands (see e.g. [3], [8], [10], [15], and [24]). Here I shall outline the four major components of this general likelihood and indicate the two likelihood models that were initially suggested to test for monogenic segregation (see [7] for a more detailed review).

Let k be the number of different genotypes that affect the phenotype. If the phenotype is monogenic, k is equal to the number of different genotypes at the locus involved; and if just two alleles are involved, k=3. I shall use the lower case letter u to denote these genotypes. If the phenotype is polygenic, we assume that the number of loci involved is infinite and that the "polygenotype" is a normally distributed random variable. I shall use the capital letter G to denote genotype in this situation. In each case the subscripts F and M will denote the father and mother, respectively.

The first component of the general likelihood is the joint genotypic distribution of mating individuals. Let $\psi_u$ be the population frequency of genotype u. Then under random mating the distribution of the mating type $u_F \times u_M$ is $\psi_{u_F}\psi_{u_M}$, and for two alleles at one locus $\psi_{u_F}$ and $\psi_{u_M}$ are simply functions of the gene frequencies as indicated in (1). The distribution of the mating $G_F \times G_M$ under random mating is $\psi_{G_F}\psi_{G_M}$ $= \phi(G_F,\sigma_G^2)\phi(G_M,\sigma_G^2)$, using the notation

$$\phi(x,\sigma^2) = \frac{1}{\sigma\sqrt{2\pi}} \exp\left[-\frac{1}{2}\left(\frac{x}{\sigma}\right)^2\right] .$$

Thus both $G_F$ and $G_M$ are $N(0,\sigma_G^2)$, $\sigma_G^2$ being known as the genetic variance.

If the phenotype is determined partly by a finite number of genotypes and partly polygenically, and we assume these two components of the genotype are independently distributed, then the joint distribution of the mixed mating type $u_F G_F \times u_M G_M$ is

$$\psi_{u_F G_F} \psi_{u_M G_M} = \psi_{u_F} \phi\left(G_F, \sigma_G^2\right) \psi_{u_M} \phi\left(G_M, \sigma_G^2\right) .$$

The second component of the likelihood describes the relationship between phenotype and genotype. Let the distribution of phenotype z given genotype u be denoted by $g_u(z)$, given polygenotype G by $g_G(z)$, and given the mixed genotype uG by $g_{uG}(z)$. For example, suppose z is a dichotomous variable, 1=affected and 0=unaffected. Then for the simple recessive disease considered earlier, for which z=1 when u=<u>aa</u> and z=0 when u=<u>AA</u> or <u>Aa</u>, we have the three conditional distributions

$$\begin{aligned} g_{AA}(0) &= 1 & g_{Aa}(0) &= 1 & & & g_{aa}(0) &= 0 \\ & & & & \text{and} & & & \\ g_{AA}(1) &= 0 & g_{Aa}(1) &= 0 & & & g_{aa}(1) &= 1 . \end{aligned} \tag{4}$$

The fact that every probability is either 0 or 1 is expressed genetically by saying that the disease is fully penetrant (every <u>aa</u> individual is affected) and that there are no phenocopies (no <u>AA</u> or <u>Aa</u> individual is affected). In general, of course, the probabilities need not all be 0 or 1. For a polygenically determined dichotomy, it is usually assumed that $g_G(1)$ is a cumulative normal function of G, e.g.,

$$g_G(1) = \int_{-\infty}^{(G-\theta)/\sigma_E} \frac{1}{\sqrt{2\pi}} \exp\left(-\frac{1}{2}t^2\right) dt = \int_{-\infty}^{G} \frac{1}{\sigma_E\sqrt{2\pi}} \exp\left[-\frac{1}{2}\left(\frac{x-\theta}{\sigma_E}\right)^2\right] dx .$$

The parameter $\sigma_E^2$ is called the environmental variance, but whenever the phenotype is categorical we cannot assign unique values separately to the genetic and environmental variances; it is only their relative magnitudes that are relevant. In the case of the mixed genotype uG, $g_{uG}(1)$ is similarly modelled, but with the parameter $\theta$ made dependent on u. If z is a continuous variable, it is assumed that these conditional distributions are all normal; using $\theta$ to denote a mean, we set

$$g_u(z) = \phi(\theta_u - z, \sigma_E^2)$$

$$g_G(z) = \phi(G + \theta - z, \sigma_E^2)$$

$$\text{and} \quad g_{uG}(z) = \phi(G + \theta_u - z, \sigma_E^2) .$$

The environmental variance can also be made dependent on u, and both means and variances can, in theory at least, be made dependent on covariates such as sex and age.

The third component of the likelihood summarizes the transmission of genotypes from one generation to the next. Let $p_{u_F u_M u}$ be the probability that the mating type $u_F \times u_M$ gives rise to an offspring with genotype u. If this probability is Mendelian, we can express it as a function of a set of transmission probabilities, each defined as the probability that a parent of given genotype transmits a set of alleles, one from each locus. For two alleles at a single autosomal locus, for example, we define

$$\tau_{AA} = P\{\underline{AA} \text{ individual transmits A}\}$$
$$\tau_{Aa} = P\{\underline{Aa} \text{ individual transmits A}\}$$
$$\tau_{aa} = P\{\underline{aa} \text{ individual transmits A}\} .$$

Then under Mendelian inheritance $\tau_{AA} = 1$, $\tau_{Aa} = \frac{1}{2}$, $\tau_{aa} = 0$ and

$$\begin{aligned} p_{u_F u_M AA} &= \tau_{u_F} \tau_{u_M} \\ p_{u_F u_M Aa} &= \tau_{u_F}(1-\tau_{u_M}) + \tau_{u_M}(1-\tau_{u_F}) \qquad (5) \\ p_{u_F u_M aa} &= (1-\tau_{u_M})(1-\tau_{u_F}) . \end{aligned}$$

The analogous distribution for polygenic inheritance is

$$p_{G_F G_M G} = \phi\left(G-(G_F+G_M)/2, \sigma_G^2/2\right) ,$$

and for the mixed genotype we assume independent transmission of the components, so that

$$p_{u_F G_F \; u_F G_M \; uG} = p_{u_F u_M u} \, p_{G_F G_M G} .$$

The manner in which the pedigrees are sampled comprises the fourth and last component of the likelihood, and I shall consider just two sampling schemes - random sampling and the following method of sampling pedigrees through probands: there is a function of the phenotype, $\pi(z)$, that defines the probability that an individual becomes a proband and hence brings the whole pedigree into the sample. (In practice the probability of becoming a proband may also depend on other factors, such as age, race, or place of residence; see [8] for a suggested model to deal with these situations. In addition, pedigrees are sometimes sampled in stages - for example, second degree relatives of probands may be examined only if the intervening first degree relative is affected; a heuristic approach to analyzing such data has been presented in [13]). Returning to the example of a recessive disease, the derivation of (3) used the function

$$\pi(1) = \pi$$
$$\pi(0) = 0 \;. \tag{6}$$

Note, however, that (3) is the appropriate likelihood only if $\pi$ is known. If $\pi$ is an unknown parameter that has to be estimated, it is best estimated from the joint distribution of phenotypes and proband statuses in the sample. If the sibship of size s contains r affected children of whom t are probands, the joint likelihood, conditional on the sibship containing at least one proband, is

$$\binom{s}{r} p^r (1-p)^{s-r} \binom{r}{t} \pi^t (1-\pi)^{r-t} / [1-(1-\pi p)^s], \tag{7}$$

$$r=1,\ 2,\ \ldots\ ,\ s;\ t=1,\ 2,\ \ldots\ ,\ r.$$

Whenever $\pi(z)$ depends on unknown parameters it is preferable, in order to make maximum use of the information available in the sample, to base inferences on a joint likelihood of this nature [11]. To do this it will be convenient to define an ascertainment function $\alpha(z,b)$, the probability that an individual with phenotype z has proband status b (b=1 if the individual is a proband, b=0 if not), as follows:

$$\alpha(z,0) = 1 - \pi(z)$$
$$\alpha(z,1) = \pi(z) \;.$$

With the components defined as above, it is easy to write down an expression for the likelihood of any pedigree, however complex its structure, if only k genotypes are involved. But whether or not the expression can be simplified to make it computationally feasible, a subject I shall not go into here, depends very much on the complexity of the pedigree. For a pedigree of n individuals, let I be the set of individuals with both parents in the pedigree, and let M be the set of unrelated individuals "marrying into" the pedigree. We do not allow the possibility that an individual has just one parent in the pedigree, so that every individual is in either I or M. (This is not a real restriction, since we can always include a parent with a missing value of z assigned. A missing value anywhere in the pedigree is handled by the simple expedient of setting all g-functions for that individual equal to unity, reflecting the fact that such an individual's missing phenotype does not alter the likelihood.) Let the phenotype and genotype of the i-th individual be $z_i$ and $u_i$, respectively. Then the likelihood of a randomly sampled pedigree is simply

$$L_0 = \sum_{u_1=1}^{k} \sum_{u_2=2}^{k} \cdots \sum_{u_n=1}^{k} \prod_{i=1}^{n} p(u_i) g_{u_i}(z_i) \;, \tag{8}$$

where

$$p(u_i) = \begin{cases} P_{u_F\, u_M\, u_i} & \text{if } i \in I \\ \psi_{u_i} & \text{if } i \in M \end{cases}$$

and $u_F$ and $u_M$ are the genotypes of the parents of i. The summation is over the $k^n$ possible genotype combinations for the n individuals. If the pedigree is sampled via probands as indicated above, then $L_0$ is multiplied by a correction for ascertainment to become

$$L_0 \prod_{i=1}^{n} \alpha(z_i b_i) \ /(1-\beta) \ , \tag{9}$$

where $\beta$, the probability that the pedigree contains no probands (i.e., the probability that it is not sampled) is given by

$$\beta = \sum_{z_1} \cdots \sum_{z_n} L_0 \prod_{i=1}^{n} [1-\pi(z_i)] \ , \text{ if } z \text{ is discrete} \ ,$$

and

$$\beta = \int_{-\infty}^{\infty} \cdots \int_{-\infty}^{\infty} L_0 \prod_{i=1}^{n} [1-\pi(z_i)] \ dz_n \ \ldots \ dz_1 \ , \text{ if } z \text{ is continuous.}$$

These likelihoods correspond to the first model suggested by Elston and Stewart [9] to test for monogenic segregation. Their suggestion was to parametrize the Mendelian probabilities $p_{u_F u_M u_i}$ for two alleles at one locus in terms of the three transmission probabilities (5); then, under a model in which these transmission probabilities are arbitrary parameters lying between 0 and 1, test the null hypothesis that they are Mendelian - i.e.,

$$H_0 : \begin{cases} \tau_{AA} = 1 \\ \tau_{Aa} = \frac{1}{2} \\ \tau_{aa} = 0 \ . \end{cases} \tag{10}$$

Now consider a sibship of s children whose parents are both known to have genotype Aa; for this sibship the likelihood (8) becomes

$$\sum_{u_1=1}^{k} \sum_{u_2=1}^{k} \cdots \sum_{u_s=1}^{k} \prod_{i=1}^{s} p_{Aa\ Aa\ u_i} g_{u_i}(z_i) \ . \tag{11}$$

Assume further the distributions (4), appropriate for a fully penetrant recessive disease with no phenocopies, so that

$$p_{Aa\ Aa\ AA}\, g_{AA}(0) = p_{Aa\ Aa\ AA}$$
$$p_{Aa\ Aa\ Aa}\, g_{Aa}(0) = p_{Aa\ Aa\ Aa}$$
$$p_{Aa\ Aa\ aa}\, g_{aa}(1) = p_{Aa\ Aa\ aa}$$

and all other similar products in (11) are 0. It follows, noting that $\sum_u p_{Aa\ Aa\ u} = 1$, that (11) reduces to

$$p_{Aa\ Aa\ aa}^{r}(1-p_{Aa\ Aa\ aa})^{s-r} ,$$

where r is the number of affected (z=1) children. Apart from the constant multiplier, which is irrelevant, this is simply the binomial probability (2); and putting (from (5))

$$p_{Aa\ Aa\ aa} = (1-\tau_{Aa})(1-\tau_{Aa}) ,$$

we see that the null hypothesis $p_{Aa\ Aa\ aa} = \frac{1}{4}$ is identical to the null hypothesis $\tau_{Aa} = \frac{1}{2}$ . Thus we see that (8) and (10) comprise a generalization of classical segregation analysis. Similarly, if we assume the sampling scheme given by (6) and that there are t probands in the sibship, for this same situation (9) reduces to (7), apart from a constant multiplier.

The other model suggested by Elston and Stewart [9] is one in which there is both polygenic and monogenic inheritance, these components acting addditively, and under this model we test the null hypothesis that the monogenic component is absent. Provided none of the individuals in the pedigree is inbred, the likelihood under this model can be expressed, using the notation developed so far, as

$$L_m = \int_{G_1}\int_{G_2}\cdots\int_{G_n}\sum_{u_i=1}^{k}\sum_{u_2=1}^{k}\cdots\sum_{u_n=1}^{k}\prod_{i=1}^{n} p(u_i)f(G_i)g_{u_iG_i}(z_i) \qquad (12)$$

where

$$f(G_i) = \begin{cases}\phi\left[G_i-(G_F+G_M)/2,\sigma^2/2\right] & \text{if } i \in I\\ \phi(G_i,\sigma_G^2) & \text{if } i \in M ,\end{cases}$$

$G_F$ and $G_M$ are the polygenotypes of the parents of i, and $\int_{G_i}$ indicates the integral from $-\infty$ to $\infty$ of everything following it with respect to $G_i$. In this model it is assumed that the probabilities $p_{u_Fu_Mu_i}$ are Mendelian; and the likelihood for the null hypothesis that monogenic segregation is absent is simply the likelihood of the pedigree assuming pure polygenic inheritance, i.e.

$$L_p = \int_{G_1}\int_{G_2}\cdots\int_{G_n}\prod_{i=1}^{n} f(G_i)g_{G_i}(z_i) .$$

This model was called the "mixed model" by Morton and MacLean [20], who extended it by allowing for a sibling environmental correlation. More recently Lalouel and Morton [13] have eliminated the sibling environmental correlation from this model, but instead have allowed the ratio $\sigma_G^2/(\sigma_G^2+\sigma_E^2)$ , the polygenic heritability, to be generation-dependent.

## COMPARISON AND SYNTHESIS OF THE MODELS

Although both models have the same main purpose, the detection of monogenic segregation in family data, this purpose is achieved by very different means. In the first model, which has been called the generalized major gene model, monogenic segregation corresponds to the null hypothesis, which is accepted by default if it is not rejected. This can happen if the data contain insufficient information about the transmission probabilities, and to guard against this possibility one should check that the data contain sufficient information at least to reject the null hypothesis that there is no transmission from one generation to the next, i.e., $H_0 : \tau_{AA} = \tau_{Aa} = \tau_{aa}$ . In the mixed model, on the other hand, monogenic segregation is detected by rejecting a null hypothesis.

Since the generalized major gene model does not allow for the possibility of polygenic transmission, the presence of such a component may be interpreted by the model as the presence of monogenic segregation, or it may affect the estimated transmission probabilities to such an extent that a monogenic mechanism, acting in concert with a polygenic mechanism, is not detected. The mixed model does not have this disadvantage, but it does have the disadvantage that all transmission from one generation to the next is assumed to be either monogenic or polygenic: any environmentally caused transmission that is not confounded with a polygenic mechnism may therefore tend to be interpreted as monogenic segregation. The generalized major gene model, on the other hand, allows for a variety of environmental transmission mechanisms, especially if the transmission probabilities are allowed to be sex-dependent [4].

MacLean et al. [16] demonstrated by simulation studies that under the mixed model much more information is available if a quantitative trait is analyzed, rather than if the quantitative trait is first converted to a dichotomous phenotype by dividing the continuous distribution at a threshold value; and this can be expected to be true under the generalized major gene model as well. Unfortunately, however, this extra information is easily misinterpreted, because of the model's assumption that, conditional on the major genotype, the phenotype is normally distributed. An overall non-normal population distribution of the phenotype can only be accommodated under the mixed model by the presence of a monogenic mechanism, so that any such non-normality in the sample data will tend to be interpreted by this model as the presence of monogenic segregation. The generalized major gene model, on the other hand, can accommodate a population distribution that approximates a mixture of three normal distributions without assuming any transmission from one generation to the next. But any polygenic mechanism that gives rise to a non-normal population distribution will tend to be interpreted as a monogenic mechanism by either model; for this reason the scale on which the phenotype is measured, or how it is transformed prior to analysis, may be of crucial importance.

It is clear from the above discussion that in many respects the two models are complementary with respect to power and robustness. A more general model that combines features of both models can thus be expected to be more useful than either. Such a model has been proposed [2, 14]: the mixed model described above with the probabilities $p_{u_F u_M u_i}$ expressed as functions of unknown transmission probabilities. More recently Bonney [1] has proposed a similar model that avoids the computational problem caused by the integrals in (12). Initial experience with all these models is promising, but again there is the possibility that any polygenic mechanism that gives rise to a non-normal population distribution will be interpreted as monogenic segregation [5]. Transformation of the data to a dichotomy, or to make the overall sample distribution as normal as possible, will overcome this difficulty; but only at the expense of greatly reducing power to detect the presence of monogenic segregation. In any case it must be understood that there are limitations to making causal inferences from observational, as opposed to experimental, data [12]; for this reason segregation analysis should only be considered a first step, always to be followed by much more detailed genetic analysis.

## REFERENCES

1. G. E. BONNEY. On the statistical determination of major gene mechanisms in continuous human traits: regressive models, Am. J. Med. Genet. 18 (1984) pp. 731-749.

2. C. R. BOYLE. and R. C. ELSTON. Multifactorial genetic models for quantitative traits in humans, Biometrics 35 (1979) pp. 55-68.

3. C. CANNINGS, E. A. THOMPSON and M. H. SKOLNICK. Probability functions on complex pedigrees, Adv. Appl. Prob. 10 (1978) pp. 26-61.

4. F M. DEMENAIS and R. C. ELSTON. A general transmission probability model for pedigree data, Hum. Hered. 31 (1981) pp. 93-99.

5. L. J. EAVES. Errors of inference in the detection of major gene effects on psychological test scores, Am. J. Hum. Genet. 35 (1983) pp. 1179-1189.

6. R. C. ELANDT-JOHNSON. Segregation analysis: An overview, In Proceedings of the 8th International Biometric Conference, L. C. A. Corsten and T. Postelnicu (eds.), Constanta Romania, Academieii Republicii Socialiste Romania, pp. 313-323, 1974.

7. R. C. ELSTON. Segregation analysis, Adv. in Hum. Genet. 11 (1981) pp. 63-120.

8. R. C. ELSTON and E. SOBEL. Sampling considerations in the gathering and analysis of pedigree data, Am. J. Hum. Genet. 31

(1979) pp. 62-69.

9. R. C. ELSTON and J. STEWART. A general model for the genetic analysis of pedigree data, Hum. Hered. 21 (1971) pp. 523-542.

10. R. C. ELSTON and K. C. YELVERTON. General models for segregation analysis, Am. J. Hum. Genet. 27 (1975) pp. 31-45.

11. W. J. EWENS. Aspects of parameter estimation in ascertainment sampling schemes, Am. J. Hum. Genet. 34 (1982) pp. 853-865.

12. O. KEMPTHORNE. Logical epistemological and statistical aspects of nature-nurture data interpretation, Biometrics 34 (1978) pp. 1-23.

13. J. M. LALOUEL and N. E. MORTON. Complex segregation analysis with pointers, Hum. Hered. 31 (1981) pp. 312-321.

14. J. M. LALOUEL, D. C. RAO, N. E. MORTON and R. C. ELSTON. A unified model for complex segregation analysis, Am. J. Hum. Genet. 35 (1983) pp. 816-826.

15. K. LANGE and R. C. ELSTON. Extensions to pedigree analysis. I. Likelihood calculations for simple and complex pedigrees, Hum. Hered. 25 (1975) pp. 95-105.

16. C. J. MacLEAN, N. E. MORTON and R. LEW. Analysis of family resemblance. IV. Operational characteristics of segregation analysis, Am. J. Hum. Genet. 27 (1975) pp. 365-384.

17. N. E. MORTON. Segregation and linkage, In Methodology in Human Genetics, J. Burdette (ed.), Holden-Day, San Francisco, pp. 17-52, 1962.

18. N. E. MORTON. Models and evidence in human population genetics, In Genetics Today, S. J. Geerts (ed.), Proceedings of the XIth International Congress of Genetics, Pergamon Press, Oxford, pp. 935-951, 1964.

19. N. E. MORTON. Segregation analysis, In Computer Applications in Genetics, N. E. Morton (ed.), University of Hawaii Press, Honolulu, 129-139 (1969).

20. N. E. MORTON and C. J. MacLEAN. Analysis of family resemblance. III. Complex segregation analysis of quantitative traits, Am. J. Hum. Genet. 26 (1974) pp. 489-503.

21. C. A. B. SMITH. A test for segregation ratios in family data, Ann. Hum. Genet. 20 (1956) pp. 257-265.

22. C. A. B. SMITH. A note on the effects of method of ascertainment on segregation ratios, Ann. Hum. Genet. 23 (1959) pp. 311-323.

23. A. G. STEINBERG. Methodology in human genetics, J. Med. Educ. 34 (1959) pp. 315-334.

24. E. A. THOMPSON and C. CANNINGS. Sampling schemes and ascertainment, In The Genetic Analysis of Common Diseases: Applications to Predictive Factors in Coronary Heart Disease, C. F. Sing and M. Skolnick (eds.), Alan R. Liss, New York, pp. 363-382, 1979.

# Genetic Epidemiology: Models of Multifactorial Inheritance and Path Analysis Applied to Qualitative Traits

*John P. Rice*

Abstract. Methods used in Genetic Epidemiology to model familial resemblance are described. Emphasis is given to qualitative traits in which affection is based on an underlying continuous liability scale on which affected individuals correspond to those with deviant scores. The Multifactorial Model, in which genetic and environmental factors act additively to determine liability, is parameterized in terms of the correlations in liability between relatives and prevalences in males and females. Path analysis is used to partition the liability distribution into components and resolve the sources of familial resemblance. Approaches to take into account ascertainment (sampling families through affected individuals) and variable age of onset are outlined. The incorporation of ancillary covariates in the analysis of family data is considered. Finally, broader issues relating the assumptions and methods of Genetic Epidemiology to those of other approaches in the study of chronic diseases are discussed.

## INTRODUCTION

A consistent finding for many chronic diseases is that cases tend to cluster within families. In terms of risk prediction the presence of illness in family members can be more significant than even premorbid characteristics of the individuals themselves. For example, the relative risks for developing schizophrenia with one or both parents schizophrenic have been estimated to be 14 and 46, respectively, and to be 65 when an identical co-twin is schizophrenic [1]. Although geneticists tend not to consider familial clustering in terms of relative risks and odds ratios, strong associations underscore the rationale for the family as the unit of observation even when genetic hypotheses are not the major focus of investigation.

---

Department of Psychiatry and the Division of Biostatistics in the Department of Preventive Medicine, Washington University School of Medicine and The Jewish Hospital of St. Louis. Supported in part by USPHS grants MH-37685, MH-31302, MH-25430 and AA-03539.

The burgeoning field of genetic epidemiology [2-4] has focused on the inheritance of common disease in man. Inheritance is used in its broad sense to include both genetic and environmental (cultural) transmission. Cultural transmission results from parents imparting to their offspring certain customs and preferences concerning diet, attitude or social climate [5-12]. In addition, attention is given to shared environmental effects for, say, siblings who are reared contemporaneously, and who have increased similarity due to non-transmissible factors.

Recognizing that environments cannot be randomized (as in animal work), that family members share environmental as well as genetic sources of resemblance, and that a major goal in the analysis of common diseases is to quantify and understand environmental similarity, it is necessary to formulate complex models that include both genetic and nongenetic types of variation and that allow for ancillary biological and environmental covariates. This modeling has as its roots the traditions of quantitative genetics and multifactional inheritance that follow from the classical work of Fisher [13], rather than from the traditions of epidemiology. However, methods in the latter discipline are becoming more important in understanding the time-place clustering of disease within families.

In what follows, we emphasize one particular model used in genetic epidemiology (the Multifactorial Model) and discuss the differences and difficulties associated with a family study as compared to a random sample or case-control design. The article of Elston in this volume considers the single major locus model and the analysis of large pedigrees. Accordingly, we do not attempt to describe the myriad of models and approaches utilized in genetic epidemiology, but rather attempt to highlight a few basic approaches.

## LIABILITY/THRESHOLD CONCEPTS AND GENETIC MODELS

We assume that the observed trait (called the phenotype) is qualitative, and refer to individuals as affected or unaffected. Often, affected individuals may be subclassified as mild or severe, or subclassified according to clinical picture. It is assumed that there is a single continuous variable X, termed the liability to develop the disorder, on which all relevant genetic and environmental factors act additively.

In the basic formulation of the Multifactorial Model [14-17] it is assumed that X is normally distributed with mean 0 and variance 1, $X \sim N(0,1)$, and that there is a threshold S as in Figure 1A with individuals with liability scores above S being affected. Alternatively, there may be multiple thresholds [16] as in Figure 1B with individuals with scores between threshold values representing milder phenotypic classes of affection.

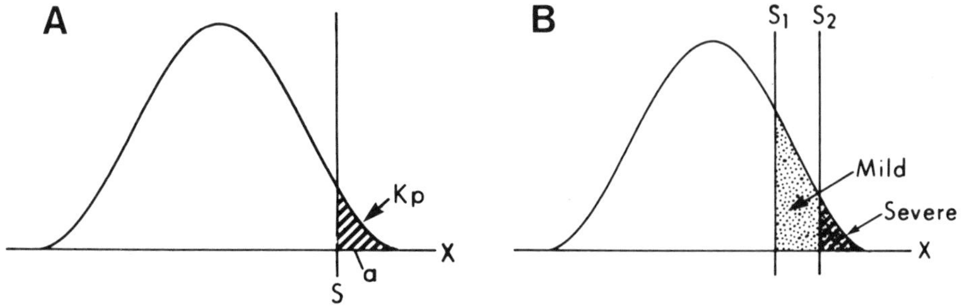


Figure 1. Liability distribution X with: (A) single threshold S and mean liability of affected individuals denoted by a; and (B) two thresholds $S_1$ and $S_2$ used to model severity.

With one threshold, the lifetime morbid risk K (also referred to as the "population prevalence" or simply "prevalence" in the genetics literature) is given by:

$$K = \int_S^{\infty} \phi(x)dx$$

where $\phi$ is the density of the standard normal random variable. The mean a and variance $\sigma^2$ of the liability of affected individuals are given by

$$a = \phi(S)/K$$

and

$$\sigma^2 = 1 - a(a-S).$$

The above concept of an abrupt threshold may be replaced by that of a risk function [17-18]. Let R(x) denote the probability that an individual with liability score x is affected. The prevalence in the population is then given by

$$K = \int_{-\infty}^{\infty} R(x)\,\phi(x)dx.$$

Note that the abrupt threshold model above can be formulated using a risk function which is a step function with $R(x) = 0$ if $x < S$, and $R(x) = 1$ if $x \geqslant S$.

Curnow and Smith [17] suggest a cummulative normal risk function $R(x) = \Phi\{(x-\mu)/\sigma\}$. Let $Z \sim N(\mu, \sigma^2)$ be independent from X and consider $Y = X + Z$. Then the probability that $Y > \mu$ equals the probability that $Z > (\mu - X)$, which is $\Phi\{(x-\mu)/\sigma\}$. That is, the abrupt threshold model for the variable Y is mathematically equivalent to the cummulative normal risk model for the variable X.

In the Multifactorial Model, familial resemblance is quantified by the correlations in liability between family members. As noted in the section on path analysis, these correlations may be parameterized in terms of the effects of genes alone (the polygenic model) or in terms of cultural transmission models. A key assumption is that the

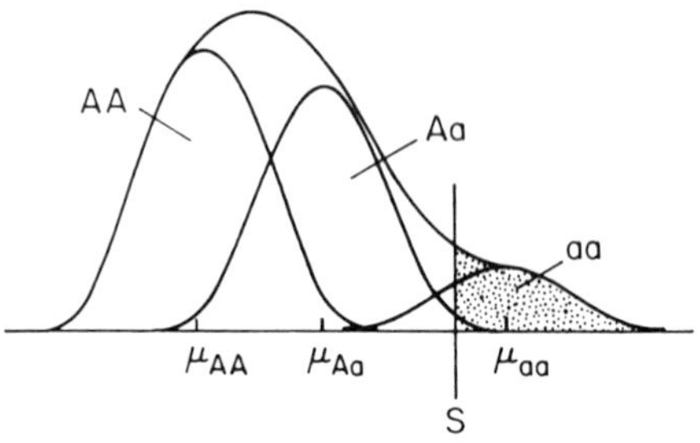


Figure 2. Liability distributions resulting from a single major locus with genotypic means $\mu_{AA}$, $\mu_{Aa}$, $\mu_{aa}$. Note the incomplete penetrance of the genotypes and the skewed composite distribution.

joint distribution in liability of family members is multivariate normal. Since X is unobserved it suffices that there is a transformation that achieves this.

One way that the normality assumption can fail is that there is a gene of major effect. That is, suppose there were a locus with two alleles, A and a, where locus refers to the position of a gene on a chromosome and allele refers to one of the alternative genes at that locus. Since humans have two copies of each (autosomal) chromosome, there are three possible genotypes: AA, Aa, aa. If the liability is the sum of effects due to this major gene g and a normally distributed residual $\xi$, $X = g + \xi$, then the distribution in the population will be as depicted in Figure 2.

Let q denote the frequency of the allele a in the population. Under the assumption of random mating, the genotypes will occur in the binomial proportions $(1-q)^2$, $2(1-q)q$, and $q^2$. The penetrances of the genotypes, $f_1$, $f_2$, $f_3$, are defined as the probability that individuals of genotypes AA, Aa, aa, respectively, are affected. Accordingly, the model is described in terms of the four parameters $q, f_1$, $f_2$, $f_3$. If $\xi$ is uncorrelated between family members, this model is referred to as the Single Major Locus (SML) Model [16,19-20]. Since the liability distributions of siblings, conditioned on parental genotypes, are assumed independent, the likelihood of a large pedigree may be computed in a straightforward manner. Moreover, Elston and Yelverton [21] included non-Mendelin transmission parameters to allow for a broad class of alternatives against which to test for a single locus.

The Mixed Model allows for a single major locus with a multifactorial background. Here we assume that the joint distribution of $\xi$ among family members, conditioned on their genotypes, is multivariate normal. In the model of Morton and McLean [22], the background was polygenic (although, they did allow for a common environment of rearing for siblings). Whereas, their approach was for nuclear families, Ott [23] described pedigree analysis for a polygenic background, but his approach is limited to small pedigrees (about size 10) by numerical considerations.

Lalouel and Morton [24] introduced the concept of a pointer, a person external to a nuclear family who leads to its ascertainment, and enables analysis of pedigrees by breaking them into their constituent nuclear parts. The non-Mendelian transmission parameters of Elston and Yelverton [21] have been incorporated into the Mixed Model [25] and a computer program POINTER is available which implements these procedures.

Accordingly, there are three basic models used in genetic epidemiology to model familial resemblance. The first is the Multifactorial Model in which the liability to manifest the disorder is the cumulative effect of many risk factors of small effect. The second is the Single Major Locus model in which there is a gene of major effect (in the sense that there is a wide separation in the mean liability of homozygous AA and aa individuals), and familial resemblance is accounted for by Mendelian transmission. However, there is environmental variation within a genotype that accounts for the reduced penetrance (i.e., not everyone with the same genotype has the same phenotype) of that locus. Thirdly, there is the Mixed Model in which there is a major single locus with a heritable background. Other approaches that involve two locus models, or that involve genetic linkage between a major locus for the trait and marker loci will not be discussed here.

It is important to emphasize here that consideration of genetic effects is meaningful only within the context of a given environment or range of environments. For example, suppose that a herd of cattle is given a uniformly poor diet and that the variation in their weight is completely due to genetic differences. In this case, the heritability of weight would be 100%. That is, the variation in the trait is totally under genetic control. If the herd was then given a uniformly rich diet, the mean weight might change dramatically due to this environmental change and the heritability in the new environment could take on any value. In the case where there is variation in the environment, then the environmental variation can be evaluated while controlling for genetic variation. The above models are an attempt to either detect a major locus (and subsequently identify the biological substrate corresponding to relevant gene products) or to model the transmission within families to elucidate environmental risk factors in a family study design.

## PATH ANALYSIS

Path analysis was introduced by Wright [26] as a tool for evaluating the interrelationships among variables by analyzing their correlational structure, and has been applied in genetics to determine the causes of familial resemblance. The relationship among

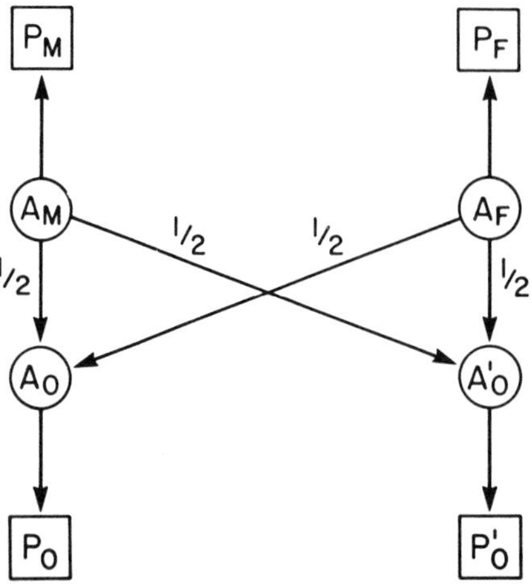


Figure 3. Path diagram of genetic transmission for the simple polygenic model. By convention, uncorrelated residuals are not displayed.

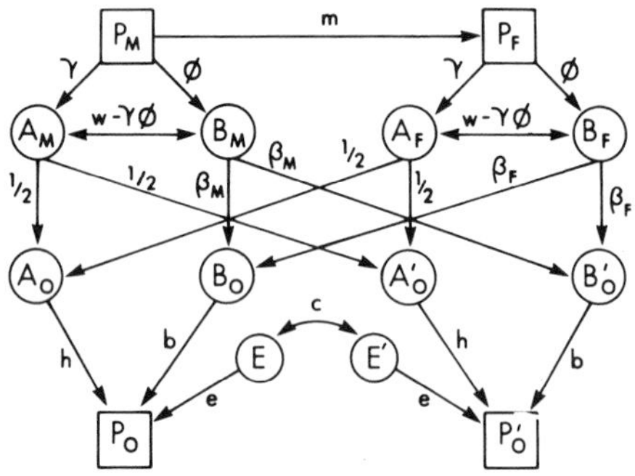


Figure 4. Path diagram depicting the sources of phenotypic resemblance between full siblings under the BETA model.

variables is depicted by a path diagram as in Figures 3-6, where each variable is assumed to have mean zero and variance one. Single-headed arrows indicate the direct influence of one (the independent) variable on another (the dependent variable) and curved double-headed arrows indicate correlations between independent variables which are otherwise unexplained in the diagram. Path coefficients (standardized partial regression coefficients) are associated with each single-headed arrow. The correlations between any two variables in the diagram may be obtained by tracing all paths connecting them with the use of a simple set of rules [27]. Alternatively, we may view path analysis in terms of a set of structural equations [28] of standardized variables.

To motivate this technique, we present three examples. The first is the simple polygenic model [27,29]. Suppose a quantitative measure $P'$ may be partitioned in terms of a genetic component $A'$ and an uncorrelated environmental component $E'$, with $P' = A' + E'$. This yields a path equation (after standardization) of

$$P = hA + eE,$$

with $h = \sigma_A/\sigma_P$ and $e = \sigma_E/\sigma_P$. The quantity $h^2$ is termed the heritability of $P'$. In terms of transmission between generations, we have

$$A_O = \tfrac{1}{2} A_F + \tfrac{1}{2} A_M + sS,$$

when F,M and O denote the father, mother and offspring, the

structural constants 1/2 reflect Mendelian laws, and S is an uncorrelated residual. The correlation between two siblings 0 and 0′ is easily computed as

$$r_{0\,0'} = \mathrm{COV}(P_0, P_{0'}) = h^2\,\mathrm{COV}(A_0, A_{0'})$$

$$= h^2\{\tfrac{1}{4}\,\mathrm{COV}(A_F + A_M + 2sS\,,\,A_F + A_M + 2sS')\}$$

$$= \tfrac{1}{2}h^2.$$

Alternatively, we could trace through the paths connecting $P_0$ and $P'_0$ in Figure 3. In this example, we assumed that the A's of parents are uncorrelated (no assortative mating), that transmission was genetic (so that we knew the structural parameters 1/2), that there was equilibrium so that the variance of A′ was identical in the two generations, that the E's were uncorrelated between individuals, and that there was no dominance (that the genes act additively, so there is no increased sibling resemblance due to genetic interactions). Much work has been done in relaxing these assumptions.

In the above model, the only source of familial resemblance is genetic in that if h = 0, then all the correlations between relatives are zero. If there were cultural transmission between parent and offspring, correlations in the residuals would result. Suppose that P′ may be partitioned as P′ = A′ + B′ + E′, where A′ denotes additive genetic effets, B′ denotes heritable cultural factors and E′ denotes environmental factors that are uncorrelated between generations, so that

$$P = hA + bB + eE.$$

We assume that the A of an offspring is determined as

$$A_0 = \tfrac{1}{2}A_F + \tfrac{1}{2}A_M + sS,$$

and that cultural transmission is modelled by the structural equation

$$B_0 = \beta_F B_F + \beta_M B_M + r_1 R_1.$$

The path coefficients $\beta_F$ and $\beta_M$ may differ with one parent having a greater impact on the child. We allow for a phenotypic correlation between mates, i.e., that there is a correlation m between $P_F$ and $P_M$, but that the partial correlations between the components of mates are zero when controlling for a mate's phenotype. These assumptions yield the regression equation

$$P_F = P_M + r_2 R_2.$$

Finally, we allow for a correlation c between the nontransmissible environments E of singleton siblings reared together. This model, termed the BETA model [9-12] contains 8 parameters - $\beta_M$, $\beta_F$, $h^2$, $b^2$, m, c, $c_{DZ}$, $c_{MZ}$, where $c_{DZ}$ and $c_{MZ}$ represent the correlations between the E's for dizygotic and monozygotic twins, respectively. General formulas for the correlation between individuals reared in a spectrum

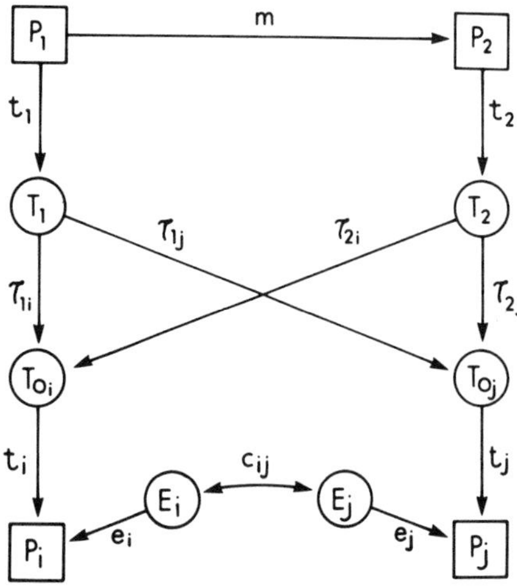


Figure 5. Path diagram for the TAU Model with Sex Effect which depicts familial resemblance for a father, mother and offspring of sexes i and j.

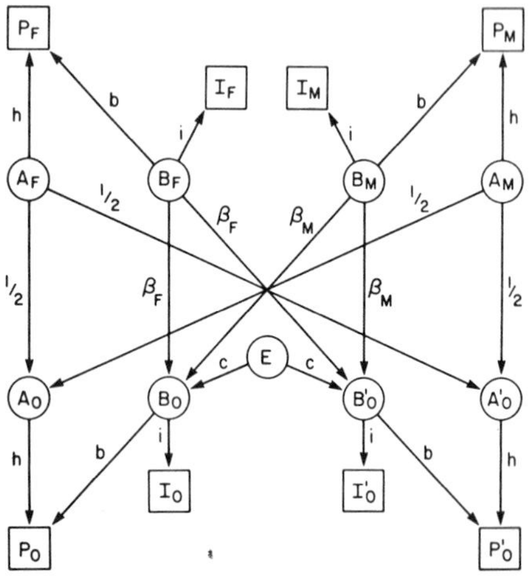


Figure 6. Path diagram for the BETA Model which includes an index of transmissible environment.

of intact, separated or extended family situations have been catalogued [11-12]. This model is similar to that used by Rao and colleagues [7,30-31]. In addition, they have incorporated environmental indices into their model that measure these latent components and that increase the ability to resolve genetic and cultural transmission.

An important observation made from the BETA model is that when $\beta_M = \beta_F = 1/2$, then all correlations between individuals reared in intact families (except MZ twins) may be expressed in terms of only $t^2 = b^2 + h^2 + 2bhw$, where w is the correlation between A and B of an individual that results from the phenotypic assortment. Accordingly, the model may not be identified in nuclear family data, so that either the use of indices or extended relationships are necessary for the identification of the model.

The final model we present is the TAU Model with Sex Effect [32-33] in which we do not explicitly separate genetic and cultural factors. Let $T_i$ denote the effects of all factors that are transmissible from a parent of sex i to an offspring and $E_i$ (uncorrelated) residual factors in sex i, where 1 = male and 2 = female. Thus

$$P_i = t_i\ T_i + e_i\ E_i.$$

It is assumed that transmission from parent to offspring is described by the path equation

$$T_{O_i} = \tau_{1i}\ T_1 + \tau_{2i}\ T_2 + r_i\ R_i.$$

Here, transmission can depend on both the sex of the parent and the sex of the offspring, so that sex specific cultural mechanisms can be considered. It is possible to model maternal effects ($\tau_{11} = \tau_{12}$; $\tau_{21} = \tau_{22}$) due to, for example, different involvement in child-rearing or effects due to uterine environment, or cross sex effects ($\tau_{11} = \tau_{22}$; $\tau_{12} = \tau_{21}$) due to the importance of gender identification or sex role modeling. In the case of polygenic transmission, all the $\tau_{ij}$'s would be 1/2.

For qualitative traits [33-34], the prevalence of the trait, or male and female prevalences, become additional parameters of the path model and determine the correlations in liability.

When dealing with multiple liability distributions (such as for males and females), care must be taken in considering the standardization of variables in the path models. For example, it is possible that on a common, unstandardized liability scale $X'$ that males and females have identical $T_1'$ and $T_2'$ components, but that the variances of $E_1'$ and $E_2'$ differ, so that the path parameters $t_1$ and $t_2$ will differ. In this case, we would expect the $\tau_{ij}$'s to be independent of sex. Likewise, before standardization, the means of the two sexes may differ either from a systematic cultural bias which differentially applies to one sex, or from systematic biological differences. If there were a single threshold $S'$ for $X'$, than $S_1$ and $S_2$ may differ due to mean difference or from difference in variances on $X'$, although the source of the difference in prevalence may be reflected in the pattern of parent-offspring correlations.

Accordingly, path analytic models offer an explicit way to model familial resemblance in the multifactorial model. When numerous types of relatives are available, it offers a way to parameterize the variance-covariance matrix in terms of relatively few parameters. The use of multigenerational data permit resolution of these models and the testing of hypotheses that can be formulated as sets of constraints on the model parameters.

The statistical aspects and considerations for the application of these genetic models are discussed below.

## STATISTICAL ISSUES AND EXTENSIONS

Consider a nuclear family consisting of a father, mother, p male and q female offspring. We assume their joint liability $(X,Y,Z_1,\ldots,Z_p,W_1,\ldots,W_q)$ has a multivariate normal distribution with mean vector $\mu' = (0,\ldots,0)$ and variance - covariance matrix $\Sigma$. The probability of a particular phenotypic configuration is then computed through integration of the multivariate normal density function. Let $F_{pq}(r,s,M)$ denote a family with r out of p affected males, s out of q affected females and with parental phenotypes denoted by M.

In many situations, it is desirable to sample families according to the disease status of family members to enrich the sample with affected individuals. The traditional method for doing this [35-36] is to choose affected index cases (probands) and then bring their family into the study. We consider below the analysis of nuclear families ascertained using this method. Alternatively, pedigrees may be sampled using a sequential sample scheme [37], or pedigrees can be broken into their constituent nuclear parts and an approximate treatment of ascertainment may be done [24] by conditioning on the index cases (pointers) external to these nuclear parts. When there is one proband per pedigree, a relatively simple approach may be used [38].

Sampling using the proband method. Let $\pi_1$ and $\pi_2$ denote the probability of selecting an affected male and affected female, respectively, as a proband. Let $\tilde{F}_{pq}(r,s,M,a,b|asc)$ denote a family (conditional on ascertainment) with a male probands and b female probands. We wish to express the probability of observing $\tilde{F}$ in terms of the probabilities of random families and $\pi_1$ and $\pi_2$. We assume here that ascertainment is through affected offspring.

Note that the probability of ascertaining a family $F_{pq}(r,s,M)$ is simply

$$\alpha_{rs} = 1 - (1-\pi_1)^r(1-\pi_2)^s,$$

so that the probability of ascertaining a family with p male and q female offspring is

$$P(asc) = \sum_{s=0}^{q} \sum_{r=0}^{p} \sum_{M} P(F_{pq}(r,s,M))\alpha_{rs}. \qquad (1)$$

The probability of observing a male and b female probands, given that the family has r affected males and s affected females and that the family has been ascertained is given by

$$\beta_{rs}(a,b,|a+b>0) = \frac{\binom{r}{a}\binom{s}{b}\pi_1^{a}(1-\pi_1)^{r-a}\pi_2^{b}(1-\pi_2)^{s-b}}{\alpha_{rs}}$$

for $0 \leq a \leq r$, $0 \leq b \leq s$, and $a+b>0$. We assume that probands are independently sampled and that their distribution is a truncated product of binomial distributions. Thus,

$$P(\tilde{F}_{pq}(r,s,M,a,b|asc)) = \frac{P(F_{pq}(r,s,M)\alpha_{rs}\beta_{rs}(a,b|a+b>0)}{P(asc)}$$

Accordingly, given a set of parameters $\theta$ to be estimated, where $\theta$ includes the correlations in liability or a set of path coefficients which parameterize $\Sigma$, and includes $\pi_i$ if the families are sampled using the proband method, the log likelihood of the sample is proportional to the sum of the logs of the probabilities computed in terms of $\theta$. This sum is then maximized to obtain maximum likelihood parameters estimates $\hat{\theta}$.

Likelihood Conditional on Proband. When the probability of ascertainment is small (i.e. the number of probands is small relative to the number of affected individuals in the sampling frame), then we expect precisely one proband per ascertained family. If we compute the probability of a family conditioned on the proband's status, we have

$$P(\tilde{F}_{p-1,q}(r,s,M|\text{male proband}) \; \frac{P(F_{pq}(r+1,s,m))}{K_1} \times \frac{r+1}{p}$$

$$P(\tilde{F}_{p,q-1}(r,s,M|\text{female proband}) = \frac{P(F_{pq}(r,s+1,M))}{K_2} \times \frac{s+1}{q},$$

where $K_1$ and $K_2$ denote the proportion of affected males and females, respectively, in the population. Elston and Sobel [38] have shown that these are the limiting expressions obtained by letting $\pi \to 0$. The situation where $\pi \to 0$ is termed single ascertainment and in practice is the usual setting in family studies of common diseases. This is important since the denominator of P(asc) in equation (1) involves a summation over all possible families of a given sibship size, and this becomes problematic when, for example, age effects are considered since each family will have a different age structure so that a new P(asc) needs to be computed for each family.

Variable Age of Onset. Many diseases display a variable age of onset so that censoring must be taken into account in applying the above models. Among individuals observed to be unaffected, we distinguish between those who will become affected (susceptible individuals) and those who will never become affected. Indeed, the lifetime morbid risk $K_L$ has traditionally been an important parameter in genetic expidemiology and included explicitly in model building. In some applications the value of $K_L$ is known a priori (offspring of affected parents for a rare dominant disorder such as Huntington's disease have $K_L$ = 50%), and in many situiations $K_L$ is well characterized from population studies prior to family studies. Risch [30] reviews the early methods for age correction and advocates a maximum likelihood approach.

It is necessary to consider the relationship between liability and the probability of being censored at a given age. Falconer [15] considers various mechanisms that account for variable age of onset. At one extreme, liability may increase monotonically with age, so that an individual's liability score is equal to the threshold value at the time of onset. In this case, onset classes would correspond to the multiple threshold model (Figure 1B) with early onset cases corresponding to individuals with deviant liability scores. At the other extreme, the likelihood of being censored may be independent of the liability score in susceptible individuals. These models can be distinguished by including age at onset of the proband as a covariate in determining the morbid risk in a relative.

Let T denote the time to onset (as measured from birth) in susceptible individuals, and let $\eta_i\ (t;\theta_1)$ and $H_i\ (t;\theta_1)$ denote the density and distribution functions for T, where $\theta_1$ denotes the parameters of the distribution. Let $K_{iL}$ denote the life-time risk to an individual of sex i, so that the prevalence at age in sex i is

$$K_{ia} = H_i(a;\theta_1)K_{iL}.$$

For the Multifactorial Model with random censoring, we let $P_L$ refer to lifetime probabilities which are expressed in terms of a set of lifetime correlations and thresholds and correspond to the limiting probabilities as the family members pass through the period of risk. For a pair of unaffected relatives of ages $\underline{a}=(a_1,a_2)$, we would compute their probability as

$$P_L(U,U) + \{1-H(a_1;\theta_1)\}\ P_L(A,U) + \{1-H(a_2;\theta_1)\}P_L(U,A)$$

$$+\{1-H(a_1,a_2;\theta_1)\}P_L(A,A).$$

That is we allow for an unaffected individual to be susceptible with onset greater than his observed age. The ages of onset in a susceptible pair may not be independent, in which case a bivariate onset distribution must be considered.

In general, as in [40], let F be a family of size m with $k_1$ affected individuals and let the ages at observations be $\underline{a} = (a_1,..,a_m)$. If F' is one of the possible lifetime possibilities for F, ordered so that the first $k_1$ individuals are affected and the next $k_2$ individuals are susceptible, $0 \leq k_2 \leq m-k_1$, then define $C_{F'}$ by

$$C_{F'} = \int_{-\infty}^{a_1} \cdots \int_{-\infty}^{a_k} \int_{a_{k_1+1}} \cdots \int_{a_{k_1+k_2}} \eta(X_1,\ldots,X_{k_1+k_2};\theta_1)\ dx_1 \ldots dx_{k_1+k_2},$$

where $\eta$ is the joint density function for age of onset.

Then $P(F|\underline{a}) = \sum_{F'} |_L\ (F')\ C_{F'}$.

In the case of single ascertainment, the likelihood

$$L(\tilde{F},\underline{b}\,|\,\text{proband},\underline{a}) = L(\underline{b}\,|\,\tilde{F},\text{proband},\underline{a})L(\tilde{F}\,|\,\text{proband},\underline{a}),$$

where $L(\underline{b}|\tilde{F},\text{proband},\underline{a})$ is the joint likelihood of onset of the affected individuals in the family.

If practice, it is usually assumed that age of onset is non-familial so that $\eta$ is given as the product of its marginal densities. Again, the function H $(x;\theta_1)$ may be known from previous studies of affected individuals, so that simultaneous estimation of $\theta$ and $\theta_1$ may be avoided.

In this case of random censoring, we have

$$\frac{K_{R_{ia}}}{K_{ia}} = \frac{K_{R_{iL}}}{K_{iL}}$$

That is, the ratio of the risk to a relative at a specific age divided by the prevalence in the population at that age is an invariant and does not depend on the age of onset of the proband.

We have defined T to be measured from birth. If there is differential mortality for affected individuals, then historical information is needed for those who are censored by death [41]. In many studies probands are identified by treatment seeking behavior, and if there is a time lag between onset of illness and treatment seeking, then it is necessary to incorporate demographic information to account for this [42]. Accordingly, the incorporation of variable age of onset into a family analysis can be complicated and must be guided by the characteristics of the disease studied and the method of sampling used to obtain families.

## COVARIATES

The qualitative liability/threshold approach seems to be appropriate for many phenotypes and to reflect clinical observation. In addition to the qualitative diagnostic information, measures of biochemical, psychosocial and environmental variables may be available on each family member, and a major goal in analysis is to understand the relationship between these covariates and the risk of disease. Since the covariates themselves may be familial, a familial study design is potentially rich in information; however, the multivariate nature of the data and the non-random method of ascertainment must be taken into account. We describe three approaches to the use of covariates.

<u>Standard Statistical Approaches</u> The logistic regression and Cox proportional hazards models can be used as convenient ways to evaluate the importance of covariates using standard software. Although the parameterization in terms of the above models is not used, these techniques can be viewed as exploratory ways to guide the application of the genetic/family analysis. For example, Rice and colleagues [43] examined the risk of affective disorder in the siblings of probands using the Cox model. Affection in the father and mother, attributes of the proband, and attributes of the sibling were included as covariates. Interestingly, a prominent effect due to birth cohort of the sibling was detected. Also, the presence of

illness in the mother was found to predict illness in an offspring, whereas paternal illness did not.

In this analysis, families with multiple siblings of the proband were treated as independent observations. This will provide consistent parameter estimates, but tests of hypotheses will be biased. However, much of the dependence between siblings may be controlled by inclusion of the parental covariates. Alternative approaches using multivariate survival analysis are included in this volume.

Indices in Path Analysis. Rao and colleagues [4,7,30] have advocated the use of indices (measures of latent path components, such as of B in Figure 6). It is assumed that the index I has a linear regression.

$$I = i\,B + \ell L,$$

and that the residual L is uncorrelated with other variables in the model. The correlations of the indices between relatives become observations in the model, as well as the biserial correlations between liability and index.

In general, the index may be assumed to measure other path components, and likelihood ratio tests used to explore its validity. Rice and colleagues [10] explored the use of SES (Socioeconomic Status) as an index of home environment relevant to IQ scores. They found the simple regression model not to fit, with SES having significant correlations with components other than B. In general, multivariate path analysis [44] may be used, although it has only been applied to quantitative phenotypes.

Covariates in Genetic Models The multifactorial model described above explicitly included the covariate sex in its formulation, and this permits testing hypotheses concerning the sources of a sex difference ($K_{1L} \neq K_{2L}$) for a disease [32-33]. The Mixed Model may be viewed as having latent covariates. In the situation where genetic markers are used as covariates in a linkage study, here is in general no association between the marker and disease at the population level, but within families the loci for the marker and disease tend to be transmitted as a unit due to proximity on the same chromosome.

For a quantitative measure Z, one approach is to assume that (after transformation of Z) the liability X and Z have a bivariate normal distribution [45], and furthermore, that the joint distribution within families is multivariate normal. For the mixed model with $X = g + \xi$, Lalouel and Morton [24] assumed that $\xi$ and Z have similar distributional properties. Under these assumptions, the joint distribution in liability , conditional on the vector of Z values in the family, is again multivariate normal with mean and variance-covariance matrix given by

$$V_{12}V_{22}^{-1}(Z^* - U_2)$$

$$V_{11}-V_{12}V_{22}^{-1}V_{21},$$

where $U_2$ is the mean vector for $Z = (Z_1,\ldots,Z_m)$, $V_{ij}$ correspond to the blocked variance-covariance matrix for $(\underline{X},\underline{Z})$, and $Z^*$ is the vector of covariate values.

In general, there is a great deal more information in a quantitative scale (like height) versus a dichotomized scale (like tall versus not tall). This strategy of finding quantitative scales correlated with liability is a way to utilize quantitative information as well as to detect possible risk factors. This suggests another approach that has been used to some extent in genetic epidemiology. The parametric models can be used to give quantitative risk predictions in unaffected individuals. That is, given diagnostic information on relatives, a transmission model gives an estimate of risk to that relative. These risk figures can then be used to examine potentially important covariates. This has been done in case-control settings by comparing offspring of affected parents versus offspring with no family history.

## DISCUSSION

Family studies offer a strategy to resolve heterogeneity at two levels. The first is to resolve whether heterogenous subforms represent the same underlying familial process. For example, the lack of cross-aggregation of early-onset, insulin dependent diabetes in the families of late-onset, non-insulin dependent diabetic probands (and vice versa) point to etiologic heterogeneity. This is confirmed by the presence of HLA associations with only the former type of diabetes. In general, the multiple threshold approach can be used to assess the relationship between putative subforms of illness [46]. This approach has been particularly important in psychiatry [47]for defining and validating nosological categories.

The other type of heterogeneity results when multiple underlying pathways lead to similar phenotypes. Geneticists distinguish between cases and phenocopies, individuals who have undistinguishable clinical pictures but who do not reflect the same underlying genetic /familial process. If phenocopies are non-familial, then the transmission models may be modified to include this possibility and familial aggregation used to statistically discriminate between true cases and phenocopies. Indeed, a major difficulty in detecting relevant covariates and understanding their relationship to etiology can be heterogeneity in the population of cases studied. Moreover, for many common diseases there are likely several subforms that are each due to the expression of a single genetic locus. Resolution of this heterogeneity will enhance investigation of the residual cases.

Much of the above treatment deals with generalizing genetic models to allow for environmental similarity between relatives. One of the most important goals of family studies is detecting relevant environmental factors and determining their role in the transmission and development of complex phenotypes. Models that allows only for random environmental effects may be inappropriate for this task. In this regard, many of the approaches described in this volume that use survival analysis and related techniques would be fruitful in family studies. Farewell [48] describes the use of surviving fractions in the analysis of time dependent data. This would permit having lifetime morbid risk (which may have, for example, a logistic regression on a vector of covariates) modelled explicitly. The time to onset in susceptible individuals may then be modelled using some of the techniques that have proven so successful in epidemologic studies.

## REFERENCES

[1] I.I. GOTTESMAN and J. SHIELDS. Schizophrenia: The Epigenetic Puzzle. Cambridge Univ. Press, (1982) Cambridge.

[2] C. SING and M. SKOLNICK. Genetic Analysis of Common Diseases: Application to Predictive Factors in Coronary Disease. Alan Liss (1979) New York.

[3] N.E. MORTON and C.S. CHUNG. Genetic Epidemiology. Academic Press (1978) New York.

[4] D.C. RAO, R.C. ELSTON, L.H. KULLER, M. FEINLEIB, C. CARTER. Genetic Epidemiology of Coronary Heart Disease: Past, Present, and Future. Alan Liss (1984) New York.

[5] S. WRIGHT. Statistical methods in biology. Proc. Am. Stat. Assoc. 26 (1931) pp. 155-163.

[6] L.L. CAVALLI-SFORZA and M.W. FELDMAN. Models for cultural inheritance. I. Group mean and within group variation. Theor. Popul. Biol. 4 (1973) pp. 42-55.

[7] D.C. RAO, N.E. MORTON, S. YEE. Resolution of cultural and biological inheritance by path analysis. Am. J. Hum. Genet. 28 (1976) pp. 228-242.

[8] L.J. EAVES. The effect of cultural transmission on continous variation Heredity 34 (1976) pp. 41-57.

[9] J. RICE, C.R. CLONINGER, T. REICH. Multifactorial inheritance with culture transmission and assortative mating. I. Description and basic properties of the unitary models Am. J. Hum. Genet. 30 (1978) pp. 618-643.

[10] J. RICE, C.R. CLONINGER, T. REICH. The analysis of behavioral

traits in the presence of cultural transmission and assortative mating: Applications to IQ and SES. Behav. Genet. 10 (1980) pp. 73-92.

[11] C.R. CLONINGER, J. RICE, T. REICH. Multifactorial inheritance with cultural transmission and assortative mating. II. A general model of combined polygenic and cultural inheritance. Am. J. Hum. Genet. 31 (1979) pp. 176-198.

[12] C.R. CLONINGER, J. RICE, T. REICH. Multifactorial inheritance with cultural transmission and assortative mating. III. Family structure and the analysis of separation experiments. Am. J. Hum. Genet. 31 (1979) pp. 366-388.

[13] R.A. FISHER. The correlation between relatives on the supposition of Mendelian inheritance. Tr. R. Soc. Edinburgh 52 (1918) pp. 399-433.

[14] D.S. FALCONER. The inheritance of liability to certain diseases, estimated from the incidence among relatives. Ann. Hum. Genet., London 29 (1965) pp. 51-76.

[15] D.S. FALCONER. The inheritance of liability to diseases with variable age of onset, with particular reference to diabetes mellitus. Ann. Hum. Genet. 31 (1967) pp. 1-20.

[16] T. REICH, J.W. JAMES, C.A. MORRIS. The use of multiple thresholds in determining the mode of transmission of semi-continuous traits. Ann. Hum. Genet. London, 36 (1972) pp.163-184.

[17] R.N. CURNOW and C. SMITH. Multifactorial models for familial disease. J.R. Statis. Soc. A 138 (1975) pp. 131-169.

[18] J.H. EDWARDS. Familial predispositions in man. Brit. Med. Bull. 25 (1969) pp. 58-64.

[19] R. ELSTON and M.A. CAMPBELL. Schizophrenia: Evidence for the major gene hypothesis. Behav. Genet. 1 (1971) pp. 3-10.

[20] R.C. ELSTON. Major locus analysis for quantitative traits. Am. J. Hum. Genet. 31 (1979) pp. 655-661.

[21] R.C. ELSTON and K.C. YELVERTON. General models for segregation analysis. Am. J. Hum. Genet. 27 (1975) pp. 31-45.

[22] N.E. MORTON and C.J. MACLEAN. Analysis of family resemblance. III. Complex segregation of quantitative traits. Am. J. Hum. Genet. 26 (1974) pp. 489-503.

[23] J. OTT. Maximum likelihood estimation by counting methods under polygenic and mixed models in human pedigrees. Am. J. Hum. Genet. 31 (1979) pp. 161-179.

[24] J.M. LALOUEL and N.E. MORTON. Complex segregation analysis with pointers. Hum. Hered. 31 (1981) pp. 312-321.

[25] J.M. LALOUEL, D.C. RAO, N.E. MORTON R.C. ELSTON. A unified model for complex segregation analysis. Am. J. Hum. Genet. 35

(1983) pp. 816-826.

[26] S. WRIGHT. Correlation and causation. J. Agric. Res. 20 (1921) pp. 557-585.

[27] C.C. LI. Path Analysis - A Primer. Boxwood Press (1975) Pacific Grove, CA.

[28] O.D. DUNCAN. Introduction to Structural Equation Models. Academic Press (1975) New York.

[29] L.L. CAVALLI-SFORZA and W.F. BODMER. The Genetics of Human Populations. W.H. Freeman (1971) San Francisco.

[30] D.C. RAO, N.E. MORTON, S. YEE. Analysis of family resemblance. II. A linear model for familial correlation. Am. J. Hum. Genet. 26 (1974) pp. 331-359.

[31] D.C. RAO, N.E. MORTON, C.R. CLONINGER. Path analysis under generalized assortative mating. I. Theory. Genet. Res., Camb. 33 (1979) pp. 175-188.

[32] J. RICE, C.R. CLONINGER, T. REICH. General causal models for sex differences in the familial transmission of multifactorial traits: An application to human spatial visualizing ability. Social Biology 27 (1980) pp. 36-47.

[33] J. RICE, P. NICHOLS, I.I. GOTTESMAN. Assessment of sex differences for qualitative multifactorial traits using path analysis. Psychiatry Research 4 (1981) pp. 301-312.

[34] D.C. RAO, N.E. MORTON, I.I. GOTTESMAN, R. LEW. Path analysis of qualitative data on pairs of relatives: Application to schizophrenia. Hum. Hered. 31 (1981) pp. 325-333.

[35] N.E. MORTON. Genetic tests under incomplete ascertainment. Am. J. Hum. Genet. 11 (1959) pp. 1-16.

[36] R.C. ELANDT-JOHNSON. Probability models and statistical methods in genetics. John Wiley and Sons: (1969) New York.

[37] E.R. THOMPSON and C. CANNINGS. Sampling schemes and ascertainment. The Genetic Analysis of Common Diseases: Application of Predictive Factors in Coronary Heart Disease. Alan Liss (1979) New York.

[38] R.C. ELSTON and E. SOBEL. Sampling considerations in the gathering and analysis of pedigree data. Am. J. Hum. Genet. 31 (1979) pp. 62-69.

[39] N. RISCH. Estimating morbidity risks with variable age of onset: Review of methods and a maximum likelihood approach. Biometrics 39 (1983) pp. 929-939.

[40] J. RICE and T. REICH. Familial analysis of qualitative traits under multifactorial inheritance. Genetic Epidemiology 2 (1985) pp. 301-315.

[41] W.D. THOMPSON and M.M. WEISSMAN. Quantifying lifetime risk of

psychiatric disorder. J. Psychiat. Res. 16 (1981) pp. 113-126.

[42] R.C. HEIMBUCH, S. MATTHYSSE, K.K. KIDD. Estimating age-of-onset distributions for disorders with variable onset. Am. J. Hum. Genet. 32 (1980) pp. 564-574.

[43] J. RICE, T. REICH, N.C. ANDREASEN et al. Sex-related differences in depression: Familial evidence. J. Affec. Dis. 7 (1984) pp. 199-210.

[44] G.P. VOGLER. Multivariage path analysis of familial resemblance. Genetic Epidemiology 2 (1985) pp. 35-53.

[45] C. SMITH, and N. MENDELL. Recurrence risk from family history and metric traits. Ann. Hum. Genet. 37 (1974) p 275.

[46] T. REICH, J. RICE, C.R. CLONINGER, R. WETTE, J. JAMES. The use of multiple thresholds and segregation analysis in analyzing the phenotypic heterogeneity of multifactorial traits. Ann. Hum. Genet., London, 42 (1979) pp. 371-390.

[47] D. GOODWIN and S. GUZE. Psychiatric Diagnosis, 2nd ed. Oxford University Press (1979) New York.

[48] V.T. FAREWELL. A model for a binary variable with time-censored observations. Biometrika 64 (1977) pp. 43-46.

## SECTION 6
Models for Cancer Screening and for Carcinogenesis

The two papers in this section describe methods for the modelling and evaluation of cancer screening data, and methods for the modelling and extrapolation of carcinogenesis data.

Nick Day and Steve Walter present recent work on the evaluation of cancer screening programs. Cancer incidence and prevalence data are shown to lead to estimates of screening test sensitivity and of the duration of the detectable preclinical period under some simple, but stringent, assumptions. Both cohort and case-control data are considered for such estimation. The criteria for evaluating a cervical cancer screening program, which primarily detects premalignant lesions, are compared with those for evaluating a breast cancer screening program, which primarily detects small but invasive cancers.

Krewski, Murdoch and Dewanji consider mathematical models for carcinogenesis. Both classical multistage models and pharmacokinetic models are described. Certain challenging problems in the analysis of carcinogenesis data are discussed, including the problem of inference on tumor incidence rates based on mortality data and the largely non-mathematical problem of low dose extrapolation.

# Screening for Cancer of the Breast and Cervix—Estimating the Duration of the Detectable Preclinical Phase

*N. E. Day* and S. D. Walter***

Abstract. Mass screening for breast and cervical cancer has been shown to be beneficial, reducing mortality from the disease in the former and both mortality and incidence in the latter. Models of the disease process and the effect of screening are helpful in estimating the benefits of alternative screening strategies, given the results from a particular screening programme. Such models are described and emphasis is placed both on the design of case-control studies to provide the information necessary for parameter estimation, and on case-control estimation procedures. Data are presented from screening programmes for both types of cancer, with estimates of the various relevant parameters, and the implications for screening policies are discussed.

## INTRODUCTION

The only cancers for which solid epidemiological evidence exists for the value of mass screening programmes are those of the breast and of the cervix. The questions that are now of interest concern the relative value of different screening policies, especially to decide who should be screened and how often. Two parameters of particular relevance are the sensitivity of the screening test and the distribution of the duration of the detectable preclinical phase (DPCP), a duration to be referred to as the sojourn time. The nature of the lesion at which screening is aimed, and so the effect of early detection, is different for the two cancers. For cancer of the cervix, the great majority of the preclinical lesions are precancerous, and can be treated to prevent progression to malignancy. The remainder are early invasive or microinvasive lesions for which the prognosis is good, and which (if treated) lead to virtually no excess mortality. In a typical screening programme, the former would outnumber the latter by about ten to one [1]. For breast cancer, however, almost all the lesions detected are invasive malignancies, predominantly at an early stage, but nevertheless associated with an appreciable excess mortality. The cases that arise during a screening programme can be expressed graphically as in Figure 1, in which two types of lesions are distinguished, those arising as interval cancers between screens, and

*International Agency for Research on Cancer, Lyon, France
**McMaster University, Hamilton, Ontario, Canada

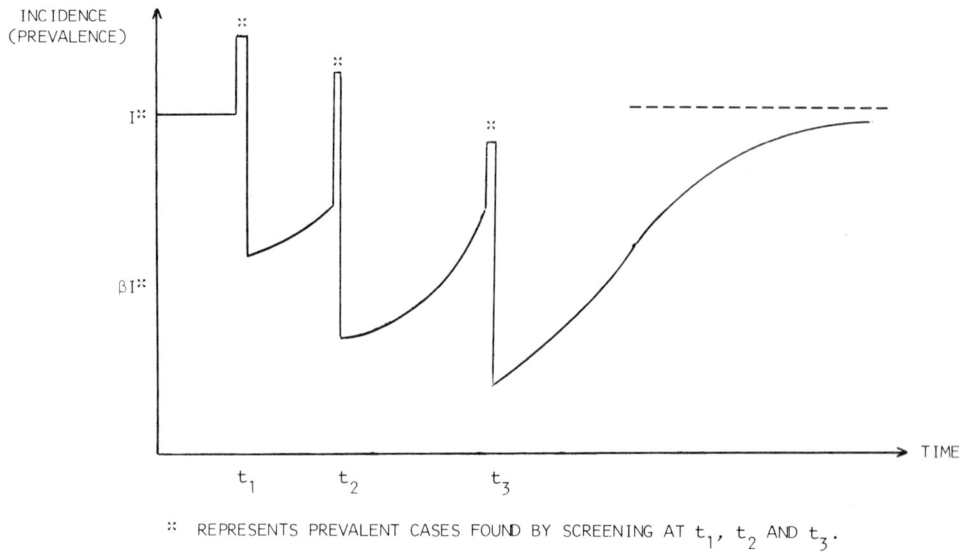


Figure 1. Theoretical effect of screen on incidence and prevalence, by time. * represents cases found by screening at $t_1$,$t_2$ and $t_3$.

those detected at screening. If the screen-detected lesions are pre-cancerous, then the benefit of a screening programme can be evaluated simply in terms of the cumulative incidence of interval cases, since these are the lesions with associated excess mortality; the evaluation is made in terms of a comparison to the cumulative incidence in the same period among a comparable unscreened group. On the other hand, if the screen-detected lesions are themselves invasive cancers, then the benefit of a screening programme has to take account of their excess mortality. The two situations will be considered separately here.

Before turning to the estimation of the various parameters, we shall briefly recapitulate the formulation of a model relating the incidence and prevalence rates of Figure 1 to the rate of progression of the disease and the characteristics of the screening test.

We assume that a steady state has been achieved, and that in the cohort of women under study the incidence of the relevant cancer in the absence of screening is $I^*$. Then if $\beta$ denotes the false negative rate and f(y) the density function of the sojourn time distribution, we can derive, as shown earlier [2] expressions for the prevalence of lesions detected at each successive screen and the incidence of interval cases. With n screens occurring at time periods $t_1,\cdots,t_n$, the incidence of interval cancers occurring at time $t(>t_n)$ is given by

$$I_n(t) = I^* \sum_{i=0}^{n} \beta^{n-i} \int_{t-t_{i+1}}^{t-t_i} f(y)dy \qquad (1)$$

with $t_0 = -\infty$ and $t_{n+1} = t$, and the prevalence at the $n^{th}$ screen is given by

$$P_n = (1-\beta)\, I^* \sum_{i=1}^{n} \beta^{n-i} \int_{t_n-t_i}^{\infty} \min(y-(t_n-t_i), t_i-t_{i-1})\, f(y)dy \quad . \qquad (2)$$

This expression for the prevalence assumes that all lesions detected at screening would progress eventually to clinical cancers at the end of the DPCP. Note that if f(y) is suitably defined, it can allow for the probability of a certain proportion of the preclinical lesions which progress only after a very long time; this subset of lesions might be regarded in effect as non-progressive, if the end of the DPCP is defined to occur after the anticipated time of death (due to some other cause) for the patient. If the screening test is not fully specific for those lesions that will progress, then the expression for $P_n$ will have to be modified accordingly. If $\alpha_n$ is the predictive value of a positive test at $n^{th}$ screen (thus allowing different values at each screen), then the observed prevalence will be $P_n/\alpha_n$ rather than $P_n$.

The incidence of interval cancers will of course not be altered since, by definition, they have progressed. It is clear that using information only on the interval cases to estimate $\beta$ and f(y) enables one to obtain independent estimates of $\alpha_1$ to $\alpha_n$. An example will be discussed later in the paper.

With this formulation, we are now in a position to discuss alternatives to the estimation procedures based on complete follow-up data described in earlier publications.

2. The use of case-control data for parameter estimation. The data provided by case-control studies permit the estimation of relative risks rather than absolute rates, so that the formulation given in the previous section needs modification. For the interval cancers, the modification is trivial, one is estimating the ratio of incidence rates, and the rate in the unscreened, $I^*$, can be taken as baseline. The relative risk at time t for someone screened n times at $t_1, \cdots, t_n$ is given by

$$r_n(t) = \sum_{i=0}^{n} \beta^{n-i} \int_{t-t_{i+1}}^{t-t_i} f(y)dy \quad . \qquad (3)$$

For the prevalence rates at successive screens, one can only estimate the ratio of the prevalence rates (in fact the odds ratio of prevalence rates) at successive screens. Taking the prevalence rate at the first screen as baseline, one can then estimate the prevalence ratios $pr_i = P_i/P_1$, which are expressed in terms of the sensitivity and the sojourn time distribution.

We now consider, for incidence and prevalence ratios separately, what observations one will make and how these will be combined into a likelihood function for parameter estimation. To eliminate nuisance parameters related to changing risk with age and calendar time, it is convenient to match each incident case by a control with the same date of birth. Specifically, for an incident case the relevant screening history consists of all tests up to the time of diagnosis (not screen based by definition). The relevant screening history for the control or matched set of controls consists of tests undergone during the same time period, i.e., up to the date of diagnosis of the case.

When defining the screening history it is important to note that only negative screening tests are relevant. For cancers where screening detects early invasive disease, a positive test leads (should lead) to diagnosis and treatment. The screening history is then the times of all negative tests before diagnosis. When screening detects precancerous conditions, positive test results may not lead to any action other than further screening. Since the interval in which we are interested is that between the start of the DPCP and clinical disease, it is clear that positive screening tests, indicating that entry to the DPCP has already occurred, are irrelevant in this approach to estimating the sojourn time distribution. The relevant screening history therefore consists of the times of all negative tests up to the first positive test, or the diagnosis of malignancy, whichever is the earlier. There may be practical difficulties in defining a negative test, an extended discussion for cervical cancer is given elsewhere [3,4]. A few of the controls may also have had positive screening tests. Their screening history clearly has to be treated in identical fashion.

The data derived from the incident cases will then consist of a series of matched sets, each set consisting of a case and several controls ($R_i$ in the $i^{th}$ set). If $H_{ij}$ represents the screening history of the $j^{th}$ member of the $i^{th}$ set (with j=0 representing a case) and if Z is an indicator variable, with Z=2 for a control and Z=0 for an incident case, then the conditional probability of the $i^{th}$ set is given by

$$\frac{\Pr(H_{i0}|z=0)\prod_{j=1}^{R_i}\Pr(H_{ij}|z=2)}{\sum_{\ell=0}^{R_i}\Pr(H_{i\ell}|z=0)\prod_{j\neq\ell}\Pr(H_{ij}|z=2)} .$$

Using Bayes theorem one can write

$$\Pr(H_{ij}|z=\ell) = \frac{\Pr(z=\ell|H_{ij})\ \Pr(H_{ij})}{\sum_{\text{all } H} \Pr(z=\ell|H_{ik})\ \Pr(H_{ik})} .$$

Making this substitution in the conditional probability expression above, we see that all terms involving $\Pr(H_{ij})$ cancel, and one is left with

$$\frac{\Pr(z=0|H_{i0}) \prod_{j=1}^{R_i} \Pr(z=2|H_{ij})}{\sum_{\ell=0}^{R_i} \Pr(z=0|H_{i\ell}) \prod_{j\neq\ell} \Pr(z=2|H_{ij})} .$$

Since the probability of being an incident case is virtually zero, we can take $\Pr(z=2|H_{ij})$ as equal to unity, so that the expression reduces to

$$\frac{\Pr(z=0|H_{i0})}{\sum_{\ell=0}^{R_i} \Pr(z=0|H_{i\ell})} . \qquad (4)$$

The quantities $\Pr(z=0|H)$ are given by expression (1) for $I_n(t)$.

It is interesting to note in passing that if an unconditional approach had been adopted, the likelihood would have contained terms involving $\Pr(H_{ij})$, the probability of each observed screening history. These probabilities are nuisance parameters, and their removal by conditioning is a considerable simplification.

For the screen-detected cases, one is estimating the odds ratio of prevalence rates. It is, therefore, clear that the controls have to consist of individuals who have been screened with a negative result. In order to remove the effects of age and secular trends in incidence, it is convenient to take as matched controls for each case included in the study individuals born at the same time and screened at the same time as the corresponding case is diagnosed. One then compares the prior screening history in terms of the number of previous negative tests and the dates on which they occurred. The contribution of each matched set to the overall conditional likelihood function can then be derived in similar fashion to that of the incident matched sets. Putting the indicator variable Z=1 for a prevalent (screen-detected) case, and using $H_{ij}$ to represent the screening history of the $j^{th}$ individual in the $i^{th}$ matched set (with j=0 representing the case), then the contribution of the $i^{th}$ set is given by

$$\frac{\Pr(z=1|H_{i0})}{\sum_{\ell=0}^{R_i} \Pr(z=1|H_{i\ell})}, \qquad (5)$$

where the probabilities are given in terms of expression (2).

If the predictive values of a positive test are not 100%, and vary between screens, then further parameters have to be added as described earlier. For breast cancer, however, it appears that the predictive value is almost 100% and expression (5) can be used (it should be noted that by predictive value for breast cancer we mean, in this setting, the probability that a screen-detected lesion confirmed histologically as breast cancer would progress to a clinical cancer. It is not the probability that a positive screening test, e.g., a positive mammogram, will lead to a positive biopsy). For cervical cancer, the predictive value of a diagnosis of dysplasia or even carcinoma in-situ is not well estimated and the use in this context of all precancerous lesions would not be helpful. The question is discussed in the section on cervical cancer.

One can now combine terms of the form given by expressions (4) and (5) to obtain the overall likelihood function, expressed in terms of $\beta$ and the parametrization of the function f(y) one has chosen to adopt. The ideas in this section are discussed at length elsewhere [5,6].

3. Incorporation of covariate information. It has been assumed that all individuals in the same matched set are at the same underlying risk, i.e., that $I^*$ is constant. In many situations information will be available on covariates which are known to influence risk and the incorporation of this information into the analysis will improve the resulting inferences on $\beta$ and f(y). A simple approach is through the addition of a multiplicative term in the underlying rate $I^*$. If a vector of covariates takes the value $\underset{\sim}{x}_{ij}$ for the $j^{th}$ of the $i^{th}$ set, and if $\underset{\sim}{\alpha}$ represents the corresponding vector of log relative risks, then one can express the underlying incidence of this individual, $I^*_{ij}$, as

$$I_{ij}^* = I_i^* \exp(\underset{\sim}{\alpha}'\underset{\sim}{x}_{ij})$$

where $I_i^*$ is the baseline rate for the $i^{th}$ matched set to which the relative risks refer. Expression (4) then becomes

$$\frac{\exp(\underset{\sim}{\alpha}'\underset{\sim}{x}_{i0})\Pr(z=0|H_{i0})}{\sum_{\ell=0}^{R_i} \exp(\underset{\sim}{\alpha}'\underset{\sim}{x}_{i\ell})\Pr(z=0|H_{i\ell})} \tag{6}$$

and expression (5) is modified in similar fashion to give

$$\frac{\exp(\underset{\sim}{\alpha}'\underset{\sim}{x}_{i0})\Pr(z=1|H_{i0})}{\sum_{\ell=0}^{R_i} \exp(\underset{\sim}{\alpha}'\underset{\sim}{x}_{i\ell})\Pr(z=1|H_{i\ell})} \; . \tag{7}$$

4. Application to screening for cervical cancer. Two difficulties arise for cancer of the cervix, first that the potential of preinvasive lesions for progression to malignancy is unclear, and second that women never screened tend to be at considerably elevated risk as compared to women who elect to be screened; the latter appears to be a selection bias effect. There is, therefore, considerable advantage in restricting studies aimed at estimating $\beta$ and $f(y)$ to invasive lesions among women screened at least once. The case series will then consist of both incident and screen-detected invasive cancers. In many programmes, the latter type of case will predominate (see [ 3 ]). One cannot, however, use the likelihood expression (5) for the matched sets containing screen-detected cases, since the sojourn time of the preclinical invasive state is different from and much shorter than the sojourn time of the total DPCP. One approach would be to partition the DPCP into two stages, preinvasive and preclinical invasive and estimate the parameters of the distribution of the two phases separately. The distribution entering into expression (4) would be that of the sum of the two sojourn times, the distribution entering into expression (5) would be that of the preclinical invasive phase sojourn time. This approach is being explored by Dr. Brookmeyer of Johns Hopkins University.

An alternative approximate approach is based on the assumption that the invasive preclinical phase is short compared to the total sojourn time. This assumption is based on the finding from screening programmes [1] that less than 10% of screen-detected lesions (including severe dysplasia and CIS, but not including moderate or mild dysplasia) are invasive. The prevalence rate of invasive preclinical lesions is then well approximated proportionally by the incidence of clinical lesions. The constant of proportionality occurs in both numerator and denominator in the terms of the likelihood function and so disappears.

The approach then is to treat the invasive preclinical lesions in the design phase as if they were prevalent, choosing controls screened negative at the same time as the case was screened positive, but in the analysis use expression (4) or (6) for incident cases.

TABLE 1

Approximate estimate of the cumulative distribution function of the sojourn time for the preclinical lesions of cervical cancer

| Time in months | Cumulative probability* | 95% confidence interval |
|---|---|---|
| 36 | 0.125 | 0.08 - 0.19 |
| 48 | 0.19 | 0.13 - 0.28 |
| 60 | 0.36 | 0.25 - 0.53 |
| 72 | 0.28 | 0.17 - 0.48 |
| 120 | 0.63 | 0.29 - 1.00 |

*Based on independent estimates in each time period, so that the values do not necessarily increase monotonically with time.

This approach has been used on data from the screening programme in north-east Scotland [3] and is now being applied to data from a number of programmes in Europe and Canada. A pooled estimate of the cumulative distribution function of f(y) is given in Table 1. For the Aberdeen data, an exponential distribution gave, surprisingly, a good fit [5], with mean sojourn time of some 25 years, and a false negative rate of 2.4%. The joint confidence region for these two parameters, however, is wide (Figure 2). Figure 2 refers to the proportion of lesions with sojourn time less than 5 years, rather than the mean of the sojourn time distribution, since the former is of more direct interest for screening purposes. The implications for screening policies are given in Table 2. Since reduction in risk of invasive cervical cancer is the aim of screening, the figures in Table 2 indicate the overall benefit of different screening policies.

TABLE 2

Percentage reduction in the cumulative rate of invasive cervical cancer over the age range 35-64, with different frequencies of screening

| Screening every: | Percentage reduction in the cumulative rate* | Number of tests |
|---|---|---|
| 1 year | 93.3 | 30 |
| 2 years | 93.3 | 15 |
| 3 years | 91.4 | 10 |
| 5 years | 83.9 | 6 |
| 10 years | 64.2 | 3 |

*Assuming a screen occurs at age 35, and that a previous screen had been performed.

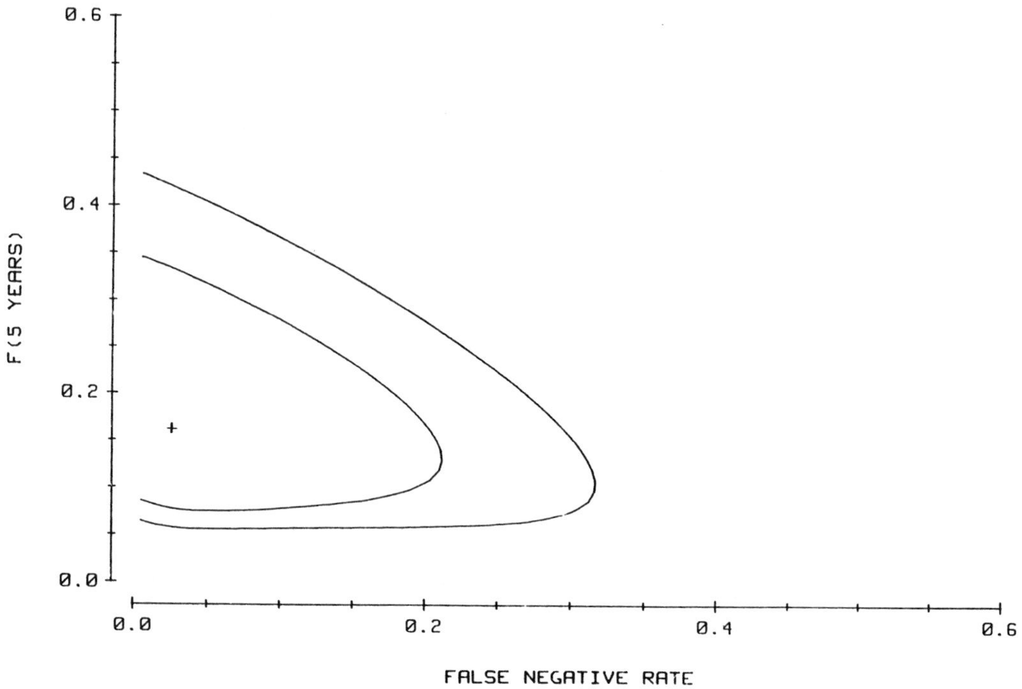


Figure 2. 95% and 80% joint confidence region for proportion with sojourn times less than 5 years [F(5 years)], and the false negative rate (β), based on an exponential model.

5. Application to screening for breast cancer. Most of the currently available information on the incidence rate of interval cancers and the prevalence rate at successive screens comes from centrally organized screening programmes, consisting of randomized studies in New York (the HIP study) [7] and Sweden [8], and mass screening programmes in The Netherlands (Utrecht and Nijmegen [9-11]). For this reason, since all the screening records are available in computer readable form, analyses have been based on the entire cohort rather than a sample selected for the case-control approach.

Analysis of the cohort data requires estimation of f(y), β and $I^*$. Estimates of these three parameters are highly correlated, and use of external rates to fix $I^*$ is beneficial. For randomized studies in which breast cancer rates in the non-compliers have been ascertained, unbiased estimates of $I^*$ are available from the control group. This procedure was used with the HIP and Swedish data, improving the stability of the estimates of β and f(y).

Analysis of the HIP material using the approach developed here has been published [12], and indicated that an exponential distribution for the sojourn time fitted well, with a mean of 1.6 years, and a false negative rate of 0.18. Data were not available to examine the effect of age on these parameters. The predictive value of a positive test result appeared close to 100%. The Utrecht programme, using as screening modality both mammography and physical examination as in the HIP but taking advantage of advances in the quality of film, yielded a mean sojourn time of 2.5 years and a false negative rate close to zero [13]. An exponential distribution again gave a good fit. The programme in the Swedish counties of Kopparberg and Ostergotland, from which results on mortality have recently been published [8], used only single-view mammography as screening modality. Estimates of $\beta$ and the exponential parameter $\lambda$ of $f(\cdot)$ are given in Table 3. The fit is reasonably good. One can see that although $\beta$ is close to zero in all age groups, $\lambda$ varies with age. The sojourn time is almost twice as long after age 50 as before age 50. For women over 50 years of age, the Swedish results agree closely with those from Utrecht.

The implications for the effectiveness of different screening strategies are less directly obtainable in this situation than with cervical cancer screening, and assumptions have to be made relating lead time to improvements in survival. With an exponential sojourn time distribution, the lead time distribution is also exponential and independent of the time already spent in the DPCP for a particular case. Since the overall benefit of screening, i.e., the reduction in mortality, is derived entirely from the screen-detected cases, one can express the relative benefits of different screening strategies in terms of the proportion of cases one would expect to be screen-detected.

TABLE 3

Preliminary estimates of the sojourn time distribution and sensitivity of breast cancer screening using single view mammography

| Age group at entry to study | False negative rate | Mean of sojourn time distribution |
|---|---|---|
| 40-44 | 0 | 1.67 |
| 45-49 | 0 | 1.44 |
| 50-54 | 0 | 2.27 |
| 55-59 | 0.08 | 3.33 |
| 60-64 | 0.11 | 3.57 |
| 65-69 | 0 | 1.96 |

Table 4 compares the proportion of cases one would expect to be screen-detected, with different screening intervals, using estimates from the HIP study and from the Utrecht programme.

Table 4

Expected number of cases screen-detected in the first six years of screening, after the first screen and including the last screen

| Frequency of screening | Percentage of cases screen-detected | |
|---|---|---|
| Screening interval (in years) | Using parameters from HIP study* | Using parameters from Utrecht study** |
| 1 | 70 | 82 |
| 2 | 53 | 69 |
| 3 | 42 | 58 |
| 6 | 24 | 38 |

* $\beta = 0.18$ $\lambda = 0.62$ [12]
** $\beta = 0$ $\lambda = 0.4$ [13]

Although one would expect the reduction in mortality to increase as the proportion of cases screen-detected increases, the form of the relationship is not necessarily linear and will depend on the relationship of lead time gained with improved survival. This topic requires further attention. It would seem, however, that improvements have occurred in screening techniques since the HIP study was launched in the early 1960's.

REFERENCES

[1] G. JOHANNESSON, G. GEIRSSON, N.E. DAY and H. TULINIUS. Screening for cancer of the uterine cervix in Iceland 1965-1978. Acta Pathologica Scandinavia, 61, (1982), pp. 199-203.

[2] N.E. DAY and S.D. WALTER. Simplified models for screening: estimation procedures from mass screening programmes. Biometrics, 40, (1984), pp. 1-14.

[3] J.E. MACGREGOR, S. MOSS, D.M. PARKIN and N.E. DAY. A case-control study of cervical cancer screening in northeast Scotland. Br. Med. J., 290, (1985), pp. 1543-1546.

[4] IARC WORKING GROUP, Summary chapter. In: Miller, A.B. and Day, N.E. eds, Screening for Gynaecological Cancer (IARC Scientific Publications No. 76), Lyon, International Agency for Research on Cancer (in press).

[5] R. BROOKMEYER, N.E. DAY and S. MOSS. Case-control studies for the estimation of the natural history of preclinical disease from screening data. Statist. Med. (in press).

[6] A.J. SASCO, N.E. DAY and S.D. WALTER. Case-control studies for the evaluation of screening. J. Chron. Dis. (in press).

[7] S. SHAPIRO, W. VENET, P. STRAX, L. VENET and R. ROESER. Ten-to-fourteen year effect of screening on breast cancer mortality. J. Natl. Cancer Inst., 69, (1982), pp. 349-355.

[8] L. TABAR, A. GAD, L.H. HOLMBERG, U. LJUNGQUIST, C.J.G. FAGERBERG, L. BALDETORP, O. GRONTOFT, B. LUNDSTROM, J.C. MANSON, G. EKLUND, N.E. DAY and F. PETTERSSON. Reduction in breast cancer mortality by mass screening with mammography: first results of a randomized trial in two Swedish counties. Lancet, i, (1985), pp. 829-832.

[9] F. DE WAARD, H.J.A. COLLETTE, J.J. ROMBACH, E.A. BAANDERS-VAN HALEWIJN and C. HONING. The DOM project for the early detection of breast cancer, Utrecht, The Netherlands. J. Chron. Dis., 37, (1984), pp. 1-44.

[10] H.J.A. COLLETTE, J.J. ROMBACH, N.E. DAY and F. DE WAARD. Evaluation of screening for breast cancer in a non-randomized study (the DOM project) by means of a case-control study. Lancet, i, (1984), pp. 1224-1226.

[11] A.L.M. VERBEEK, J.H.C.L. HENDRIKS, R. HOLLAND, M. MRAVUNAC, F. STURMANS and N.E. DAY. Reduction of breast cancer mortality through mass screening with modern mammography: first results of the Nijmegen project 1975-81. Lancet, i, (1984), pp. 1222-1224.

[12] S.D. WALTER and N.E. DAY. Estimation of the duration of a pre-clinical disease state using screening data. Am. J. Epidemiol., 118, (1983), pp. 865-886.

[13] N.E. DAY, S.D. WALTER and B. COLLETTE. Statistical models of disease natural history: their use in the evaluation of screening programmes. In: Prorok, P.C. and Miller, A.B., eds, Screening for Cancer. I - General Principles on Evaluation of Screening for Cancer and Screening for Lung, Bladder and Oral Cancer, Geneva, International Union Against Cancer (UICC Technical Report Series No. 78), pp. 55-70.

# Statistical Modeling and Extrapolation of Carcinogenesis Data

*D. Krewski[1,2], D. Murdoch[1], and A. Dewanji[1]*

Mathematical models of carcinogenesis are reviewed, including pharmacokinetic models for metabolic activation of carcinogenic substances. Maximum likelihood procedures for fitting these models to epidemiological data are discussed, including situations where the time to tumour occurrence is unobservable. The plausibility of different possible shapes of the dose response curve at low doses is examined, and a robust method for linear extrapolation to low doses is proposed and applied to epidemiological data on radiation carcinogenesis.

## INTRODUCTION

The etiology of many chronic diseases involves complexities associated with the fact that many such diseases are multi-causal in nature, with disease progression subsequently being modulated by a variety of dietary, hormonal, immunological and other physiological factors. In the past, particular attention has focused on the case of carcinogenesis which may occur following long-term exposure to low levels of environmental carcinogens.

In this paper, mathematical models of carcinogenesis are reviewed in section 2, including the multi-stage model with time dependent exposure patterns. Special attention is paid to pharmacokinetic models for metabolic activation, which may be required to convert the toxic precursor to its active form.

In section 3, maximum likelihood methods for fitting such models to epidemiological data are also considered, including those cases in which the time to tumour occurrence may not be directly observable. Dose response models which may be used to describe the

---

[1] Environmental Health Directorate
Health Protection Branch
Health & Welfare Canada
Ottawa, Ontario
CANADA K1A 0L2

[2] Dept. of Mathematics & Statistics
Carleton University
Ottawa, Ontario
CANADA K1S 5B6

effects on response of increasing exposure are also considered.

Because humans are generally exposed to low levels of environmental toxicants, the extrapolation of carcinogenesis data obtained at higher exposure levels inducing observable rates of response is considered in section 4. A number of arguments have been advanced which suggest that dose response curves for carcinogenesis may be linear at low doses. In section 4, the biological plausibility of this assumption is examined in detail. A robust method for linear extrapolation to low doses is proposed, and its properties examined by computer simulation. An application of this procedure to epidemiological data on radiation induced stomach cancer is also given.

## MATHEMATICAL MODELS OF CARCINOGENESIS

### 2.1. Time to Tumour Models

Let $T$ denote time to tumour occurrence and $d$ denote the corresponding level of exposure or dose. Define

$$\begin{aligned} P(t;d) &= \Pr\{T \leq t;\ d\} \\ &= 1 - \exp\{-\int_0^t \lambda(u;d)\,du\} \\ &\simeq \Lambda(t;d) \end{aligned} \qquad (2.1.1)$$

for small $d$ and $t$, where $\Lambda(t;d)$ and $\Lambda(t;d) = \int_0^t \lambda(u;d)du$ denote the hazard and the cumulative hazard functions respectively. Different forms of $P(t;d)$, or, equivalently, $\lambda(t;d)$, which may be used to model the time to tumour distribution as a function of exposure are discussed briefly below.

#### Multi-Event Models

Suppose that a tumour arises as a result of the occurrence of a number of fundamental biological events. In this case, $T = \max\{T_1,\ldots,T_k\}$, where the $T_i$ are independent random variables with cumulative hazard rate $\Lambda_i$, corresponding to the times at which the different events occur. Then

$$\begin{aligned} P(t;d) &= \prod_{i=1}^{k} [1-\exp\{-\Lambda_i(t;d)\}] \\ &\simeq \prod_{i=1}^{k} \Lambda_i(t;d) \quad \text{for small } d \text{ and } t \\ &= \{\prod_{i=1}^{k} \psi_i(d)\}t^k , \end{aligned} \qquad (2.1.2)$$

if $\lambda_i(t;d) = \psi_i(d)$ for $i=1,\ldots,k$. This latter constant hazard assumption leads to a Weibull distribution for $T$ with hazard rate $k(\prod_{i=1}^{k}\psi_i(d))t^{k-1}$.

## Multi-Stage Models

Suppose that a tumour occurs when the $k$ events occur in order, and that the hazard rate for the $i^{th}$ event is given by $\lambda_i(t) = \alpha_i+\beta_i d(t)$, where $d(t)$ denotes the dose at time $t$ [7]. If a tissue is comprised of a large number $n$ of cells acting independently, then the probability of tumour occurrence by time $t$ somewhere in the tissue is approximately $1-\exp\{-H(t)\}$, where

$$H(t) = \int_0^t\int_0^{u_k}\int_0^{u_{k-1}}\cdots\int_0^{u_2}\prod_{i=1}^{k}[a_i+b_i d(u_i)]du_1\cdots du_{k-1}du_k. \tag{2.1.3}$$

(This result obtains under the conditions that $\alpha_i n^{1/k}\to a_i$, $\beta_i n^{1/k}\to b_i$, and $\lambda_i\to 0$ uniformly in any finite interval.)

For constant exposure $d(t) = d$, this reduces to the usual multistage model with

$$H(t) = \frac{t^k}{k!}\prod_{i=1}^{k}(a_i+b_i d). \tag{2.1.4}$$

Moolgavkar & Venzon [32] and Moolgavkar & Knudson [31] have applied specialized two-stage models of this type which also allow for tissue growth.

## Relative and Additive Risk Models

Cox [5] postulated a regression relationship for the hazard rate at time $t$ of the form

$$\lambda(t;d) = \lambda_0(t)\exp\{\underset{\sim}{Z}(t)\underset{\sim}{\beta}\}, \tag{2.1.5}$$

where $\lambda_0(\cdot) > 0$ is an unspecified baseline hazard function, $\underset{\sim}{\beta}$ is the vector of regression parameters, and $\underset{\sim}{Z}(t)$ is the row vector of covariates which may depend upon both time $t$ and dose $d$. If $\underset{\sim}{Z}(t)$ is time-independent, then this model is of the proportional hazards form.

In contrast, Thomas [36] suggests an additive risk model where the hazard function has the general form

$$\lambda(t;d) = \lambda_0(t) + \gamma(\underset{\sim}{Z}(t)\underset{\sim}{\beta}), \tag{2.1.6}$$

where $\gamma$ is a suitably chosen function; for example, $\gamma(\underset{\sim}{Z}(t)\underset{\sim}{\beta}) = \underset{\sim}{Z}(t)\underset{\sim}{\beta}$.

### Other Models

Other general failure time models have been reviewed by Kalbfleisch et al. [18]. For example, in the compartmental models developed by Matis and Wehrly [29] and Hartley et al. [14], the transformation of a normal cell to a cancerous cell takes place with probability proportional to the concentration of the carcinogen in the compartment it occupies. Assuming that the flow between compartments follows linear kinetics, the cumulative hazard function for this transformation is of the proportional hazards form

$$\Lambda(t;d) = g(d)H(t), \tag{2.1.7}$$

where $g$ is a positive convex function of dose, and $H$ is a positive non-decreasing function of time. Because different models may predict notably different risks at low levels of exposure, extrapolation methods which are robust against model misspecification are considered in section 4.

## 2.2 Pharmacokinetic Models for Metabolic Activation

In many cases, some form of metabolic activation may be required to convert the toxic precursor to its active form. Pharmacokinetic models for metabolic activation are typically composed of many steps, each of which follows a simple kinetic law. These may be illustrated by considering elimination of a substance $X$ from the body.

Under zero order kinetics, elimination takes place at a constant rate, regardless of the amount in the body. Thus, in the absence of uptake or any other route of elimination, the concentration $[X]$ of $X$ varies according to

$$\frac{d[X]}{dt} = -k , \tag{2.2.1}$$

where $k > 0$ is the rate constant of the reaction. First order or linear kinetics occur when the rate of elimination is proportional to concentration, with

$$\frac{d[X]}{dt} = -k[X]. \tag{2.2.2}$$

In order to model saturable pathways, Michaelis-Menten kinetics are used, where

$$\frac{d[X]}{dt} = -\frac{k[X]}{1 + S[X]} \tag{2.2.3}$$

$(S \geq 0)$. For small concentrations (or where the saturability $S = 0$), this behaves like first order kinetics with rate constant $k$. For large concentrations this approximates zero order kinetics with maximum flow of $k/S$.

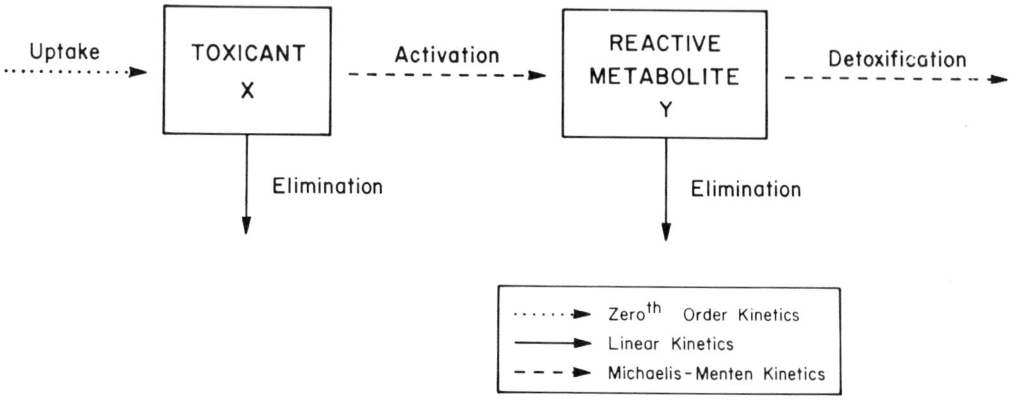


Figure 1 A Simple Pharmacokinetic Model for Metabolic Activation

Consider the simple pharmacokinetic model for metabolic activation of a particular toxicant shown in Figure 1. Here, the target organism is exposed to the toxin at a constant rate $d$. (This could be the case, for example, with the inhalation of atmospheric pollutants.) Once absorbed into the body, the toxin $X$ may be either eliminated from the body or activated to its reactive form $Y$. The reactive metabolite may then be eliminated or detoxified.

We assume that the elimination both of $X$ and $Y$ follows first order linear kinetics, with rate coefficients $k_x$ and $k_y$ respectively. Activation and detoxification, on the other hand, are assumed to be enzymatically mediated processes following saturable Michaelis-Menten kinetics with parameters $(k_a, S_a)$ and $(k_d, S_d)$ respectively. Under these conditions, the compartmental model in Figure 2 satisfies the system of nonlinear differential equations

$$\frac{d[X]}{dt} = d - k_x[X] - \frac{k_a[X]}{1+S_a[X]} \tag{2.2.4}$$

and

$$\frac{d[Y]}{dt} = \frac{k_a[X]}{1+S_a[X]} - \frac{k_d[Y]}{1+S_d[Y]} - k_y[Y]. \tag{2.2.5}$$

Under the steady state condition $d[X]/dt = 0$, (2.2.4) may be solved to yield

$$[X] = \frac{dS_a - k_a - k_x + \sqrt{(dS_a - k_a - k_x)^2 + 4dk_xS_a}}{2k_xS_a}. \tag{2.2.6}$$

A similar expression for the concentration $[Y]$ of the reactive metabolite as a function of the level of exposure $d$ may be obtained by solving (2.2.5) with $[X]$ replaced according to (2.2.6) [26].

This simple model may be used to illustrate the varied impact of

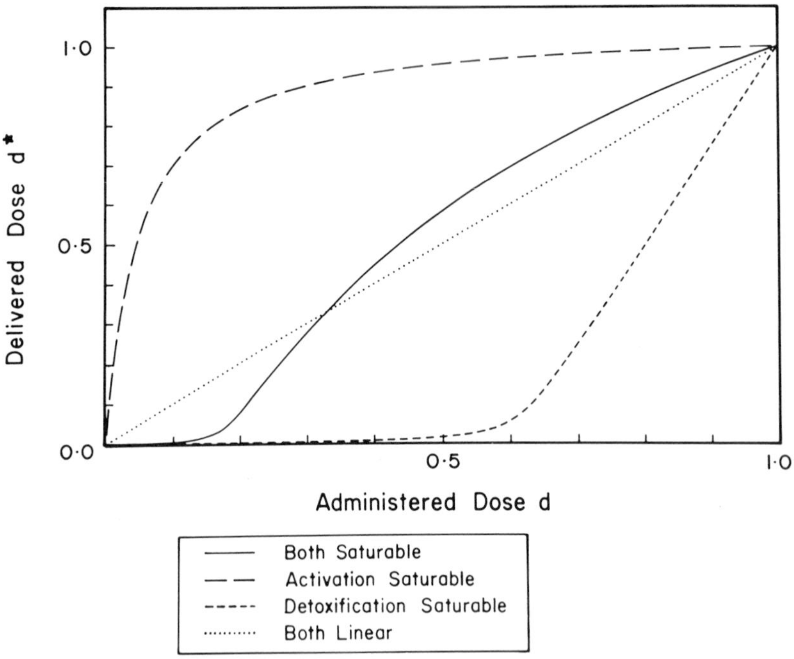


Figure 2 Relationship Between the Dose $d^*$ Delivered to the Target Tissue and the Administered Dose d with Saturable Activation and Detoxification

saturation effects on the relationship between the dose $d^* = [Y]$ delivered to the target tissue and the exogeneous level of exposure d (Figure 2). (The pharmacokinetic parameters leading to these particular examples are given in Table 1.) Note that in all four examples, $d^*$ is proportional to d at low doses.

TABLE 1

Pharmacokinetic Parameters for Models with Saturable Activation and Detoxification.[1]

| Model | $S_a$ | $k_y$ | $k_d$ | $S_d$ | Low Dose Slope |
|---|---|---|---|---|---|
| Linear | 0 | .0909 | 0 | 0 | 1 |
| Both Saturable | 0.1 | .0205 | 4.1 | 328 | .022 |
| Activation Saturable | 1 | .0048 | 0 | 0 | 19 |
| Detoxification Saturable | 0 | .0355 | 19.0 | 342 | .0048 |
| Apparently Linear | 0 | .0908 | 10 | $10^5$ | .0090 |

[1] $k_x = .05$ and $k_a = .005$ for all 5 models.

# ESTIMATION

## 3.1. Competing Risks

In most epidemiological studies, not all individuals will develop tumours during the course of the investigation. For example, some may die of other causes called competing risks, or survive tumour-free until the end of the study without responding and are thus censored. More generally, censoring may occur at any point in time during the course of the study at which an individual is lost to follow-up. In this section, different methods of incorporating competing risks and their applicability with censored failure time data are discussed.

### Cause Specific Hazard Functions

Let $T$ denote the time to either tumour occurrence or death from competing risks, and let $J$ indicate the type of failure which has occurred. ($J=1$ indicates the occurrence of a tumour and $J=2$ indicates death from competing risks.) The cause specific hazard function for the $j^{th}$ failure type is

$$\lambda_j(t;d) = \lim_{\Delta t \downarrow 0} \frac{P\{T \in (t,t+\Delta t],\ J=j;\ d \mid T \geq t\}}{\Delta t}, \tag{3.1.1}$$

($j=1,2$). The likelihood contribution $C$ from a response of type $j$ can be written as

$$C = \lim_{\Delta t \downarrow 0} \frac{P\{T \in (t,t+\Delta t],\ J=j;\ d\}}{\Delta t} \tag{3.1.2}$$

$$= \lambda_j(t;d)\exp\{-\Lambda(t;d)\}, \tag{3.1.3}$$

where $\Lambda(t;d) = \Lambda_1(t;d) + \Lambda_2(t;d)$, with $\Lambda_j(t;d) = \int_0^t \lambda_j(u;d)du$ for $j=1,2$. For a censored observation, the likelihood contribution is

$$C = P(T > t;d) = \exp\{-\Lambda(t;d)\}. \tag{3.1.4}$$

Without further assumptions, observations on $(T,J)$ with likelihood contributions given by (3.1.3) and (3.1.4) at a given dose $d$ allow estimation of only the $\lambda_j(t;d)$, or functions thereof [33].

### Latent Failure Time Models

Another approach to incorporation of competing risks presumes the existence of latent response times $T_1$ and $T_2$ for the failure time of interest and the time to death from competing risks. In this case, $T = \min\{T_1,T_2\}$ and $J = \{j : T_j = T\}$. The model specifies a joint survival or multiple decrement function

$$Q(t_1,t_2;d) = P\{T_1 > t_1, T_2 > t_2;d\}. \tag{3.1.5}$$

The cause specific hazards in (3.1.1) can be written as

$$\lambda_j(t;d) = -\frac{\partial}{\partial t_j} \log Q(t_1,t_2;d)\Big|_{t_1=t_2=t} \qquad (3.1.6)$$

for $j=1,2$, and are uniquely identifiable with data of the type $(T,J)$. However, $Q(t_1,t_2;d)$ cannot be estimated without further assumption [37]. Under the assumption of independence between $T_1$ and $T_2$, (3.1.5) factors as

$$Q(t_1,t_2;d) = Q_1(t_1;d)Q_2(t_2;d), \qquad (3.1.7)$$

where $Q_j(t;d) = P(T_j > t;d)$. Consequently, the marginal hazard function for $T_j$ can be defined as

$$h_j(t;d) = \lim_{\Delta t \downarrow 0} \frac{P\{T_j \in (t,t+\Delta t];\ d \mid T_j \geq t\}}{t}$$

$$= -\frac{\partial}{\partial t} \log Q_j(t;d)\ , \qquad (3.1.8)$$

for $j=1,2$. Under independence, it is easily seen that

$$\lambda_j(t;d) = h_j(t;d), \qquad (3.1.9)$$

(see [19] p.174). In this case, the likelihood contributions in (3.1.3) and (3.1.4) reduce to $h_j(t;d)Q_1(t;d)Q_2(t;d)$ and $Q_1(t;d)Q_2(t;d)$ respectively, which allows the estimation of $h_j(t;d)$ or $Q_j(t;d)$.

Although methods based on the cause specific hazards and latent failure time models may appear to be equivalent with the independence assumption in light of (3.1.9), the notion of independent competing risks only applies within the context of latent failure time models. The disadvantage of the latent failure time models lies in the interpretation of the marginal survival function $Q_j(t;d)$, which is presumed to give the probability that $T_j > t$ in the impossible situation in which all other types of response are removed.

## 3.2. Unobservable Failure Times

Consider the compartment model for oncogenesis shown in Figure 3. Here, S denotes the start of the period of observation, T the time of tumour onset, $D_{CR}$ death from competing risks, and $D_T$ death from tumour. Let $X_1$ represent the time of the first event (tumour onset, or death by competing risks without tumour) and $X_2$ represent the time of the second event (death from tumour, or death by competing risks with tumour present). We let $J_1$ be an indicator of the outcome for the first event defined by

$$J_1 = 1 \quad \text{if } X_1 \text{ corresponds to tumour onset,}$$

$$= 2 \quad \text{if } X_1 \text{ corresponds to death by competing risks.}$$

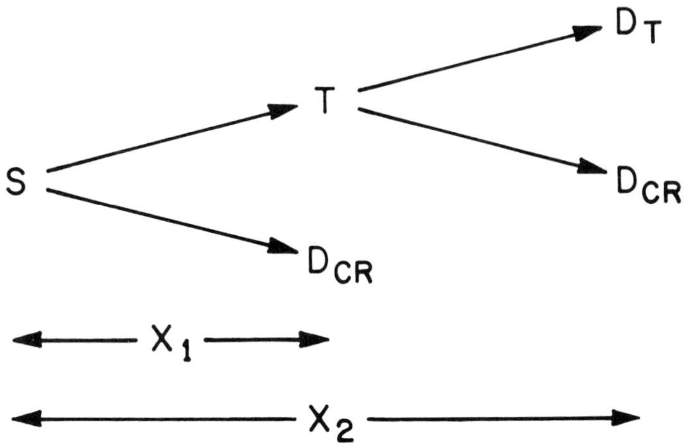


Figure 3 A Compartmental Model for Carcinogenesis

If $J_1 = 2$, the second event does not occur. Similarly, define

$$J_2 = 1 \quad \text{if} \quad X_2 \quad \text{corresponds to death from tumour,}$$
$$\quad = 2 \quad \text{if} \quad X_2 \quad \text{corresponds to death by competing risks.}$$

The model can be specified in terms of the cause specific transition intensity functions

$$\lambda_j(u) = \lim_{\Delta u \to 0} (\Delta u)^{-1} P\{X_1 \in [u, u+\Delta u),\ J_1 = j \mid X_1 \geq u\}, \tag{3.2.1}$$

and

$$\lambda_{1j}(t|u) = \lim_{\Delta t \to 0} (\Delta t)^{-1} P\{X_2 \in [t, t+\Delta t), J_2 = j \mid X_1 = u, J_1 = 1, X_2 \geq t\}, \tag{3.2.2}$$

for $j=1,2$. Let

$$Q_j(u) = \exp\{-\int_0^u \lambda_j(v)dv\}, \tag{3.2.3}$$

and

$$Q_{1j}(t|u) = \exp\{-\int_u^t \lambda_{1j}(v|u)dv\}, \tag{3.2.4}$$

for $j=1,2$. The survival function for the first event is given by

$$S_1(t) = \exp\{-\int_0^t (\lambda_1(u)+\lambda_2(u))du\}$$
$$= Q_1(t)Q_2(t), \tag{3.2.5}$$

while the conditional survival function for the second event given tumour onset at time $u$ is

$$S_2(t|u) = \exp\{-\int_u^t (\lambda_{11}(v|u)+\lambda_{12}(v|u))dv\}$$

$$= Q_{11}(t|u)Q_{12}(t|u). \qquad (3.2.6)$$

The overall survival function is then given by

$$S(t) = S_1(t) + \int_0^t \lambda_1(u)S_1(u)S_2(t|u)du. \qquad (3.2.7)$$

Let $N_2(t)$ denote the number of deaths from competing risks without tumour at time $t$, $N_3(t)$ denote the number of censored individuals at time $t$, and $N_{1j}(t)$ denote the number of deaths at time $t$ with tumour present and $J_2 = j$ $(j=1,2)$. For purposes of likelihood construction, consider the case of death from competing risks at time $t$ with tumour present. In this case, the probability of surviving tumour-free up to time $u$ $(0 < u < t)$ is $S_1(u)$ and, conditional upon this, the probability of tumour development in $(u,u+du]$ is $\lambda_1(u)du$. This is followed by post tumour survival up to time $t$ which, conditional on tumour development at time $u$ occurs with probability $S_2(t|u)$; conditional upon this, the probability of dying from competing risks in $(t,t+dt]$ is $\lambda_{12}(t|u)dt$. Thus, the likelihood contribution for this event is given by

$$C = \int_0^t \lambda_1(u)S_1(u)\lambda_{12}(t|u)S_2(t|u)du. \qquad (3.2.8)$$

Similarly, the likelihood contribution for an individual lost to follow-up at time $t$ is $C = S(t)$. The full likelihood function can be written as

$$L = \prod_t [(\lambda_2(t)S_1(t))^{N_2(t)} \prod_{j=1}^{2} \{(\int_0^t \lambda_1(u)S_1(u)\lambda_{1j}(t|u)S_2(t|u)du)^{N_{1j}(t)}\}\cdot (S(t))^{N_3(t))}], \qquad (3.2.9)$$

where the first product is over the observed death and censoring times [18].

For fatal tumours, $\lambda_{11}(t|u)$ is very large for $u < t$, and $\lambda_{11}(t|t)S_2(t|t) = 1$, with $N_{12}(t) \approx 0$. For nonfatal or incidental tumours, $\lambda_{11}(t|u) \approx 0$ with $N_{11}(t) \approx 0$. Since the form of the likelihood function simplifies considerably in both of these limiting cases [18], the analysis becomes simpler ([10],[19] p.168-169, [30]).

Other possible simplifications may be based on the Markov $(\lambda_{11}(t|u) = \lambda_{11}(t))$, or the semi-Markov $(\lambda_{11}(t|u) = \lambda_{11}(t-u))$ assumptions for the conditional intensity functions of the time to death from tumour given the time to tumour onset [11]. In the former case, the conditional intensity function is a function of the time on study, whereas in the latter, it is a function of the time since tumour onset.

Within the context of a multiple decrement model, independence between the time to death from competing risks and the time to tumour onset as well as the time to death from tumour is often assumed. Within this framework, let X, Y and Z denote the time to tumour onset, time to death from tumour, and time to death from competing risks respectively. Here X(Y) denotes the latent time to tumour onset (death from tumour) if Z is observed without (with) tumour. Under the independent multiple decrement model, the hazards $\lambda_j(\cdot)$ and $\lambda_{1j}(\cdot|\cdot)$ (j=1,2) reduce to the corresponding marginal hazard functions with $\lambda_{12}(t|u) = \lambda_2(t)$, for all $u \leq t$. The likelihood contribution (3.2.8) now becomes

$$C = \left(\int_0^t \lambda_1(u)Q_1(u)Q_{11}(t|u)\,du\right) \times (\lambda_2(t)Q_2(t))$$

$$= (S_Y(t)-S_X(t)) \times f_Z(t) \qquad (3.2.10)$$

where $S_X(\cdot)$, $S_Y(\cdot)$ and $S_Z(\cdot)$ are the marginal survival functions and $f_X(\cdot)$, $f_Y(\cdot)$ and $f_Z(\cdot)$ are the marginal densities of X, Y and Z respectively. Similarly, the likelihood contribution for an individual lost to follow-up at time t is $C = S_Y(t)S_Z(t)$.

The full likelihood (3.2.9) now factors as

$$L = \prod_t \Big\{ \Big[ (Q_1(t))^{N_2(t)} \left(\int_0^t \lambda_1(u)Q_1(u)\lambda_{11}(t|u)Q_{11}(t|u)\,du\right)^{N_{11}(t)} \times$$

$$\left(\int_0^t \lambda_1(u)Q_1(u)Q_{11}(t|u)\,du\right)^{N_{12}(t)} \left(Q_1(t)+\int_0^t \lambda_1(u)Q_1(u)Q_{11}(t|u)\,du\right)^{N_3(t)} \Big]$$

$$\times \Big[ (\lambda_2(t))^{N_2(t)+N_{12}(t)} (Q_2(t))^{N_2(t)+N_{11}(t)+N_{12}(t)+N_3(t)} \Big] \Big\}$$

$$= \prod_t \Big\{ \Big[ (S_X(t))^{N_2(t)} (f_Y(t))^{N_{11}(t)} (S_Y(t)-S_X(t))^{N_{12}(t)} (S_Y(t))^{N_3(t)} \Big] \times$$

$$\Big[ (f_Z(t))^{N_2(t)+N_{12}(t)} (S_Z(t))^{N_{11}(t)+N_3(t)} \Big] \Big\}. \qquad (3.2.11)$$

It follows from (3.2.11) that the only identifiable aspects of the process are the marginal distributions of X, Y and Z, or functions thereof, such as the tumour mortality and prevalance functions [27]. In most cases, the second part of (3.2.11) involving only Z is of little interest and hence ignored.

For fatal tumours, the likelihood function (3.2.11) reduces to the Kaplan-Meier [20] form, and can be analyzed accordingly. For incidental tumours, the first part of (3.2.11) takes the form of binomial likelihood, and has been considered by Hoel & Walburg [16].

In many situations, the cause of death is unknown; $J_2$ is then not observable. In this case, the second event becomes the time to death with tumour present, with total conditional intensity function $\lambda_{DT}(t|u) = \lambda_{11}(t|u) + \lambda_{12}(t|u)$. McKnight & Crowley [30] and Dewanji & Kalbfleisch [11] consider this case, and note that the tumour onset distribution is not identiable without knowledge of tumour lethality.

A parametric approach to analysis of such data would be to parametrize $S_X$, $S_Y$ and $S_Z$ as

$$S_X(t) = \exp\{-\alpha t^{\gamma}\}, \tag{3.2.12}$$

$$S_Y(t) = \exp\{-\alpha\rho t^{\gamma}\}, \tag{3.2.13}$$

and

$$S_Z(t) = \exp\{-\mu t^{\nu}\}, \tag{3.2.14}$$

where $\alpha, \gamma, \mu, \nu \geq 0$, and $\rho$ is the lethality parameter with $0\leq\rho\leq 1$ and $\rho = 0$ (or 1) for incidental (fatal) tumours. As noted above, however, the joint distribution for X and Y is not generally identifiable in this case. However, a joint distribution for X and Y satisfying the restriction $\{X \leq Y\}$ can be constructed using the margins given by (3.2.12) and (3.2.13) [38].

In laboratory studies, (3.2.9) can be analyzed using the method of Dewanji & Kalbfleisch [11] with interim sacrifice plans. The likelihood function (3.2.11) has been considered by Kodell et al. [23], Dinse & Lagakos [13] and Turnbull & Mitchell [38] from the non-parametric point of view. Kodell & Nelson [22] consider three independent Weibull distributions for X, Y-X and Z, and estimate the related parameters by direct maximisation of the likelihood function. Dinse [12] notes that under independence or a slightly weaker condition called 'representativeness' [28] the prevalence function, $1-(S_X(t)/S_Y(t))$, and the mortality function, $S_Y(t)$, are both identifiable when the cause of death is known for at least some subjects.

### 3.3 Dose Response Curves

In the cause specific hazard framework, $P_1(t;d) = 1-\exp\{-\int_0^t \lambda_1(u;d)du\}$, considered as a function of d, may be considered as a dose response curve in the absence of competing risks. Since $P_1(t;d)$ does not have a probabilistic interpretation, a dose response curve may be defined in terms of $P_1^*(t;d) = P(X_1 \leq t, J_1=1;d)$, the probability of observing a tumour in the presence of competing risks. Note that

$$P_1^*(t;d) = \int_0^t \lambda_1(u;d)Q_1(u;d)Q_2(u;d)du$$

$$= \int_0^t P_1(u;d)\lambda_2(u;d)Q_2(u;d)du+P_1(t;d)Q_2(t;d), \qquad (3.3.1)$$

where the last equality is obtained by using integration by parts [18]. The corresponding dose response curve in the multiple decrement model would be

$$1-S_X^*(t;d) = \int_0^t \lambda_1(u;d)Q_1(u;d)(1-P_2(u;d))du$$

$$= \int_0^t \lambda_1(u;d)Q_1(u;d)du-\int_0^t \lambda_1(u;d)Q_1(u;d)P_2(u;d)du$$

$$= (1-S_X(t;d))-\int_0^t f_X(u;d)(1-S_Z(u;d))du, \qquad (3.3.2)$$

[25].

Under a low dose proportional hazards assumption for tumour occurrence (that is, $P_1(t;d) = H(t)g(d)$, for low doses), it is easily seen from (3.3.1) that, at a fixed time $t$, $P_1^*(t;d)$ is proportional to $P_1(t;d)$ provided that the distribution of death from competing risks without tumour is independent of the dose $d$, at least in the low dose region. Under these conditions, the shape of the dose response curve at low doses will be the same regardless of whether $P_1$ or $P_1^*$ is used. The same conclusion follows from (3.3.2) with the multiple decrement model.

## LINEAR EXTRAPOLATION

### 4.1. Low Dose Linearity

Let $P(d)$ denote the probability of a response at dose $d \geq 0$ at a fixed time $t$. Assuming that $P''(d)$ is bounded on some interval $[0,D]$, a simple expansion of $P(d)$ about zero shows that the excess risk

$$\Pi(d) = P(d) - P(0) \qquad (4.1.1)$$

will be nearly linear at low doses provided $0 < P'(0) < \infty$. Crump et al. [6] suggested that spontaneously occurring lesions may be thought of as arising due to the existence of an effective background dose $\Delta > 0$, with test agent acting by simply adding an amount $d \geq 0$ to the existing environmental dose. Under these conditions, we may write $P(d) = F(d+\Delta)$ so that $P'(0) > 0$ provided only that $F(d)$ is strictly increasing in $d$ for all $d > 0$. This argument is appealing in that no assumptions are necessary concerning the form of F save that it is strictly increasing, and has often been invoked as a justification for linear extrapolation. Low dose linearity will obtain with pharmacokinetic models comprised entirely of linear and Michaelis-Menten components, provided that the probability of tumour occurrence is proportional to the delivered dose at low levels of exposure [26].

It is not inconceivable that the dose response curve may be non-linear at low doses. Sublinearity or convexity can occur with certain arbitrary tolerance distributions [40], or with the multi-stage model in which the transition intensity function for at least one of the stages is a quadratic or other strictly convex function of dose [39]. If second order kinetics is involved in metabolic activation [15], sublinearity can also occur.

For certain mechanisms of carcinogenesis, it has been suggested that a threshold in the dose response curve may well exist [17]. These include indirect nongenotoxic mechanisms such as recurrent cytotoxicity, physical irritation, hormonal imbalances, alterations in immunological or nutritional status, and increased stress. Shank & Barrows [35], for example, describe a mechanism of liver tumour induction which may be due to the toxic effects of high doses of hydrazine.

Cornfield [4] proposed a simple pharmacokinetic model which predicts a threshold in the dose response curve in steady state under conditions of irreversible deactivation. As pointed out by Brown et al. [3], however, this result does not hold under non-equilibrium conditions, nor does it hold if the deactivation process is reversible.

Supralinearity or convexity at low doses can in theory occur in a heterogeneous population containing a large number of highly sensitive individuals. For example, consider a population comprised of individuals whose response probability is given by

$$P(d|\lambda) = 1 - \exp(-\lambda d), \qquad (4.1.6)$$

where the low dose slope parameter $\lambda > 0$ is randomly distributed according to some distribution $F$. The population dose response curve is then given by the mixture

$$P(d) = \int_0^\infty P(d|\lambda)dF(\lambda). \qquad (4.1.7)$$

As shown in the Appendix, (4.1.7) will be linear if $E(\lambda) < \infty$ and supralinear if $E(\lambda) = +\infty$.

Mixing heterogeneous individuals in a population can have other effects on the low dose shape of the dose response curve. Brown [2] gives an example of a low dose quadratic curve based on a mixture of individual dose response curves with varying thresholds. Hoel [15] describes a mixture of low-dose quadratic distributions that is low-dose linear. More general results of this type are given in Krewski et al. [26].

Taken as a whole, these arguments suggest that low dose linearity may be a reasonable assumption on which to base estimates of risk associated with low levels of exposure to carcinogenic agents. (The example of supralinearity arising from heterogeneity in the population requires the questionable assumption that the individual low dose slopes are unbounded.) Even if a threshold hypothesis could be supported, there remains the problem of determining the minimum of the individual thresholds, a minimum which could be near zero and difficult to determine. Similarly, the degree of sublinearity in the intermediate situation would be hard to assess. Linear extrapolation, however, may still be used to obtain an upper bound on the low dose risk in these cases.

### 4.2. Robust Linear Extrapolation

Under the assumption of low dose linearity, low dose extrapolation of carcinogenicity data effectively involves estimating the slope

$$\beta = \lim_{d \downarrow 0} \frac{P(d) - P(0)}{d} \tag{4.2.1}$$

of the dose response curve at the origin. In the absence of any information concerning the functional form of $P(d)$, a reasonable estimator of $\beta$ could be based on the secant

$$\beta_\delta = \frac{P(\delta) - P(0)}{\delta} \tag{4.2.2}$$

for some small level of exposure $\delta > 0$, since $\beta_\delta \to \beta$ as $\delta \to 0$. As discussed below, the different methods of linear extrapolation which have been proposed in the literature are all essentially based on this concept.

These procedures may be conveniently described in terms of the estimator $\hat{P}(d)$ of $P(d)$ and the dose $\delta$ at which the secant is calculated. The observed response rates $\hat{p}_i = x_i/n_i$ may be used to estimate $p_i = P(d_i)$ at the available doses $d_i$ $(i=0,1,\ldots,k)$. Under the condition that $P(d)$ is strictly increasing in $d$, any non-monotonicity in the observed response rates could be smoothed out using isotonic regression [1]. If it is further assumed that the dose response curve has at most one inflection point, sigmoidal regression [34] may be similarly used to obtain a smoothed estimator satisfying this constraint. Finally, a parametric model may be assumed, and the parameters estimated by the method of maximum likelihood as discussed previously.

The dose $\delta$ at which the secant $\beta_\delta$ is to be evaluated could be chosen to be the lowest dose $d_1$. Since it is possible that $\hat{p}_1 < \hat{p}_0$, a better choice might be the lowest dose $d_i$ for which $\hat{p}_i > \hat{p}_0$. Another possibility is to choose the smallest secant from those doses in the low dose region. (Operationally, this may be defined as those doses at which the observed response rate is not significantly greater than in the control.) Finally, if a parametric model is used, $\delta$ could be taken as that dose for which the estimated excess risk $\hat{\Pi}(\delta) = \pi$, with $\pi$ chosen small enough so as to lie in the low dose region yet large enough so that the particular parametric form assumed for $P(d)$ is not critical.

If interval estimates of $\beta$ are to be calculated in addition to point estimates, the method by which the confidence limits are to be obtained also needs to be specified. For estimators based on the observed data, this will generally involve the use of some form of binomial confidence limits, with some adjustments to the individual confidence coefficients in those cases where more than one dose may be involved. Confidence limits for procedures based on parametric models are generally based on the asymptotic distributions of the corresponding maximum likelihood estimators or on the distribution of the likelihood function itself [8].

While a detailed comparison of all the linear extrapolation procedures proposed to date is currently underway [24], one approach in particular appears promising. This method essentially selects the minimum (positive) secant $\beta_\delta$ over those doses at which the observed response rate is not significantly greater ($p < .05$) than that in the unexposed group. By using only the observed response rates and evaluating the secant at one of the experimental doses in the low dose region, the procedure is robust against model specification.

An upper confidence limit on the secant $\beta_\delta$ may be obtained by replacing the $\hat{p}_i$ by upper confidence limits $p_i^U$ defined as the solutions of the equations

$$\sum_{j=0}^{x_i} \binom{n_i}{j} (p_i^U)^j (1-p_i^U)^{n_i-j} = 1-(1-\alpha)^{1/(k+1)} \tag{4.2.3}$$

$(i=1,\ldots,k)$ and $\hat{p}_0$ by its lower confidence limit $p_0^L$ defined by

$$\sum_{j=x_0}^{n_0} \binom{n_0}{j} (p_0^L)^j (1-p_0^L)^{n_0-j} = 1-(1-\alpha)^{1/(k+1)}. \tag{4.2.4}$$

Because of the independence between $\hat{p}_0$ and the remaining $\hat{p}_i$, the values on the right hand sides of (4.2.3) and (4.2.5) will provide a $100(1-\alpha)\%$ upper confidence limit on the low dose slope.

In order to evaluate the properties of this procedure, we conducted a computer simulation using the four pharmacokinetically based models shown in Figure 2. Here, the probability of tumour induction

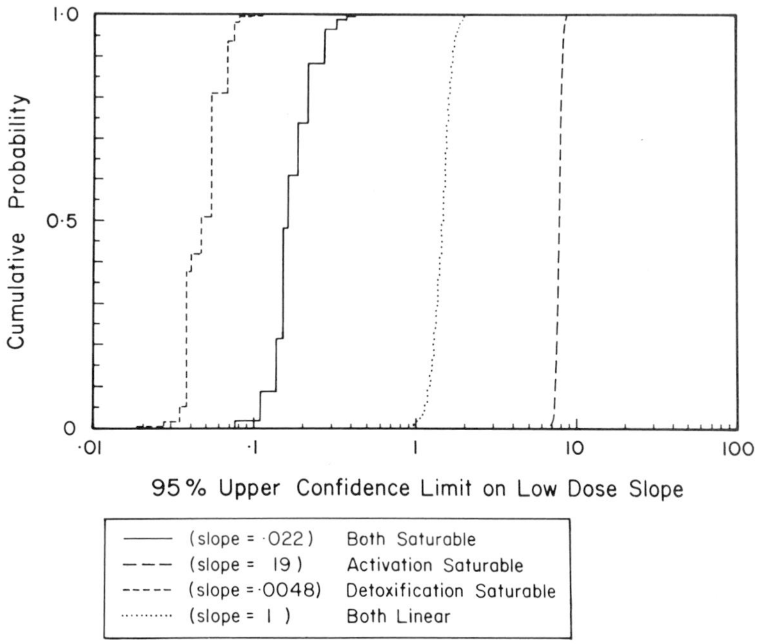


Figure 4 Empirical Cumulative Distribution Functions of Upper Confidence Limits on the Low Dose Slope with Saturable Activation and Detoxification

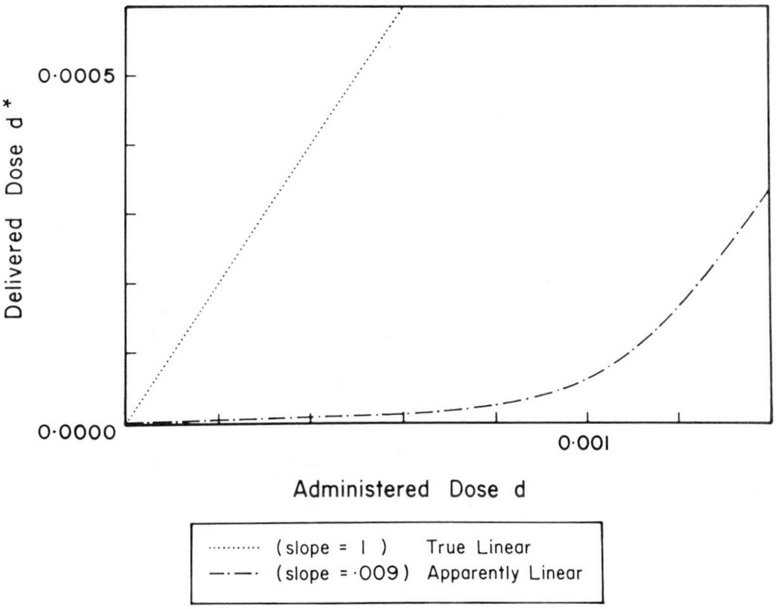


Figure 5 Relationship Between the Dose $d^*$ Delivered to the Target Tissue and the Administered Dose d with Linear and Apparently Linear Kinetics

was assumed to be related to dose using the simple exponential model $P(d) = 1-\exp(-d^*)$, where the dose $d^*$ delivered to the target tissue is related to the administered dose $d$ as in §2.2. In this study, six exposure levels $d_i=0$, 1/16, 1/8, 1/4, 1/2 and 1 were used, with 500 observations at each dose. In each case, one thousand data sets were simulated and a 95% upper confidence limit on the low dose slope calculated as described above.

The empirical distribution functions of these confidence limits are shown in Figure 4. In the "Both Linear" case, the values are tightly clustered around the true value of unity, while maintaining the desired coverage probability. In the two cases where activation is saturable, however, the upper confidence limits were always well in excess of the actual low dose slope. The serious undercoverage apparent when only the detoxification process is saturable is attributable to the extreme steepness of the dose response curve at low doses.

A second simulation was also carried out using only the case of linear kinetics and an apparently linear case in which saturation of the detoxification process occurs at very low doses. The response probabilities for these two models are almost identical at the doses used in the simulation, with the empirical distribution function for the apparently linear curve being virtually indistinguishable from that shown in Figure 4 for the linear case. However, since the low dose slope is much less than one in the apparently linear case (Figure 5), linear extrapolation can overestimate the low dose slope even with an apparently linear dose response curve.

TABLE 2

Deaths from Stomach Cancer in A-bomb Survivors in Hiroshima and Nagasaki [21].

| Group(i) | Dose (rads) | Mean Dose ($D_i$) (rads) | Group Size ($n_i$) | No. of deaths ($x_i$) | Proportion Dying ($\hat{p}_i$) |
|---|---|---|---|---|---|
| 0 | 0 | 0. | 31581 | 708 | .02242 |
| 1 | 1 - 9 | 3.4 | 23073 | 473 | .02050 |
| 2 | 10 - 49 | 21.8 | 14942 | 340 | .02275 |
| 3 | 50 - 99 | 70.6 | 4225 | 91 | .02154 |
| 4 | 100 - 199 | 142.4 | 3128 | 64 | .02046 |
| 5 | 200 - 299 | 243.6 | 1381 | 32 | .02317 |
| 6 | 300 - 399 | 345.3 | 639 | 17 | .02660 |
| 7 | 400 + | 526.4 | 887 | 29 | .03269 |

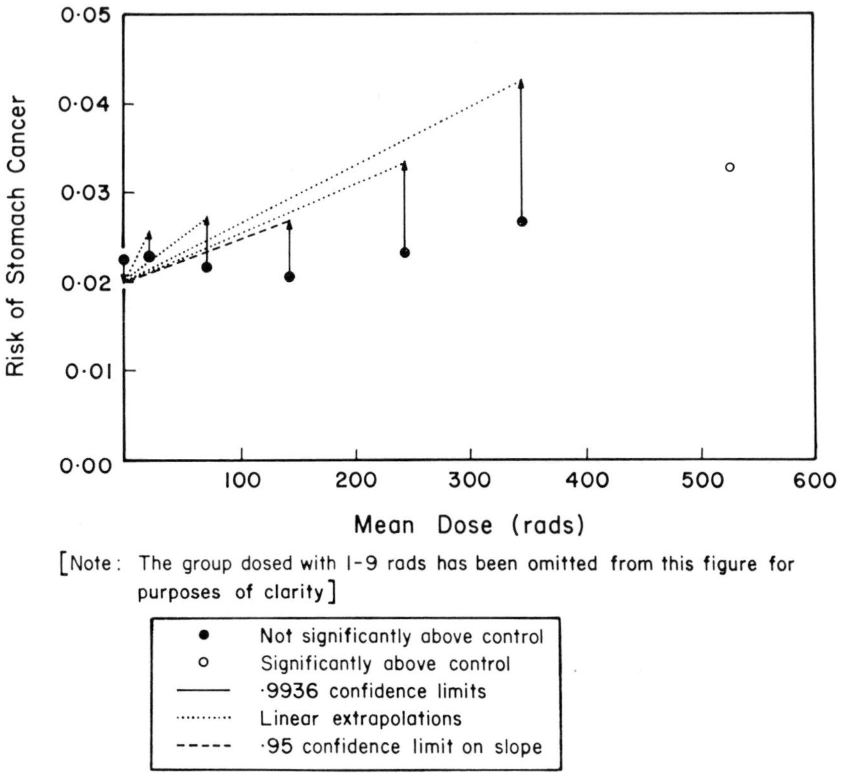


Figure 6 Risk of Stomach Cancer from Radiation in A-bomb Survivors and Upper Confidence Limit on the Low Dose Slope

As a practical example of the application of this technique, consider the data on the occurrence of stomach cancer in A-bomb survivors from Hiroshima and Nagasaki (Table 2) originally reported by Kato & Schull [21] and discussed by Day [9]. The only dose group with response significantly higher than control is the 400+ rad group. Secants from the $(.95)^{1/8} = .9936$ upper confidence limits on the other groups to the .9936 lower confidence limit on the control response are shown in Figure 6. The smallest slope, $4.5 \times 10^{-5}$ rad$^{-1}$, provides a 95% upper confidence limit on the low dose slope for the excess mortality due to radiation induced stomach cancer.

## CONCLUSIONS

The process of carcinogenesis is characterized by protracted latent periods, uncertain mechanisms of tumour induction, and the possible influence of a variety of modifying factors. While the different mathematical models of carcinogenesis discussed in this paper may provide adequate statistical descriptions of epidemiological data, it seems unlikely that any of these models can capture all of the complexities of the carcinogenic process.

In order to estimate potential carcinogenic risks associated with low levels of exposure, some form of reasonably robust estimation procedure, possibly providing only upper limits on low dose risks, thus seems desirable. Discounting the possibility of supralinearity in the low dose region, the simple linear extrapolation procedure discussed in this paper may prove useful in this regard.

## Appendix: Population Heterogeneity and Supralinearity

Consider a population in which the probability that a given individual responds at dose $d$ is given by

$$P(d|\lambda) = 1-\exp(-\lambda d) \tag{A.1}$$

$(\lambda > 0)$. Since the slope of the dose response curve in (A.1) at the origin is simply $\lambda$, $P(d|\lambda)$ is low dose linear.

Suppose now that the value of $\lambda$ varies among individuals in the population in accordance with some distribution $F$, reflecting the heterogeneity in individual susceptability. The population dose response curve is then given by

$$P(d) = \int_0^\infty P(d|\lambda)dF(\lambda) = \int_0^\infty [1-\exp(-\lambda d)]dF(\lambda). \tag{A.2}$$

The slope of $P(d)$ at the origin is given by

$$\lim_{d\downarrow 0} \frac{P(d)}{d} = \lim_{d\downarrow 0} \int_0^\infty \frac{(1-e^{-\lambda d})}{d} dF(\lambda). \tag{A.3}$$

Since $1-e^{-\lambda d} < \lambda d$, the dominated convergence theorem yields

$$P'(0) = \int_0^\infty \lim_{d\downarrow 0} \frac{1-e^{-\lambda d}}{d} dF(\lambda) = \int_0^\infty \lambda dF(\lambda), \tag{A.4}$$

provided the integral in (A.4) converges. Thus, if $E(\lambda) < \infty$, $P(d)$ is low dose linear.

Conversely, suppose that $E(\lambda) = +\infty$. From (A.3), for any $M > 0$ we have

$$P'(0) \geq \lim_{d\downarrow 0} \int_0^M \frac{1-e^{-\lambda d}}{d} dF(\lambda)$$

$$> \lim_{d\downarrow 0} \int_0^M \lambda(1-\lambda d)dF(\lambda)$$

$$= \int_0^M \lambda dF(\lambda) \qquad (A.5)$$

since $1-e^{-\lambda d} > \lambda d - (\lambda d)^2$. Since $M$ can be selected to be arbitrarily large, it follows that $P'(0) = +\infty$, and $P(d)$ is supralinear at low doses whenever $E(\lambda)$ is infinite.


## ACKNOWLEDGEMENTS

The authors would like to thank Mrs. Gill Murray for preparing the typescript. Figures 1-6 were drawn by Hans Metz. This research was supported in part by grant no. A8664 from the Natural Sciences and Engineering Research Council of Canada to D. Krewski.


## REFERENCES


[1] R.E. BARLOW, D.J. BATHOLOMEW, J.M. BREMNER and H.D. BRUNK, Statistical Inference Under Order Restrictions, John Wiley, New York, 1972.

[2] C.C. BROWN, Mathematical aspects of dose-response studies in carcinogenesis - the concept of thresholds, Oncology, 33(1976), pp.62-65.

[3] D. BROWN, T.R. FEARS, M.H. GAIL, M.A. SCHNEIDERMAN, R.E. TARONE and N. MANTEL, Letter to the editor and reply by J. Cornfield, Science, 202(1978), pp.1105-1108.

[4] J. CORNFIELD, Carcinogenic risk assessment, Science, 198(1977), pp.693-699.

[5] D.R. COX, Regression models and life-tables (with discussion), J. Royal Stat. Soc. Ser. B, 34(1972), pp.187-220.

[6] K.S. CRUMP, D.G. HOEL, C.H. LANGLEY and R. PETO, Fundamental carcinogenic processes and their implications for low dose risk assessment, Cancer Research, 36(1976), pp.2973-2979.

[7] K.S. CRUMP and R.B. HOWE, The multistage model with a time-dependent dose pattern: applications to carcinogenic risk assessment, Risk Analysis, 4(1984), pp.163-176.

[8] K.S. CRUMP and R. HOWE, A review of methods for calculating statistical confidence limits in low-dose extrapolation, Toxicological Risk Assessment, Vol. 1: Biological and Statistical Criteria, D.B. Clayson, D. Krewski, I. Munro, eds., CRC Press, Boca Raton, Florida, 1985, pp.187-203.

[9] N.E. DAY, Epidemiological methods for the assessment of human cancer risk, Toxicological Risk Assessment, Vol. II: General

Criteria and Case Studies, D.B. Clayson, D. Krewski, I. Munro, eds., CRC Press, Boca Raton, Florida, 1985, pp.3-15.

[10] A. DEWANJI, Analysis of incomplete failure time data, unpublished Ph.D. thesis, University of Waterloo, Waterloo, Ontario, Canada, 1984.

[11] A. DEWANJI and J.D. KALBFLEISCH, Nonparametric methods for survival/sacrifice experiments, submitted, 1985.

[12] G.E. DINSE, Nonparametric prevalence and mortality estimators with incomplete cause-of-death data, submitted, 1985.

[13] G.E. DINSE and S.W. LAGAKOS, Nonparametric estimation of lifetime and disease onset distributions from incomplete observations, Biometrics, 38(1982), pp.921-932.

[14] H.O. HARTLEY, H.D. TOLLEY and R.L. SIELKEN JR., The product form of the hazard rate model in carcinogenic testing, Statistics and Related Topics, M. Csörgő, D.A. Dawson, J.N.K. Rao and A.K.Md.E. Saleh, eds., North Holland, Amsterdam, 1981, pp.185-200.

[15] D.G. HOEL, Incorporation of pharmacokinetics in low-dose risk estimation, Toxicological Risk Assessment, Vol. 1: Biological and Statistical Criteria, D.B. Clayson, D. Krewski, I. Munro, eds., CRC Press, Boca Raton, Florida, 1985, pp.205-214.

[16] D.G. HOEL and H.E. WALBURG JR., Statistical analysis of survival experiments, JNCI, 49(1972), pp.361-372.

[17] INTERNATIONAL LIFE SCIENCES INSTITUTE, Interpretation and extrapolation of chemical and biological carcinogenicity data to establish human safety standards, Current Issues in Toxicology, H.D. Grice, ed., Springer-Verlag, New York, 1984, pp.1-152.

[18] J.D. KALBFLEISCH, D. KREWSKI and J. VAN RYZIN, Dose response models for time-to-response toxicity data, Can. J. Stat., 11(1983), pp.25-49.

[19] J.D. KALBFLEISCH and R.L. PRENTICE, The Statistical Analysis of Failure Time Data, Wiley, New York, 1980.

[20] E.L. KAPLAN and P. MEIER, Nonparametric estimation from incomplete observations, JASA, 53(1958), pp.457-481.

[21] H. KATO and W.J. SCHULL, Studies of the mortality of A-bomb survivors. 7. Mortality, 1950-1978: Part I. Cancer mortality, Radiation Research 90(1982), pp.395-432.

[22] R.L. KODELL and C.J. NELSON, An illness-death model for the study of the carcinogenic process using survival/sacrifice data, Biometrics, 36(1980), pp.267-277.

[23] R.L. KODELL, G.W. SHAW and A.M. JOHNSON, Nonparametric joint estimators for disease resistance and survival functions in survival/sacrifice experiments, Biometrics, 38(1982), pp.43-58.

[24] D. KREWSKI, M. BICKIS and D. COLIN, A comparison of statistical methods for linear extrapolation, in preparation, 1985.

[25] D. KREWSKI, K.S. CRUMP, J.H. FARMER, D.W. GAYLOR, R. HOWE, C. PORTIER, D. SALSBURG, R.L. SIELKEN and J. VAN RYZIN, A comparison of statistical methods for low dose extrapolation utilizing time to tumour data, Fundamental and Applied Toxicology, 3(1983), pp. 140-158.

[26] D. KREWSKI, D. MURDOCH and A. DEWANJI, Statistical modelling and extrapolation of carcinogenesis data, Technical Report No. 69, Laboratory for Research in Statistics and Probability, Carleton University, Ottawa, 1985.

[27] S.W. LAGAKOS, An evaluation of some two-sample tests used to analyse animal carcinogenicity experiments, Util. Math., 21B (1982), pp. 239-260.

[28] S.W. LAGAKOS and L.M. RYAN, On the representativeness assumption in prevalence tests of carcinogenicity, J. Royal Stat. Soc. Ser. C, 34(1985), pp. 54-62.

[29] J.H. MATIS and T.E. WEHRLY, Stochastic models of compartmental systems, Biometrics, 35(1979), pp. 199-220.

[30] B. MCKNIGHT and J. CROWLEY, Tests for differences in tumour incidence based on animal carcinogenesis experiments, JASA, 79(1984), pp. 639-648.

[31] S.H. MOOLGAVKAR and A.G. KNUDSON JR., Mutation and cancer: A model for human carcinogenesis, JNCI, 66(1981), pp.1037-1052.

[32] S.H. MOOLGAVKAR and D.J. VENZON, Two-event models for carcinogenesis: Incidence curves for childhood and adult tumors, Math. Biosci., 47(1979), pp. 55-77.

[33] R.L. PRENTICE, J.D. KALBFLEISCH, A.V. PETERSON JR., N. FLOURNOY, V.T. FAREWELL and N.E. BRESLOW, The analysis of failure times in the presence of competing risks, Biometrics, 34(1978), pp. 541-554.

[34] R.L. SCHMOYER, Sigmoidally constrained maximum likelihood estimation in quantal bioassay, JASA, 79(1984), pp. 448-453.

[35] R.C. SHANK and L.R. BARROWS, Toxicological effects on carcinogenesis, Toxicological Risk Assessment, Vol. 1: Biological and Statistical Criteria, D.B. Clayson, D. Krewski, and I. Munro, eds., CRC Press, Boca Raton, Florida, 1985, pp. 91-104.

[36] D.C. THOMAS, Use of auxiliary information in fitting nonproportional hazards models, SIMS Research Application Conference on Modern Statistical Methods in Chronic Disease Epidemiology, June 24-28, Alta, Utah, 1985.

[37] A.A. TSIATIS, A nonidentifiability aspect of the problem of competing risks, Proc. Natl. Acad. Sci. U.S.A., 72(1975), pp. 20-22.

[38] B.W. TURNBULL and T.J. MITCHELL, Nonparametric estimation of the distribution of time to onset for specific diseases in survival/sacrifice experiments, Biometrics, 40(1984), pp. 41-50.

[39] J. VAN RYZIN, The assessment of low-dose carcinogenicity: discussion, Biometrics, 38 Supplement(1982), pp. 130-139.

[40] T. YANAGIMOTO and D.G. HOEL, Comparisons of models for estimation of safe doses using measures of the heaviness of tail of a distribution, Annals Inst. Stat. Math., 32(1980), pp. 465-480.